KU-285-061

are to be returned on or before
dat

Perinatal Mental Health

LIVERPOOL
JOHN MOORES UNIVERSITY
AVRIL ROBARTS LRC
TITHEBARN STREET
LIVERPOOL L2 2ER
TEL. 0151 231 4022

LIVERPOOL JMU LIBRARY

3 1111 01292 7131

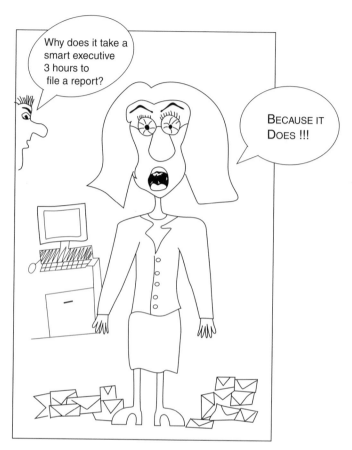

Postnatal depression

Perinatal Mental Health

A Guide for Health Professionals and Users

Jane Hanley

School of Health Science
Swansea University
Carmarthen
Wales

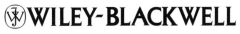

WILEY-BLACKWELL

A John Wiley & Sons, Ltd., Publication

This edition first published 2009
© 2009 John Wiley & Sons, Ltd.

Wiley-Blackwell is an imprint of John Wiley & Sons, formed by the merger of Wiley's global Scientific, Technical and Medical business with Blackwell Publishing.

Registered office
John Wiley & Sons Ltd, The Atrium, Southern Gate, Chichester, West Sussex, PO19 8SQ, United Kingdom

Editorial office
John Wiley & Sons Ltd, The Atrium, Southern Gate, Chichester, West Sussex, PO19 8SQ, United Kingdom

For details of our global editorial offices, for customer services and for information about how to apply for permission to reuse the copyright material in this book please see our website at www.wiley.com/wiley-blackwell.

The right of the author to be identified as the author of this work has been asserted in accordance with the Copyright, Designs and Patents Act 1988.

All rights reserved. No part of this publication may be reproduced, stored in a retrieval system, or transmitted, in any form or by any means, electronic, mechanical, photocopying, recording or otherwise, except as permitted by the UK Copyright, Designs and Patents Act 1988, without the prior permission of the publisher.

Wiley also publishes its books in a variety of electronic formats. Some content that appears in print may not be available in electronic books.

Designations used by companies to distinguish their products are often claimed as trademarks. All brand names and product names used in this book are trade names, service marks, trademarks or registered trademarks of their respective owners. The publisher is not associated with any product or vendor mentioned in this book. This publication is designed to provide accurate and authoritative information in regard to the subject matter covered. It is sold on the understanding that the publisher is not engaged in rendering professional services. If professional advice or other expert assistance is required, the services of a competent professional should be sought.

Library of Congress Cataloging-in-Publication Data

Hanley, Jane.
Perinatal mental health: a guide for health professionals and users / Jane Hanley.
    p. ; cm.
Includes bibliographical references and index.
ISBN 978-0-470-51068-1 (pbk.)
    1. Postpartum depression–x Nursing.   I. Title.
[DNLM: 1. Postpartum Period–psychology–Nurses' Instruction.   2. Depression, Postpartum–Nurses' Instruction.   3. Mental Disorders–Nurses' Instruction. WQ 500 H514p 2009]
RG852.H36 2009
618.7′60231–dc22

                                                                        2008044813

A catalogue record for this book is available from the British Library.

Set in 10/12 pt Sabon by Aptara® Inc., New Delhi, India
Printed in Singapore by Markono Print Media Pte Ltd

1   2009

Contents

Women's mental health: from Hippocrates to Kumar

Blessings on the hand of women!
Fathers, sons, and daughters cry,
And the sacred song is mingled
With the worship in the sky –
Mingles where no tempest darkens,
Rainbows evermore are hurled;
For the hand that rocks the cradle
Is the hand that rules the world.
William Ross Wallace 1819–1881

An overview of perinatal mental health

It is stating the obvious that childbirth is not a new phenomenon, nor has the study of it been neglected over the years. For the most part, and up until recent years, research has focused more on the actual physical side of childbearing, with little regard given to any psychological or emotional factors. There is now a growing body of researchers who suggest that there is overwhelming evidence to recommend that the good mental health of mothers be maintained during the perinatal period. This is because it is now believed that it is crucial to secure a happy outcome for the mother, her infant, and her family, and it is through this research that methods and management strategies may be discovered in order to achieve these outcomes. Despite the evidence of risk to infant development and factors which could harm the mother and her family, the study of maternal and infant mental welfare remains a subject that is often misunderstood and misrepresented.

Criticism has been levied about the weakness and lack of rigour of some pieces of research into perinatal mental health. It seems that few research projects concentrate on producing the results from randomised control trials and there are very few of the type of 'gold standard' research. The reasons for the failure to conduct rigorous research may be many, but not least that it is the overall sensitivity of the condition together with the reluctance of ethics committees to grant permission for such studies. There is apprehension that any enquiries into a mother's mental health may endanger her mental state even further by having the potential to resurrect thoughts and feelings of a mother's previously depressed state of mind. These objections make it difficult to carry out sufficient studies of research into the subject. Many of the studies, particularly of a qualitative nature, have had to be carried out retrospectively, capturing the thoughts and feelings of an event which has passed.

A recent UK Government commissioned report: the Darzi Plan –, *High Quality Care for All* (Darzi, 2008), which is set to revolutionise the vision of the future of health care, highlighted the necessity for services to be focused on individual needs, with the choice for services being centralised. It advocated integrated partnerships, maximising the contribution of the workforce and an intention to prevent policies on health inequalities and diversity. Nowhere, however, did it mention the importance of, or even refer to, perinatal mental health. Even in this enlightened document the mental health needs of mothers were overlooked. Mental health has, historically, been an area of contention when discussing the next priority for government funding. It would appear that those perceived as the more common biological diseases of cancer and the heart override any need for the solution of problems incurred in mental ill-health. The alleviation of mental illness, coupled with the stigma, remains as big a problem in the twenty-first century as it ever was, even though dealing with mental illness and its concomitant dilemmas involves a great deal of the work force and even the finances of the country.

Opinions as to whether postnatal depression is a specific disease have been debated since the time of Hippocrates. From the time of Louis Marcé (1858) the theories of its origin, ranging from hormonal (Dalton, 1985), to social (Guscott & Steiner, 1991; Oakley, 1975) have been considered and disputed. However, it is only in the last thirty years or so that in-depth study of the subject has revealed the high incidence of this distressing complaint (Gerrard *et al.*, 1993). It has been argued that there are still too many women, who, together with their families, are suffering in silence (Kelly, 1994). Recent television and newspaper coverage has stimulated some interest in postnatal depression. However, much remains to be done to educate the public at large, ensuring that a greater awareness of the prevalence of this condition and its damaging symptoms can be recognised and managed.

The debate, however, is not new. It is reputed that the incidence of postnatal depression, as a major mental disorder following childbirth, has been the subject of medical observation since the days of Hippocrates. This ancient Greek philosopher recognised that health and disease are interdependent upon the interplay between human actions and the environment of man. The customs, values, climate, diet, and modes of life and age determined the characteristics of each disease. The additional requirements which determined a person's health status included the whole of the persona and were involved with the examination in detail of a person's innermost thoughts, their speech patterns and the silences contained within them. The reasons for the mannerisms were thought to be peculiar to that person. There was intricate examination of sleeping habits to establish whether they were fitful, filled with dreams and what those dreams consisted of and when those dreams occurred.

This approach encompassed the person as a whole and recognised the importance and effect of the integration of environmental and socio-economic living conditions as well as individual and collectivist lifestyles on the health of the person. Although this philosophy is still largely advocated in primary care, and health care professionals are urged to apply this approach, this is often marginalised by the more scientific approach that is advocated by the medical profession.

An exploration of the history of the mother's mental health

In 460 BC Hippocrates described 'puerperal fever', also recognised as puerperal sepsis. The name was derived from the Latin *puer* – meaning a boy or child. It was discovered in more recent times that the condition is caused by the Streptococcus A bacterium. Symptoms include a high fever of sudden onset with resulting delirium. Hippocrates, however, credited the cause as the suppressed lochial discharge, which was transported to the brain, where it produced *'agitation, delirium and attacks of mania'*.

Over time, determining health by exploring the body and the environment became compromised as medicine strove to understand the pathology of life. Once it became possible to study cadavers, the expertise on the functioning of particular body parts provided great insight into their operative modes. Anatomical studies performed by Leonardo da Vinci determined an understanding of the locomotion of the human body.

The eleventh-century writings of the gynaecologist Trotula of Salerno noted that *'if the womb is too moist, the brain is filled with water, and the moisture running over to the eyes compels them to involuntary shed tears'*.

Descartes was a mathematician and physicist who is considered the founder of modern philosophy. In 1637 he published *Discourse on the Method* in which he expressed his disillusion with traditional philosophy and the limitations of theology. He respected the certainty of algebra and geometry but as they depended purely on hypothesis he felt it was impossible for the interpretation of reality and to determine what the world was actually like. He recognised the radical difference between the physical and mental aspects of the world and the reality of his own mind. '*I think, therefore I am.*' In 1649 *The Passions of the Soul* further suggested that the human body was split into the biological body and the psychological or spiritual mind and defined the relationship between the body brain and mind:

> Regard this body as a machine which, having been made by the hand of God, is incomparably better ordered than any machine that can be devised by man, and contains in itself movements more wonderful than those in any machine[e] ... it is for all practical purposes impossible for a machine to have enough organs to make it act in all the contingencies of life in the way in which our reason makes us act.
>
> (Descartes)

Descartes suggested that the human body is purely a vehicle for the mind and it is only able to function because the mind instructs it to do so: '*the mind is not immediately affected by all parts of the body, but only by the brain, or perhaps just by one small part of the brain, namely the part which is said to contain the "common sense".'* This philosophy gave an entirely different perspective on medicine and the regard for the mind and body working independently of each other.

Louis Marcé

In 1858, Louis Marcé recognised that recently delivered mothers and nursing mothers were prone to disturbances of the mind which, whilst they were similar to the more common forms of mental illness, were, however, different in the organic conditions amidst which they develop. He compared the various descriptions of puerperal psychosis, concentrating on the condition of the blood and its effects on *'those ailments of a special nature that affect recently delivered women'*. He considered that the important period *'is limited to the thirty or forty days in which the uterus is in the condition of a suppurating organ'*.

The functions of maternity are discussed in his *Treatise*; the dangers involved in too frequent pregnancies and repeated miscarriages are recognised and the differences in the physical and mental symptoms are exposed. Whilst discussing the types of psychosis Marcé discovers there are *'present certain differences which it is too good to highlight'*. He differentiates between general paralysis of the insane found in tertiary syphilis, and other types of psychoses. Marcé concludes his treatise by stating that *'our aim is not to study the various mental illnesses for their own sake but rather, with the help of clinical documents, seek out the special modifications which these ailments/affections undergo'*.

Twentieth century opinions and interpretations

Many twentieth-century writers have written about the effects of depression and the torment suffered by women. Sylvia Plath, the twentieth-century American writer and poet is no exception. She speaks of her tormented life, besieged by the wrath and pain of depression and as she plummeted even further into the mire, she describes the pain she experiences as:

> *Look at that ugly dead mask here and do not forget it. It is a chalk mask with dead dry poison behind it, like the death angel. It is what I was this fall, and what I never want to be again. The pouting disconsolate mouth, the flat, bored numb expressionless eyes, symptoms of the decay within. I smile, now, thinking: we all like to think we are important enough to need psychiatrists. But all I need is sleep, a constructive attitude, and a little good luck.*
>
> (Kukil, 2000, p. 155)

Her pain was so intense that she was acquainted with the awfulness of suicidal thoughts which she describes as: *'with the groggy sleepless blood dragging through my veins, and the air thick and gray with rain and the damn little men across the street pounding on the roof with pick and axes and chisels, and the acrid hellish stench of tar'* (Stevenson, 1990, p. 35).

Sylvia Plath describes her own feelings of the struggle to be creative while overwhelmed with depressive thoughts: '*You are frozen mentally – scared to get going, eager to crawl back to the womb. First think: here is your room – here is your life, your mind: don't panic*' (Plath, 2000, p. 186).

RD Laing in his definitive book *The Divided Self* describes his thoughts during his depressive psychosis as being trapped in a deep cave: '*It is getting tighter and tighter in here, I am frightened. If I get out of here, it may be terrible. More of these people would be outside. They would crush me, altogether, for they are even heavier that those in here. I think*' (p. 169).

Spalding (1988) in her book *Stevie Smith* states that Stevie had the symptoms of clinical depression, which were tiredness apathy and irritability, all of which forced her to cut one of her wrists (p. 213).

Depression in women can occur at any age, but it is that which happens at and around the time of childbirth that arouses the most interest today, not only because research is increasing, but also because that same research is uncovering facts about which society was ignorant. Societal changes and attitudes make this a challenging condition. Previously it was postnatal depression that dominated research, but this has been superseded by perinatal mental health, to include all mental health disorders that occur around the time of childbirth, both in the ante and postnatal period and up to one year following the birth of the infant. In some instances it is considered in the pre-conceptual stage.

In the early eighties, Channi Kumar, one of the definitive researchers into perinatal mental health commented that postnatal depression might seem of relatively minor clinical importance when compared with the more florid mental illnesses. However, this insidious and chronic condition that can be responsible for the impairment of both personal and family life could be substantially even more severe and longer lasting. He stressed that as it is over one hundred times greater in terms of breakdown, in purely statistical terms, postnatal depression merits very serious attention.

Depression as a concept in itself is physically inexplicable and appears too complex and difficult to understand – so much so that it is easier to use a 'standard one fits all' diagnosis. Most general practitioners (GPs) will accept the responsibility for front line psychiatry and will make commendable efforts to relieve patients of their problems. What is becoming clearer about depression, however, is not that the cure, if indeed there is one, relies on antidepressant medication, but that it requires time and patience from the GP, as well as from others who are concerned about that person. Time is a precious commodity that medical practitioners rarely have, and in today's rationing of time to patients, it becomes even more crucial that time is given to the depressed patient, and perhaps even more so to the woman who has recently given birth. It is probably reasonable to suggest that only those who have suffered from, or experienced mental illness and depression *per se* are in a position to understand what it means to feel the plethora of negative thoughts and how mental illness can be more painful than any physical pain.

Unfortunately, society demands explanations for every illness and the diagnosis of depressive conditions is not alone. The nomenclature of depression in itself is interesting. Is it a depressive 'illness'? To be ill is defined as being 'out of health', 'sick', 'unsound' or 'harmful' and illness is a state of being ill. Some philosophers have defined physical illness as a condition where organic systems do not function according to normal standards. In contrast, the problems of mentally ill individuals are located within the minds of the sufferers. Someone who is mentally disordered is simply 'out of his mind'.

Is depression a condition which is seen either as a state of physical fitness or an ailment or abnormality, as in a 'heart condition'? The word 'disease' is rarely used but it is synonymous with distress. 'Dis' implies the reversal of an action or state. Dis-ease literally means someone who is not at ease, distress someone who is overly stressed. 'Mental health disorder' appears to be the latest label. Disorder interpreted as a lack of order, disease or ailment.

Women's health and welfare in general has been taken into account by many researchers. The impact a mother has, both on and in society, is becoming more relevant. It is an interesting concept to question whether depression and in particular postnatal depression is determined by the society in which a woman lives, or whether it is indeed a physiological manifestation.

In order to pursue the notion that social expectations and evaluations influence the conception of the self and behaviour, it is pertinent to consider the various types of theoretical explanations for ill health. It was Parsons (1951) who originally considered the view of illness as a social state and provided a functionalist analysis of the sick role. This theory has been developed by sociologists and philosophers and allows conditions like postnatal depression to be viewed from a theorist's, non-medical perspective, which questions whether depression is the result of a sociological deterioration rather than a purely physical reaction?

Others have postulated that there is a fundamental distinction between physical illness and mental illness. Each type of illness is interpreted with the use of common-sense frameworks. The body is seen as a part of the physical world in which we live, and as such, it is affected by the laws of cause and effect. Things may happen but fundamentally there is no control over when and how they happen. The mind, however, is viewed in more of a cultural framework of actions, meanings and motives (Horowitz, 1982). In this way perinatal mental health may be observed as a manifestation of social difficulties, as well as a malfunction of the mental processes, since the social difficulties encountered by the mother will have an adverse effect on her mental status.

Durkheim (1858–1917) was concerned about the social processes and constraints that integrate individuals into the larger social community. His belief was that when society was strongly integrated, the individuals who were a part of it were held firmly under control, rather than being allowed to dictate the terms and conditions of that society. From this functionalist perspective, illness can be regarded as a form of social deviance, in which an individual adopts the sick role. Unlike the criminal who chooses to violate social norms, sick persons are considered 'deviant' because they have no control over their condition. The sick role is characterised by the exemption of the sick person from normal social responsibilities. Neither blame nor responsibility is attached to being sick, but sick people are expected to seek out medical attention to 'cure' the problem quickly, to enable them to return to their place in society. Postnatal depression and other mental disorders can be construed as a manifestation of an illness in that the 'patient' in this instance, though lacking any physical signs or symptoms of disease is, or appears to be, 'suffering'. This makes it clear in many if not all cases, that the sufferer requires as much sympathy and understanding for her needs as any other sick patient does, although it can be argued that consciously, and perhaps subconsciously, the woman believes she is 'sick', as do those associated with her. However, it is possible that the woman is subconsciously feigning sickness in order that she may receive that sympathy. The incumbent of a sick role is also expected to comply with the regime prescribed by a competent member of the medical profession (Abercrombie *et al.*, 1984). This obligation of conforming to the sick role ensures this role is not used as an excuse for opting out of normal social responsibilities (Morgan *et al.*, 1991).

Parsons' (1951) earlier work provides a basis for Morgan's assumption, as Parsons' concept of the sick role was based on the premise that a sick person is not in that position because they chose to be, but rather because they had it foisted upon them, either by infection or injury or some other non-deliberate external force. Parsons (1951) argues that being sick is not just experiencing the physical condition of a sick state, but it constitutes a social role, since it involves behaviour based on institutional expectations and is reinforced by the norms of society corresponding to these expectations. In the case of postnatal depression this could mean that women may seek medical permission to vacate the role of 'caring mother'. Women may on the one hand be constrained by common beliefs and facts that belong to a bygone age, that is from a functional perspective they may believe that they should stay at home to care for the child. On the other hand they may feel obliged to agree with modern day feminist thinking regarding their 'rights' to freedom and the need to accept the triple role of wife, mother and worker. Whichever way they turn it appears that women will believe themselves to be disadvantaged.

Whereas many writers have criticised the works of Parsons, some originally offered a viable alternative medical supremacy in controlling role conformity. One exception was Friedson (1970) who reformed the functionalist framework to produce the 'labelling approach' (Morgan *et al.*, 1991). In this interpretation a clear distinction was made between disease, which is regarded as a biophysical phenomenon that exists independently of human evaluation and illness, which depends on the social and medical response to disease. This theory explains illness as a deviance not as a product of individual psychology, physiology or of genetic inheritance, but of social control. In respect of this perspective, women with perinatal mental health disorders might be seen as deviant because they reject or cannot cope with the pressures of motherhood. They must therefore be given a label or diagnosis which places them in a socially acceptable category.

During the 1970s, symbolic interactionism was seen as a major alternative to functionalism. Whereas functionalist theory focuses on the influence of the larger society on the individual, symbolic interaction emphasises interpersonal forms of interaction. The intellectual roots of this paradigm are in the concept of self, as developed by Mead (1934) who argued that reflexivity (referring to self) is crucial to the self as a social phenomenon. The individual is seen as a creative, thinking organism responsible for his or her own behaviour that does not react mechanically to social processes. Social life depends on the individual's ability to imagine how they would react to other people's situations or roles. The ability to achieve this state depends on the individual's capacity for internal conversation. Mead (1934) believed that society was conceived by an exchange of gestures involving the use of symbols. Symbols impose particular meanings on objects and events and, as a result, exclude other possible meanings. Without symbols no human interaction or human society would be possible (Haralambos, 1985). However, the theory has been criticised for failing to give sufficient weight to the objective restraints on social action. In recent years, Denzin (1992) has sought to resurrect the theory by refining and developing the finer points and argues that interpretive and symbolic interactionists see society as an emergent phenomenon that it is constantly changing and, as a result, cannot be understood through grand theory. Consequently, it is believed that people are constrained by the constructions they build and inherit from the past, and that recurrent meanings and practices are produced when individuals do things together. To understand social behaviour, therefore, the focus should be on the actual, lived emotional experiences of individuals and the assumption that people create the worlds of experience they live in through the meanings gleaned through interaction. From this viewpoint new mothers would be expected to behave in a way that they have internalised. If, for some reason, their 'internalised ideals' conflict with reality, they may wish to 'opt out'.

In work by Waters (1994) it is assumed that the world is subjective and consists of creations, meanings and ideas of thinking and acting subjects. Individuals are competent and communicative agents who actively construct the social world. In order to understand the social world it is important to understand the individual's meaning of the world. The individual is not responsible for the creation of the world they were born into as that world already exists. Whatever the individual learns and absorbs about culture and values during a lifetime is achieved by their own discovery and negotiation. These are usually appropriate to the type of lifestyle familiar to them. Although certain social phenomena are intrinsic, it is argued it is possible to affect change as an ongoing process during a lifetime. Many factors affect that change and it is the decision of the individual to adopt that change. An informed choice is usually made, but those beliefs that are arguably undeniable in one culture, may be rejected or even discredited in another, and there is always the probability that a steadfastly held belief may be altered, or even dismissed, as information about that belief is changed. Hence the observation that knowledge is not value free. This idea therefore presupposes that postnatal depression is only one of the many decisions the mother might take to achieve respite, or that self-knowledge predisposes some women to hide behind a mental condition until they feel ready to resume their role in society.

This approach expands on the theory of medicalisation and regards all medical categories as social constructs, which define and give meaning to certain classes of events. The implication is not that illness is imaginary but that medicine is a form of social practice that observes, treats and tabulates the origin of illness. Foucault (1973) was a forerunner in the concept of social construction of medicine. He termed the concept the 'clinical gaze', whereby the medical approach views the body by clinical observation, physical examinations and bedside teachings. Over a period of time this gave rise to the belief in a solid invariant reality of the body, and as a result, the body was observed in a completely different way. Armstrong (1983) examined how the clinical gaze served to create new specialities and expand the remit of those specialities which had already been developed. This philosophy developed during the 1960s when practitioners started regarding the person as a whole being, not as a segment of illness or disease.

Often, however, the diagnosis of postnatal depression is made only in relation to the manifestation of certain behaviours. Socially structured predisposing factors are therefore likely to be ignored. This means that the issues, which may be causing severe stress for a mother, are ignored. Only when a medically orientated social construction is presented will the women receive attention.

A feminist perspective

Feminism and female emancipation have had a significant impact on the way women view themselves. They have created enormous inroads into the male domain, but many question whether men have accommodated women into the social world. As females have created a niche for themselves so they have exposed themselves and left themselves wide open to abuse and it has been postulated that the function of childbirth itself constitutes such abuse. Ideally, there should be no sexually based differences between men and women.

Paglia (1995) describes a woman as:

One who does not dream of transcendental or historical escape from natural cycle. Her sexual maturity means marriage to the moon, waxing and waning in lunar phases. Moon, month, menses mean the same word same world[e] ... The female body is a chthonian machine, indifferent to the spirit, which inhabits it. Organically it has one mission, pregnancy, which it may spend a lifetime staving off. Nature cares only for species, never individuals: women, who probably have a greater realism and wisdom than men because of it, most directly experience the humiliating dimensions of this biologic fact.

Therefore to emulate men in the world of work, or conversely to desire to opt out and be a mother may mean that women are unlikely to conform to everyone's construction of motherhood. This means that women may experience internal conflict between a feminist construction of proper role behaviour and their natural instincts.

These sociological perspectives all serve to determine whether women are subjected to pressures foisted upon them by society as a whole, and if this is the case, the question must be asked whether the pressures are too heavy to bear. Is the result of all these indications the 'breakdown' or manifestation of perinatal mental illness?

In recent years society has seen the disintegration of the supportive mothering role of the extended family, as grandmothers as well as mothers, seek gainful employment. Sometimes the female family members are so removed, geographically, that the support network of families becomes even more fragmented than ever. It is also recognised that this is a complex cultural phenomenon, which cannot be simplified. Another problem is that the nuclear family appears to be less relevant today than it has been in the past. Divorce is increasing and the single parent family is rapidly becoming accepted as a normal status in society. Efforts by the Government to become child friendly and provide good child care echo the sentiments of women who may have been forced to work over the past few decades by the capitalist nature of society and feminist pressures. However, good childcare is essential, and there are mothers who would prefer to care for their own children. Unfortunately, past and present Government policy appears to preclude this, and mothers are not only encouraged to resume paid employment as soon as possible, but are actively persuaded to introduce care workers to look after their children during working hours.

With obligation on women to become – at least in some cases – the sole breadwinner, it is not to be wondered that some of these women succumb to pressures of which previous generations have been unaware.

LIVERPOOL JOHN MOORES UNIVERSITY
LEARNING SERVICES

The antenatal period

2

Pregnancy as a natural phenomenon

Much attention has been given to perinatal mental health disorders and postnatal depression in particular, but until recently there was little research into the effects of the antenatal period on maternal mood. Pitt (1968) was one of the first psychiatrists to recognise the importance of an 'atypical' depression following childbirth, and deemed it as a common and important complication of the puerperium which necessitated a greater understanding. Since then, the focus of research into mothers' mental health has featured primarily on the postnatal period. It had been believed that the condition of pregnancy protected women from feelings of despondency and despair; therefore improving maternal mental health during pregnancy may stand alone as a legitimate goal.

It appears that there has been the commonly held misconception that mothers thrive and positively 'glow with health' whilst they are pregnant. Phrases describe mothers as 'blooming' or having 'fresher complexions' and 'glossy hair'. The whole demeanour of a woman with child is one of serenity and calm. It is interesting, then, to discover in the work by Evans *et al.* (2001) that the symptoms of depression are not more common or severe after childbirth than during pregnancy. The research suggested that antenatal depression affects 15–20% of mothers, which is a higher percentage than women who get postnatal depression. Characteristically, and in line with postnatal depression, it was previously thought that antenatal depression occurred in 10% of mothers (Cox & Holden, 1994), but recent studies have found the prevalence to be over a quarter of pregnant mothers (Bolton *et al.*, 1998).

Authors have acclaimed the pregnant mother as a thing of loveliness, to be admired and coveted. Mansfield (1910) in this poem captured the solicitude of infant *in utero* towards his carer as:

Her beauty fed my common earth.
I cannot see nor breathe nor stir,
but through the death of some of her.

While John Suckling (1646) wrote:

'Tis expectation makes a blessing dear:
Heaven were not heaven, if we knew what it were.

Fraser (2006) asked eleven mothers to describe their final trimester of pregnancy by completing abstract drawings and accounts of their perceptions and feelings; although there were different responses to the positive and negative aspects of their pregnancy, they all reported 'joy' as the common underlying emotion.

Research is continuing to show that many women were distressed during their pregnancy but failed to recognise it as a problem. However, anecdotal evidence from mothers who have shared their experiences on websites state: 'Crying in pregnancy was "perfectly normal" and how could I be depressed when I was so happy to be pregnant?' It is possible that women accept the differing emotions as part of the excitement or foreboding of being pregnant with the baby they either longed for or dreaded. It is also possible they are unable to recognise the source of these emotions and may explain this as being tired, anxious or lonely (Welford, 1998). The plethora of feelings which assail the mother may make it difficult to differentiate between what is normal for her, and what is different from normal because of bearing an infant.

Not only is depression common in pregnancy but it is associated with the high rates of mortality and morbidity for infants as well as mothers (Rondo *et al.*, 2003).

It is possible that hormonal changes are responsible but there is insufficient evidence to suggest this is the case. However, the biological changes of increased concentrations of sex steroids during pregnancy are known to have a direct effect on the mother's emotional state.

Pregnancy is a major life-changing event so it is not beyond the realms of possibility that women may become depressed during this period, particularly if this compounds other life stressors. The addition or untimely advent of a pregnancy may cause further stress, which in turn may become unmanageable.

The writer Maureen Lawrence (1972) portrays the feelings of depression during pregnancy, which probably encapsulate some of the commoner emotions felt by women burdened by pregnancy:

She felt lazy. The stirring of the curtains told her it was good drying weather; she must rinse out the stain, but her body felt achingly large to move. It felt like something that would burst open at a touch. She thought of what it said in the paper and in the books from the clinic. It was not just the baby. There was water, and a long chord that sometimes got fast in a knot round the baby's neck. She felt afraid. There was washing, shopping, cleaning. She felt afraid. She has to get out of bed, get down on her knees, get the case quickly, get dressed, get ready.

Perhaps her most succinct description of the trauma of pregnancy was: *'and always it was dark. She could see no end to it, except in darkness'* (p. 175).

Tokophobia

A study by Hofberg & Brockington (2000) uncovered the condition of tokophobia, a morbid fear of childbirth, which in many cases is so profound that it sometimes leads to a complete avoidance of pregnancy, even though many of the mothers admit that they would dearly love children. Such is the fear in some women that in extreme cases they are resigned to the fact that adoption or fostering is the only possible course of action for them to rear children in the future. For other women the only recourse is to remain childless and in some cases women will avoid long-term relationships which could result in childbearing. It is believed that as many as one in seven women suffer from the condition.

This intense anxiety and unreasoning dread of childbirth sometimes culminates in a fear of death, but it is their overwhelming need for a baby that in the main overcomes this. This 'dread' is also associated with anxiety, depression, post-traumatic stress disorder (PTSD) and bonding disorders. Mothers have admitted it is deeply psychologically traumatising for them, which leads to a profound disgust of childbirth. Some mothers may feel disgusted by the fact that something alien is growing inside them.

Tokophobia has been categorised into primary and secondary tokophobia.

Primary tokophobia may begin during adolescence. Girls may have normal sexual relations but this fear may be so powerful that they take extra care with contraceptive methods to avoid becoming pregnant, sometimes using several different methods at the same time. Some women have blamed their first visual images of childbirth on their perception of their own childbirth. One woman remembered watching a video of childbirth in a sex education lesson and described it as *'barbaric, like watching a horror film[e] ... I couldn't believe the amount of blood'* (Nicholas, 2007). Another mother said she felt nauseous at images portrayed at the birth. It is also possible to develop tokophobia during the pregnancy and mothers can be concerned that they will die during childbirth.

Avoidance of the act of childbirth itself is also a common symptom and it is most probable the mothers would request and prefer a Caesarean birth because, for them, it would be less gruesome. They would be allowed sedation throughout the procedure to avoid confrontation with the operation. This, too, has its drawbacks, as for some women the thought of having their stomachs cut open is fairly terrifying.

In Hofberg & Brockington's study it was found that the majority of the mothers who had primary tokophobia also suffered with postnatal depression; PTSD was endured by two of the mothers and bonding was delayed in another two cases.

Secondary tokophobia occurs in the second pregnancy following a traumatic or distressing delivery during the previous pregnancy which, understandably, makes mothers fear their forthcoming delivery. These women become pregnant again despite their overwhelming fears. In the Hofberg study some of these mothers suffered from postnatal depression, PTSD and bonding difficulties. All of them suffered from extreme anxiety during their pregnancy.

It is possible to overlook the condition and the symptoms presented because the horror and disgust of giving birth to a child remains one of society's taboo subjects. The general feeling is that all women want to experience the joy of giving birth and that it is the most natural thing in the world. For some mothers it is a pathological problem and they find it very difficult to discuss tokophobia for fear of the reaction they may have from friends, who may accuse them of being insensitive, not to mention heartless. It has been argued that mothers who give voice to their own traumatic deliveries only serve to collude with the view that mothers who have an innate fear of childbirth have no right to feel as they do. This fosters the belief that the mother with tokophobia is unique.

Some organisations (such as Birth Trauma Association) have called for greater recognition of the condition and for the understanding that the increasing prevalence of a genuine and morbid fear of pregnancy and birth is real. Obstetricians and midwives, most importantly, should be more sympathetic to the mothers' needs. There should be a greater emphasis on pain relief and more acceptance of the need for a Caesarean delivery. There is always some anxiety about giving birth, but the intensity of tokophobia means that mothers will overcompensate with their type of contraception in order to prevent pregnancy. It should be recognised as a psychological problem which requires support, not condemnation.

Mother's nutritional status and eating disorders

One survey found that one in fifty pregnant women developed an eating disorder because of the stress they encountered during the pregnancy. The main stressors were the worries about eating the correct type of food. There is no conclusive evidence to suggest that there is an increase in the number of pregnant women experiencing an eating disorder, although the pressure on women to return to their pre-pregnancy weight is increasing and that in itself could add to the risk.

For some women, the stress that surrounds the idea of their bodily state commences early in the pregnancy and reveals a distortion of their body image. Rather than seeing themselves as pregnant and carrying a baby, some mothers avoid or in some instances fail to recognise the natural process of childbearing and complain that their clothes feel tighter and increasingly uncomfortable. The tummy feels generally bloated and they are aware they are becoming fat. Any gain in weight within their social environment is seen as highly undesirable, and some women have been determined to avoid gaining any unnecessary weight during their pregnancy other than that which is recommended by obstetricians and dieticians. As the foetus grows the result is the struggle to maintain the control over weight gain. In order to achieve this, however, it is probable that some women will carefully monitor their diet and restrict their calorie intake, sometimes dangerously compromising their own health and that of their infant. This determination to control her weight is further enhanced as the woman strives to accomplish a strict and sometimes severe daily exercise routine.

For some women, the body image becomes more important than the pregnancy. In some communications women have commented that whereas being pregnant is acceptable, the inevitable weight gain is not. This is particularly so even when then they are aware of the amount of weight that could be expected to be gained throughout the pregnancy.

In some studies, contrary to any beliefs that the mother might enjoy being pregnant, some women tended to abandon any thoughts of a state of childbearing where they might blossom with health and be blissfully happy. They laboured under more critical thoughts by describing pregnancy as a state that would make them appear like a 'fat blob'. Some of the women demonstrated some insight into their behaviour, but they appeared to be under the illusion that any previous stressful behaviour about their diet and consequent need to exercise would diminish or even cease once they became pregnant. However, despite their best efforts, when they did become pregnant their obsession with body image remained just as strong.

In general, it is the more affluent and educated women who tend to exercise routinely and restrict their calories during pregnancy. They are also more anxious, stressed and not delighted by being pregnant. They rationalise their behaviour by explaining that any weight gain would cause health risks for both themselves and their foetus, but they fail to recognise that by starving themselves they are depriving their infant of essential nutrients. A further problem is that although they may be overly conscious about their weight, they sometimes appear ignorant of how much weight they should gain during the pregnancy and what foods would facilitate that gain.

Whilst some women make a conscious effort to maintain the perfect pregnant figure there are women who are gaining too much weight. Some reports have found that obese mothers were more likely to report being emotional or subjected to traumatic stress during their pregnancy. Some obese women are likely to become depressed because they are unhappy with their appearance and often complain about poor health status. However, there is little evidence to suggest that obesity in these women increases the incidence of their depressive outcomes (Atlantis & Baker, 2008; La Coursiere *et al.*, 2006; Markowitz *et al.*, 2008). Indeed, it is argued that the physiological changes in the hormone and immune systems of depressed women may cause them to become obese in the first place. As an added antithesis, the symptoms of depression often make it difficult to be fully compliant and aware of health issues. Adhering to fitness and diet regimes may be almost impossible to do. It becomes a chicken and egg scenario as it becomes difficult to manage one and the other. Exercise and techniques that help to limit or reduce stress are helpful and can manage both the depressive symptoms and the weight issues, but strict dieting may deepen the depression. The addition of antidepressants may cause a further weight gain. It is estimated that nearly 40% of pregnant women have 'big babies' where they gain more than the recommended amount of weight. The recommended weight gain is based on pre-pregnancy body mass index (BMI), which compares weight to height. It is recommended that women of normal weight should gain between 11–13.5 kg and underweight women should gain 12.5–18 kg. Overweight women should be able to limit their weight increase to 6.5–11 kg and obese women should gain about a stone during the pregnancy.

There is evidence to suggest that eating disorders in mothers affect children's growth. A further study concentrated on the effect of the growth of infants whose mothers suffered from an eating disorder and postnatal depression (Stein *et al.*, 1999). They also looked at the conditions under which growth retardation may occur. It was found that the infants of mothers with eating disorders were smaller, both in weight and length, than either of the comparison groups. There was little evidence that mothers with eating disorders preferred smaller children or were dissatisfied with their children's shape; rather, these women were highly sensitive to their children's body shape, compared with the other groups.

Several studies have found that the problem with excessive weight during pregnancy is that mothers tend not to lose the excess weight and in effect gain more weight over the ensuing years. There is increasing evidence to show that there is also the added risk of the infant gaining excessive weight during his/her early childhood.

Recent research has suggested that there should be a holistic approach to the treatment and management of depressed and clinically obese women, together with recognition that the two conditions may not be wholly isolated.

Anorexia nervosa

Anorexia nervosa is a severe emotional disorder, which seldom appears before puberty and primarily affects girls: 3% of adolescent girls. In recent years it appears to be affecting boys, too. It rarely occurs in either men or women over the age of forty.

It sometimes follows a traumatic event and is often entangled with emotional or stressful life crises. Some studies have found that dominating and controlling parents have been a factor. There is a lack of emotional attachment and often the parents find it difficult to respond to the emotional needs of their offspring. There are usually great expectations of the child, which are often unfulfilled. Some may argue that by not eating the child regains control as an act of passive revenge.

There is a large body of work that subscribes to the theory that there is a direct relationship between eating disorders and sexual abuse. In one study, 30% of the women with eating disorders reported sexual abuse. This type of abuse was prevalent among bulimics but was rare among those women who were classed as anorexic 'restrictors'. It has been suggested that a history of sexual abuse was just as common in women with psychiatric disorders as in the bulimic or anorexic women (Stieger & Zankor, 1990; Welch & Fairburn, 1994). Likewise, there are sufferers of abuse who have not experienced any bulimic episode. However, sexual abuse should not be discounted as a cause of eating disorders as excessive dieting may help the woman to regain control where sexual abuse has occurred.

There are often tentative conclusions about whether an eating disorder is more a symptom of dysfunctional family life than being strictly related to sexual abuse. This relationship is complex and is probably affected by both individual and family characteristics. It is probable that any traumatic event has the potential to lead to the development of bulimia nervosa, and the home environment may enable such traumatic events to perpetuate.

There are recorded cases of a family history, with one fifth of those suffering from an eating disorder having a relative who also has the condition. It is unclear, however, whether this is in fact hereditary, or whether it is learned behaviour. It is often reported that the adolescent becomes fixated with the populist culture that equates a slim and lean body with success and beauty. It has been argued that there are changes in the serotonin levels and the process of purging the body of the necessary nutrients may deplete the amount of trypophan, which is necessary for the production of serotonin.

There have been some reports of an association between beta-haemolytic streptococcal infection in the form of Epstein Barr virus and the development of anorexia. Other physiological components have been offered but to date the research is sparse and nothing is conclusive.

Anorexia is classified into two main types. The first is associated with extreme dieting, and in some cases a starvation diet where the minimum of food is eaten. This is not because of hunger, but as an appeasement, because they are often under pressure to eat 'something' though this may be contrary to their own belief. Some may resort to excessive exercise in order to loose any extra weight that may have been gained by eating.

The second type is called bulimia, more commonly known as 'binge' eating. This is characterised by eating and then inducing vomiting immediately afterwards or as soon as it is convenient. To expel any eaten food, despite the quantity, as rapidly and effectively as possible, the girl may resort to the use of laxatives, or in the more severe cases, enemas. Diuretics are viewed as a convenient way to loose extra fluid. This is often carried out without the knowledge of the family and often even close friends are unaware of the consequences.

The most notable indicators are severe and often rapid and sustained weight loss. This loss may be accompanied by physical symptoms. The most prominent is the irregularity and sometimes absence of menstrual periods. The hair and skin are dry and thin and the extremities, the hands and feet, are often cold, with a bluish tinge, indicating poor circulation. As the feelings of hunger are often absent, the stomach tends to feel bloated or often irritable.

It is more usual for a girl to prepare an elaborate meal for others than to enjoy the food herself. The excuse not to indulge in the meal with guests is 'when you have been cooking all day you don't really feel hungry'. Mealtimes may be scrupulously planned beforehand. The mealtime itself becomes almost ritualistic, with food being cut into small pieces and eaten slowly and deliberately, chewing each individual piece. The food may be toyed with on the plate and pushed over to one side to give the impression that more has been consumed than actually has. It is not unusual for food which should have been consumed, to be hidden during the meal to be disposed of later.

The most predominant psychological signs are a profound distortion of body image, whereby despite the extreme weight loss the girl has the false belief that she still requires to lose more weight. Other signs may include poor judgement, poor memory and feelings of depression, with a flattening of affect, poor quality sleep and a diminished interest in sex.

Management of the disorder

The condition has several risk factors during pregnancy. There is an increased risk of having a caesarean section, the infant having a low birthweight or being born prematurely. The added risk for these infants is that their prematurity may affect their neurological and physical development.

Other birth complications may also present, though studies have shown that the majority of women carry their babies to term and the infants have good Apgar scores. There is a also a greater risk of the mother having postnatal depression as the mother becomes increasingly unable to cope with the pressure and stresses of parenthood, particularly if her mental state was fragile prior to the pregnancy.

As the condition is often life threatening it is important to restore the weight that has been lost as quickly as possible and ensure that there is no further weight loss. The most effective form of management is cognitive behavioural therapy combined with antidepressants. Here complementary therapies and herbal remedies have a sound function and can help to promote appetite as well as self-esteem. In these circumstances it is not only the mother who requires help but therapy is recommended for the family. The existing feelings of guilt and anxiety need to be tackled and partners and parents, in particular, need to be aware of the gravity of the condition and understand how they may be contributing to it. The importance of support and encouragement for the mother is vital and will help recovery.

Complementary therapies and herbal remedies have an influence on increasing the appetite as well as promoting self-esteem (LaValle et al., 2000; Wheatland, 2002). Hypnotherapy has been known to have a marginal success rate.

Social influences are important too, including engaging the family in the significance of weight control and not being over critical of any weight gain that might have been achieved. Family therapy is recommended to explore any feelings of guilt and anxiety and the way in which these may inadvertently be contributing to the condition.

Treatment can sometimes be prolonged and there is no completely effective management of the condition. Recovery can often take over five years and long-term studies have found that 50–70% recover, whereas 25% will never fully recover.

Pregnancy itself poses a potential problem and often the mother may find it difficult to become pregnant again primarily because of her fertility situation. Women with an eating disorder have higher rates of spontaneous abortion or find it difficult to carry the foetus to term. Infants are often of low birthweight and there is an increased risk of birth defects. The malnourishment of the foetus is also a concern as there is often a tendency towards calcium deficiency.

There is also the added risk of the mother suffering from a relapse because of the added stress of the pregnancy and in the postnatal period the increased demands made on her by parenthood.

The fourth edition of the American Psychiatric Association's *Diagnostic and Statistical Manual of Mental Disorders* (APA, 1994) lists four criteria that an individual must meet in order to be diagnosed as anorexic, generalised as follows:

1) The individual maintains a body weight that is about 15% below normal for age, height and body type.
2) The individual has an intense fear of gaining weight or becoming fat, even though they are underweight. Paradoxically, losing weight can make this fear of gaining even worse.
3) The individual has a distorted body image. Some may feel fat all over, others recognise that they are generally thin, but see specific body parts (particularly the stomach and thighs) as being too fat. Their self-worth is based on their body size and shape. They deny that their low body weight is serious cause for concern.
4) In women, there is an absence of at least three consecutive menstrual cycles. A woman also meets these criteria if her period occurs only while she is taking a hormone pill (including, but not limited to, oral contraceptives).

Bulimia nervosa

The number of women suffering from bulimia is difficult to define, but some statistics have suggested that as many as one in three women have engaged in some sort of bulimic behaviour (Thornton & Russell, 1997).

Researchers are divided about the exact causes of bulimia and as in other eating disorders; it is probable it is the product of a number of factors. It is generally considered to be both a psychological and emotional disorder. It is possible for it to co-exist with obsessive compulsive disorder or depression.

The first cause might be attributed to low self-esteem and dissatisfaction with the body image. It may be felt that trying to lose weight quickly might restore some feelings of self-worth. Once again, cultural pressure may cause an aspiration to mimic the slim bodies of models, portrayed by the media, and fashion may also be a precursor.

It may be caused by the type of emotional stress that is activated during a traumatic experience, but paradoxically bulimia might be seen as a way to manage distress. The intake of food on an eating binge may temporarily distract the mother from her thoughts of distress and focus on the pleasure of taste and fulfilment. The act of purging can help to regain control so that weight gain does not become an additional issue.

Also, while bulimic behaviour may have started as a seemingly innocent way to lose weight, the cycle of bingeing and purging usually becomes an addictive escape from all other types of problems. It is not uncommon for women to become addicted to an illegal substance or adopt behaviours which will help them to avoid painful or distressing situations; for sufferers of bulimia the principles are the same. The bingeing and purging acts as a comfort barrier to life's disturbing events and does not have the negative connotations of alcohol or drug abuse:

> When life is OK I am OK and so are my eating habits. But sometimes the slightest thing upsets me and I have to go and find something quickly to eat. One Easter I had twelve Easter eggs and ate them all at the same time.

> I would often avoid going out for meals with friends, if there was a celebration which involved a dinner I would make excuses not to go. If I felt compelled to go I would give loads of reasons why I could not join them at the table. If that failed sit, eat and pick the most opportune moment to go to the ladies to vomit.

Some women have cited a past history of sexual abuse as one of the main causes of the disorder. The evidence for this is inconsistent when reporting the number of patients with eating disorders that have been sexually abused. The figures for bulimic women with a history of sexual abuse have been reported to range from 7% to 70%; however, the majority report that approximately 60% of bulimics have experienced some form of sexual abuse. Bulimia may be used as a way to dissociate the woman's thoughts from what was a frightening and destructive experience: 'When I was abused by my uncle I was rewarded with ice cream and sweets[e] ... I hated the thought of food and[e]' ....

There may be a genetic component, as it is believed that those who have a close relative who has, or has had, bulimia are four times more likely to develop it compared to those who do not have a relative who has had the condition. Other studies have linked it to lowered levels of brain serotonin function (Kaye *et al.*, 2008).

The word bulimia comes from the Latin word to mean 'ravenous hunger' and its history may be traced back centuries. It is described as an obsession with food, body image and weight gain. It is characterised by repeatedly overeating, or bingeing on foods. As the mother recognises the enormity of what she has consumed and why, she resorts to self-inducing vomiting either manually or with the use of a purgative. She may choose to exercise excessively in a bid to counteract the large amount of calories she has eaten. In some cases laxatives and diuretics may be used on a regular basis. The mother usually defines a fixed time when an amount of food should be eaten. This amount is larger than the average sized portion and in most cases can be seen as excessive, often exceeding 2000 calories. Often, the food consists primarily of carbohydrates and sugars. The mother may not be able to control the quantity she eats and despite wishing to stop feels compelled to finish the meal. The taste of food is irresistible and the feeling of elation after the meal is liberating. Revolted by her lack of willpower and control she will instigate the method of purging the food from her body. Once the cycle has finished she promises herself that it will never be repeated, but often it does occur again.

For the majority, this is a secret addiction which dominates their lives. Often they will avoid eating in company but if forced to will sometimes go to extraordinary lengths to conceal what they are eating. John Prescott revealed in his memoires how his bulimic episodes were generated by stress and how he tried to conceal his condition from his wife:

> *I could sup a whole tin of Carnation condensed milk, just for the taste[e] ... I thought, of course, I was being clever, and no one would ever know, but Pauline realised in the end. The signs in the toilet gave it away, and all the missing food.*
>
> (Oakeshott, 2008)

Often mothers will describe it as having a split personality, whereby one part of her is revolted by her behaviour but is unable to control it, whilst the other half takes a perverted joy in the overwhelming feeling of being satisfied. Some have resorted to stealing food off others' plates or raiding cupboards in an effort to find food.

One survey reported that for some it was the boredom, mental numbness and family dynamics which were reasons for starting and sustaining bulimia. The pressure to lose weight and the influences of the media were also listed. An interesting aspect was that it was seen as a release for physical and sexual tension. Jane Fonda, the actress, admitted to bulimia in an effort to have the perfect body and please her husband; Joan Rivers suffered from it following the death of her husband and Princess Diana during her marriage.

Consequences of bulimia

The most common problems for bulimic women include rotten teeth, constipation, bloating and other digestive disorders. The excessive vomiting often leads to temporary electrolyte imbalance. With prolonged, excessive vomiting there can be kidney damage and ultimate failure. There is also the danger of an oesophageal rupture or choking on vomit. Anaemia and hypoglycaemia are also common. There is often irregularity with the menstrual cycle or amenorrhoea.

Bulimia nervosa is more common in women of childbearing age and also carries the risk of obstetric complications, foetal abnormalities, which may include cleft palate and cleft lip and the possible onset of postnatal depression (Franco *et al.*, 2001; Morgan *et al.*, 2006). The risk of postnatal depression has not been extensively documented but there is evidence to suggest that the predictors of post and perinatal depression have been outlined by this condition and that mothers with bulimia may be more at risk of developing depression.

In most instances the menstrual cycle is often irregular, making contraception difficult, and often the pregnancy is unplanned. The knowledge that they are pregnant is the usually the precursor for some women to seek treatment for their condition. Women are concerned that their abnormal eating behaviours may cause damage to their unborn infant, and in some instances, in view of the increasing evidence, it is difficult to dispel those fears unless she agrees to some form of treatment for the bulimia. Others may be concerned about gaining weight throughout the pregnancy and the anxiety that would produce.

One study showed that when the mothers were treated for the condition the prevalence of their binge eating and self-induced vomiting reduced throughout the pregnancy and by the third trimester in all of the cases had improved and most cases had ceased altogether (Lacey & Smith, 1987). It may be argued that the physical changes caused by the pregnancy often negate the ability to continue the routine of vomiting and bingeing. However, for some of the women the symptoms returned during the postnatal period and for some women the eating disorder was more disturbed than prior to the pregnancy. A small minority of mothers admitted to being overly concerned with their infant's diet and worried that their child might be gaining too much weight. Some would regulate the amount of carbohydrates and sweet stuff to prevent any unnecessary weight gain.

There are important implications for early recognition of bulimia nervosa, in particular in understanding the perception of parenting skills, as the quality of the parent-child interactions may be altered. One study found that conflict arose because the psychopathology of the mother's eating disorder interfered with her ability to respond to her infant's nutritional needs (Stein *et al.*, 1999). All these have serious outcomes for the cognitive behaviour of the children if the mother's condition remains unmanaged. It has been suggested that all women with bulimia should be specifically assessed for postnatal depression following childbirth. There is also a need for further research into the prediction of risk, exploration of the causes and the efficacy of positive intervention and management programmes of the condition.

In 1980, the American Psychiatric Association formally recognised bulimia. The fourth edition, the *Diagnostic and Statistical Manual of Mental Disorders* (APA, 1994) lists the criteria that must be met for a diagnosis to be made. However, many bulimics will engage in the behaviour yet not meet the full diagnostic criteria for bulimia nervosa.

Studies continue to show that the body image and appearance of a woman during and after pregnancy is often as important as the pregnancy itself. The effort of a woman to control her shape and body weight by whatever means must be taken seriously, particularly if the mother chooses an eating disorder to achieve this. These women are often distressed and the purging type of eating disorder is probably more of a concern than women who restrict their intake. They are not easy to detect and therefore the ability to recognise the condition relies heavily on the skills of the health professional. However, once the mother has agreed to some form of management it is relatively straightforward and the result can help the woman to be less vulnerable to a depressive disorder postnatally.

Eating disorders sometimes mirror other major psychiatric disorders and therefore the use of antidepressants is a consideration. The most effective are the SSRIs, as one of the advantages in the case of anorexia is that fluoxetine may cause an increase in weight. However, this may also be in conflict with the mother's desire to remain slim and there is a danger the drug will not be tolerated. Imipramine has some therapeutic properties, while clomipramine may stimulate weight gain. Naturally, there is a need for nutritional supplements to support and sustain the mother's health.

Stress and anxiety during pregnancy

Several studies are emerging which look at the adverse environment this may cause for the infant (Tcixeira *et al.*, 1999). There is growing evidence that stress and anxiety have an effect on the foetus, and as a result the infant. It is unclear, however, what type of anxiety or stress is the most harmful. Clinical studies have shown that the mother's relationship with the partner has a considerable impact on her emotional state. What is becoming increasingly clear is that it is possible that the foetus's environment is modified if the mother is subjected to stress. It has been found that there is a strong correlation between the cortisol levels of the mother and her foetus.

Corticotrophin releasing hormone (CRH) is produced by the hypothalamus in response to a stressful experience. The CRH influences the pituitary gland to produce adrenocorticotrophic hormone (ACTH). This causes the adrenal gland to produce cortisol. During pregnancy the placenta then produces CRH. The levels of cortisol increase significantly and are comparable to those found in Cushing's syndrome. The high levels of cortisol, either produced in response to maternal stress or produced by stress incurred by the foetus, stimulate the placenta to produce more CRH. It is believed it is these high levels that generate the process of labour. Studies have shown that these raised levels of maternal cortisol are usually resolved by six to eight weeks post-partum.

In studies by Wadhwa *et al.* (2004) and Kammerer *et al.* (2006) it was found that the changes in the levels of the hormones influenced the mother's mood. Atypical depression and post-traumatic syndrome are associated with high levels of cortisol at parturition, followed by sudden cortisol withdrawal post-partum. As the woman's pregnancy progresses so does the maternal response to stress.

This still requires more research to understand the complexities of the process but it is known that antenatal stress can affect infants differently. Studies continue to show that if a mother experiences an episode of major depression during the early part of the pregnancy it can exert subtle effects in girls' motor functioning, whereas boys' mental and motor development appear to be more severely affected. It has also been found that high levels of stress in mothers resulted in some infants being born prematurely and/or with small heads and limbs.

There is growing literature to suggest that the physical characteristics of infants at birth (their weight and length) are influential in their future physical and mental well-being, together with predetermining the risk of developing life-limiting conditions in later life. Scientists who continue to research in this area believe that although it is unlikely that birth phenotype has this causal effect, it is more probable that the foetus's environment influences both the structure and function of physiological systems which may be responsible for health and disease. There are still many factors yet to be uncovered which would lead to a greater understanding of the processes which underpin or indeed contribute to the causes of prematurity in babies, poor child development and what might determine the process of chronic degenerative diseases in adulthood. There is undisputed evidence that pre and perinatal stress and, in particular, chronic maternal stress may exert a significant influence on the foetal and the developmental outcomes (Talge *et al.*, 2007). It has been suggested that maternal stress may develop through one or more of three major physiological pathways. These are neuroendocrine, immune/inflammatory and that found in the placental hormone – corticotrophin releasing factor (CRF). These may all play a central role in coordinating the effects of endocrine, immune/inflammatory and vascular processes on foetal and subsequent developmental outcomes. The suggestion is that maternal stress may have a direct influence on the foetus's developing biological systems. The effects of maternal stress are modulated by the nature, duration and timing of the occurrence of stress during gestation. The effects of antenatal stress on the birthweight of the baby have been found to be comparable to those of smoking and it is well documented that low birthweight is a marker for coronary heart disease in later life.

It has been postulated that other factors may influence the stress levels, one of which is the mother's dietary intake. The genetic make-up and situations that influence the infant's resilience to his/her environment are also to be taken into consideration. It is becoming increasingly clear that any intervention that would reduce the mother's stress and anxiety during her pregnancy would have a positive effect on the infant, and should reduce any problems with his/her cognitive, behavioural and emotional development. This may also have an effect on the child in later life and adulthood (Talge *et al.*, 2007) though this, like any intervention, needs further testing.

Given this positive and negative feedback it is important to ensure that there is some form of intervention during the pregnancy to alleviate, or even prevent, situations arising in the first place. The most obvious professionals are midwives and obstetricians, and significant inroads are being established to ensure that there is at least an awareness of the problem, if not actual intervention. It may be argued that midwives have always had the ability to establish good rapport with their patients and have been able to discuss the physical aspects of the pregnancy and foetus in sufficient detail. Many studies have focused on subjective measures of stress on birth outcomes rather than objective measures of these constructs. There is also an argument for assessing the constructs of maternal stress with greater accuracy, based on empirical evidence.

This emerging evidence has allowed studies to open up a whole new domain and, as in all uncharted territory, it will take time and experience to tackle the inevitable problems which may emerge. It is difficult to calculate the exact timing of interventions but it has been suggested that the third trimester of the pregnancy is of particular importance and it is probable that any support or help offered during this period of time may be effective. With so many other physical changes happening to both the mother and foetus it may be difficult to remember the psychological barriers or stressors.

This does raise the question of women who work during their pregnancy. As women age during their employment it is often a factor which is not taken into account. A woman's pregnant status is no exception and there is little guarantee that she will be spared the stresses of the job, whether she is pregnant or not. The economic situation in most households dictates that women work rather than allowing them the luxury of discontinuing. As the fabric of society changes, the mother is as likely to be single as in a partnership, and is likely to be solely dependent on her own income. It is becoming increasingly popular to remain in work for as long as is possible and so long as the woman's physical state does not pose a risk to health and safety issues.

Some employers, in education for example, will allow their staff to work right up until the date of delivery, subject to a risk assessment early in the pregnancy. The teacher is required to give 28 days notice of her intention to leave. Interestingly, in the case of ordinary absence, insurance is negotiated to provide some funds for the employment of reserve (or supply) teachers, should the illness exceed five days. In the case of a pregnancy an additional premium is taken out to provide some payment towards the cost of a reserve teacher. The financial implications are that the Department of Education pays the wages of the pregnant teacher when she leaves: full pay for two weeks, nine-tenths for four weeks and half pay for twelve weeks. Following that there is no salary, but the mother does get the Statutory Maternity Pay as well. The full wages for a supply teacher are provided for whatever time the mother is off work. If the Department fails to take out any insurance then there are no funds to help the staff. In previous years it was more acceptable to finish work at 34 weeks, six weeks before the expected date of delivery. This allowed women to become acquainted with what would be their postnatal circumstance, both on a social and environmental level.

It is improbable that one formula will suit all women. As the majority of pregnant women are working there is little to persuade them to finish work at an earlier date. They may find it more stressful to remain at home where they may be isolated from the network of work colleagues and with only the monotony of housework to alleviate the boredom.

It can be argued that there are certain aspects of society which are capable of maintaining the status quo of this type of superficiality by persuading women that they should be satisfied with the more trivial aspects of their lives. Society is fed a diet of consumerism and led to believe that the issues of fashion and fad are necessary. This ephemeral life diverts attention away from the real, more important changes in society and has the ability to persuade women not to challenge or be critical of deeper issues in the social system that influence the decisions they make. Critical theorists maintain that modern society is irrational, oppressive and takes away the basic features of life. If society accepts this knowledge then it is argued that every system is capable of social change. Critical appraisal with good quality and competitive arguments will ensure that fact emerges as well as the truth and that this will stem from a consensus of opinion. It has been postulated that an overall awareness of the barriers that prevent current change, will encourage people to aspire to make that change. Therefore if women cease to believe in the prevailing concept that a perfect and happy pregnancy is possible, without an appropriate network from society they might begin to recognise that these factors may be a threat to their own and their family's emotional well-being. As a result women may be empowered to challenge the policies and structures which currently direct and impoverish their lives.

Looking at it from a global perspective, implications for future research include consideration of the effects of stress on women in the developing world, in wars and in political conflict. Biological factors need to be better understood. Mechanisms of resilience and protective prenatal and postnatal environments are also noted as factors to be investigated, as well as the efficacy of interventions to reduce maternal stress.

Identification of antenatal depression as an indicator of postnatal depression

It can be accepted that antenatal depression is a depressive disorder, which begins in pregnancy and is often a predictor of postnatal depression.

In a survey conducted by Stanley *et al.* (2006) on midwives and community nurses, they found that the health professionals had less emphasis than the mothers on the value of continuity of care in pregnancy and in promoting disclosure of mental health problems. Community midwives appeared less confident than health visitors in detecting and responding to mothers with symptoms of antenatal depression. However, both groups of professionals also had little knowledge of relevant community services. The coordination and collaboration was limited and contact with mental health services was lower than might have been anticipated. As might be expected, it was the general practitioner who was viewed as the key person in the management of the depression, but despite this some mothers felt the GP did not respond, or was not as sympathetic as they would have anticipated.

The problem with detecting antenatal depression is who will be able to screen expectant mothers most effectively? The obvious answer is the midwife, who is the primary provider of antenatal care. In a study on antenatal depression Stanley *et al.* (2004) identified that over three-quarters of the midwives recognised they had cared for a mother with antenatal depression. Stewart & Henshaw (2002) have identified midwives as the key health professionals to predict and detect any mental health disorder. However, what little evidence there is has shown that midwives, although recognising and willing to embrace the emotional and mental health of women, are still reluctant to do so because of the increase in their work and caseloads.

Midwives routinely ask three questions at the booking clinics. At the pregnant woman's first encounter with a midwife she is asked if she has any family history of perinatal mental illness or if there are details of a past or present severe mental illness. If the woman responds that she has, then the type or treatment by psychiatrist or specialist mental health team is noted.

There is always the danger, as in diagnosing postnatal depression, that the expectant mother will not reveal any mental health problems for fear of any probable consequences. The most likely scenario is that they believe they will be reported to social services and their child will be removed from them. Another more common misconception is that if they disclose, in any way, any history of mental illness this may result in negative attitudes of health professionals, coupled with the stigma of being labelled as 'mad'.

Motherhood is supposed to be a joyous fulfilling event which mothers should accept gladly. Pregnancy is often a slow debilitating process. Movement becomes more difficult, and there are an increasing number of restrictions on what the woman can and cannot do, ensuring that even simple household chores become tiresome burdens. This is just the consequence of carrying a child and until we achieve the brave new world where children are born in bottles, it will continue to remain so. There is also the distinct possibility that once the child is born everything else will have to change.

The GP is in an impossible position. A battery of tests may not be as useful as it appears to be. Phrases like, 'Pull yourself together,' or 'Don't worry, everybody gets it and it will go away,' are futile because there is the remote possibility that it will not. The GP is forced into the decision to accept the responsibility for the woman and might probably decide to prescribe an antidepressant. The information may be available that the woman is exhibiting signs of a reduction in the flow of serotonin, which is one clinical explanation for the onset of depression. However, there does not appear to be any great clarity in whether the decline in serotonin is preceded, or followed by, the onset of the depression.

It is presumed that the woman consulted the GP because doctors are supposed to make sick people better. The doctor may be reasonably sure that the depression will eventually subside, but is still left with a depressed patient who needs to be helped. Antidepressants may work, or at least appear to work. This raises the question that if the depressive condition is self-limiting, was it the prescription that performed the cure, or was it time?

One further reason for visiting the GP is that s/he is the gatekeeper to the entire system and, as such, is licensed to prescribe drugs. S/he may prescribe drugs because the law has given the medical profession the right to do so. Those laws, put in place a century or more ago, were meant to control the supply of potentially dangerous medications, long before antidepressants were thought of, although depressive conditions have been recorded for well over a century. The doctor facing a depressed patient is thus almost as much a victim as the patient. As the prime carer in a team of associated health care professionals only the doctor can prescribe this medication and will be the person who will be held liable should anything go wrong. With the present growth of litigation this has placed the GP in a difficult position.

Screening tools

Antenatal screening tools have been developed to predict depression after birth. In a study by Austin & Lumley (2003), however, it was found that there were no screening tools that met the criteria for routine application in the antenatal period. The study suggests that the current use of screening tools should be considered carefully. It was found that many of them have a high proportion of false positives amongst women who are identified as 'at risk' and a proportion of women identified as 'low risk' who go on to develop depression. They argued that even if an excellent screening tool was devised then its application would have to be tempered and those applying it would need to be aware that not all the mothers likely to become depressed may be targeted. One criticism was that when the screening aspects of the studies were examined most of the sample sizes were too small for sensitivity and specificity. Attempts at developing a predictive index have been elusive.

The Edinburgh Postnatal Depression Scale (EPDS, see Appendix 2) has been validated for use in the antenatal period. Although there is some contention about the use in the postnatal stage, there has been little debate about its use in the antenatal stage. Buist *et al.* (2006) found that routine screening with the EPDS is acceptable to most women and health professionals. However, it was felt that with sensitive explanation, along with staff training and support, it is essential in implementing depression screening.

The NICE Guidelines (2007) recommend that midwives use the following questions during the woman's visit to the antenatal booking clinic:

- Is there a past or present severe mental illness?
- Has there been previous treatment by a psychiatrist or specialist mental health team?
- Is there a history of perinatal mental illness?

Other screening tools include:

- Post Partum Depression Scale (PPDS) developed by Beck & Gable (2001). This is a 35 item questionnaire, simply written and easy to complete and specifically designed for new mothers.
- Edwards *et al.* (2008) found that antenatal screening for psychosocial risk factors was useful in identifying socio-economic deprivation and other problems during the antenatal period, but was not useful as a predictor of postnatal depression.

Risk factors for mothers

Studies have shown that socio-economic deprivation, unemployment and poverty expose mothers to antenatal depression (Bolton *et al.*, 1998). As found in mothers with postnatal depression, poor social support, lack of a supportive partner and marital disharmony are also risk factors (Johanson *et al.*, 2000). A previous episode of depression is also likely to indicate a possible reoccurrence of depressive symptoms (Spinelli, 1997).

Although there are few studies there is also evidence to suggest that domestic violence increases the risk of antenatal depression. The Research Centre on Violence, Abuse and Gender Relations recognises there has been no detailed research into why men attack their pregnant partners, but in some cases men appear to deliberately want to cause the woman to miscarry her child. The most likely reason was that the woman was at her most vulnerable and unable to retaliate or defend herself. It is a recorded fact that domestic violence increases with marriage, when a woman has children and when she is pregnant. This, like any abuse, leads to major changes in the woman's psychological needs and can have more of an adverse outcome than if the woman was not pregnant.

There is evidence that sexual abuse as a child might predispose women to become depressed when they are pregnant. The inability to control these physical and emotional changes may reflect the similar feelings of being abused. A history of sexual abuse may be associated with an aversion to routine obstetric care. This in turn might be allied to primary tokophobia. It is possible that the trauma of a vaginal delivery may cause a resurgence of memories of abuse. This in turn may contribute to secondary tokophobia.

Poor parenting role models are also a risk factor, as in postnatal depression the lack of support from family and friends may have a serious negative impact. For the single expectant mother, the experience of family anger and rejection may only compound the problem. The vital role that families play in supporting the pregnant woman to make the transition to motherhood is recognised in many studies, not only those concerned with perinatal mental health. It is a distinct role but one that can be complemented by health professionals and multidisciplinary agencies.

Unplanned pregnancy was also noted a risk factor in the Swedish study conducted by Rubertsson *et al.* (2003). It may be argued that the expectant mother may experience a period of enjoyable relative freedom, which contrasts favourably with being at school or being at home. She might have married or chosen to cohabit with a partner, if only because that could give her freedom from home. Freedom is not simply economic liberation, it is also social liberation. One of the consequences can mean a pregnancy, either accidental or deliberate. If that pregnancy is not terminated either by accident or design, itself a traumatic decision that sometimes has equally formidable consequences, then within nine months a child is going to appear.

Pregnant mothers and bipolar disorder

All women with a history of bipolar disorder should be aware of the risks of pregnancy and should be advised of the importance of effective contraception. A pregnancy and any future pregnancies should be planned in consultation with a psychiatric specialist, with an in-depth discussion of the treatment options, the risks and the benefits. The requirements of each woman are tailored to her individual needs and as a result, treatment may vary from woman to woman. Treatment may include the continuation of existing medication or changing to an alternative medication which is known to have fewer side effects. In the case of lithium or valproate, the dosage may be reduced or a slow release formula prescribed as an alternative. In some instances lithium may be discontinued prior to the pregnancy and the original dosage reintroduced immediately following delivery. Consideration must be given to the maternal physiological changes that occur and this may necessitate a change in dosage. The glomerular filtration rate increases during pregnancy and this can cause any drug treatment to be excreted more rapidly. This causes serum levels to fall and thus the woman may require higher doses of medication to prevent a relapse. Following the delivery these changes reverse and thus there is a risk of higher serum levels which may cause side effects if the doses are not reduced (Goodwin, 2003). Carbamazepine and valproate are associated with congenital abnormalities which include neural tube defect, facial dysmorphobia, cleft lip and palate, cardiac defects, digital hypoplasia and nail dysplasia.

The reality for one mother was never to become pregnant again following the birth of her first child. Her episode of bipolar disorder was so traumatic – not for her as she enjoyed the moments of excessive elation, but for her family who suffered the interminable chaos and disruption that her behaviour caused.

Pregnant women and suicide

The risk of maternal suicide during normal pregnancy is low but should not be discounted. Probably one of the major risks of depression in pregnancy is suicide and, rarely, infanticide. SSRIs are implicated in the increased risks of both suicide and violence (Breggin, 2001; 2003).

It may be argued that pregnant women are just as likely to experience suicidal thoughts as non-pregnant mothers; however, it would appear they are less likely to carry them out. Studies have found very few cases of suicide and in a study by Appleby (1991) it was found that only 5% committed suicide. It is postulated that pregnancy involves a behavioural inhibitory factor (Marzuk *et al.*, 1997) which is caused by the production of serotonin. The blood levels of the pregnant mother have been shown to have higher levels of this chemical, and it is understood that the foetus also produces this serotonin. Perhaps it is this which guards against self-harm and acts as a protective factor against suicide.

Causes for contemplating suicide may be multi-factorial but obstetric or physical problems during pregnancy may also have adverse effects. Women may be overwhelmed by morning sickness or persistent back pain, which may exacerbate any feelings of low self-esteem. Problems with infertility and difficulty in conceiving or previous miscarriages can cause severe anxiety in pregnancy, as the mother needs constant reassurance that her foetus is healthy and developing well.

A Swedish study (Mittendorfer-Rutz *et al.*, 2005) made the interesting discovery that the probability of committing suicide may be determined genetically. Following the progress of teenage mothers it was found that their offspring had a two-fold increase in having a propensity to attempting suicide. There is also an indication that infants born under 2 kg in weight and less than 47 cm in length were more likely to be prone to suicidal urges. The study did not claim to have definitive answers to the reasons for a propensity to a suicidal nature, but did stress the importance and the influence of maternal health.

A question might be raised as to whether a mother who attempts suicide could be found guilty of the attempted murder of her foetus.

Pregnant mothers and substance misuse

Studies have shown that over 90% of pregnant women take prescription or non-prescription drugs, illicit drugs or use social drugs (tobacco and alcohol) at some time during pregnancy. Mothers who are likely to suffer from depression are amongst those who may misuse drugs and alcohol in particular. There is little doubt that any substance misuse has the ability to harm the foetus. Approximately 2–3% of all birth defects result from the use of drugs other than alcohol.

The most common obstetric problems with opiate addiction, particularly heroin and cocaine, are miscarriage, stillbirth and retarded growth *in utero* that ultimately leads to a low birthweight, premature labour and withdrawal symptoms after birth. Withdrawal of heroin causes the smooth muscle to contract, which leads to spasm of the placental blood vessels. This results in reduced placental blood flow and is the cause of reduced birthweight in babies.

The use of cocaine as a recreational drug does not have the adverse outcomes compared with those of a frequent and heavy user. The drug is a powerful constrictor of blood vessels which increases the risk of adverse outcomes in the pregnancy. These may include separation of the placenta, retarded cerebral growth, poor development of organs, poor development of limbs, and intra-uterine death.

It is known that tobacco has significant harmful effects on the foetus, but as cannabis is often smoked in conjunction with tobacco it is difficult to ascertain which is the main cause. There is a risk of a reduction in the infant's birthweight or an increased risk of Sudden Infant Death Syndrome (SIDS).

It is difficult to predict the damage alcohol consumption is capable of in pregnancy, even where low levels are consumed. It is reported that high levels of consumption of alcohol, particularly binge drinking, result in a reduction in infant birthweight and may cause a minority of infants to present with Foetal Alcohol Syndrome. Features of this include a reduction in all parameters of growth, particularly the head circumference. This has consequences for neural development, central nervous dysfunction and the characteristic dysmorphic facial features.

Benzodiazapines

Benzodiazepines were originally developed as muscle relaxants, but when their efficacy for calming anxiety was noted they became excessively prescribed for relieving anxiety and stress. They are tranquillisers, which are mood altering drugs. Those in most common use are Valium, temazepam and Librium but the group benzodiazapines also contain the familiar names of Rohypnol (flunitrazepam) Dalmane (flurazepam) and Mogadon (nitrazepam)

There are no reports of any benefit from prescribing a substitute for Valium during pregnancy, but equally there is no reliable evidence that sole use of benzodiazapines affects pregnancy outcomes. The overuse of tranquillisers is frequently associated with medical and social problems, which, as the evidence has shown, is associated with poorer pregnancy outcomes.

Use of benzodiazapines in pregnancy causes withdrawal symptoms in the infant, which can be particularly severe if more than one drug is abused. There is further evidence to show that there is a slightly increased risk of a cleft palate.

The amphetamines are a group of sympathomimetic drugs that are used to stimulate the central nervous system. Members of this group include amphetamine, dextroamphetamine, and methamphetamine. Appetite suppression and an aim to control weight gain are the main reasons for taking these drugs. Ecstasy has been associated with the dance and club culture, taken primarily by youngsters and provides the ability and energy to stay alert, awake and participate in the dancing. A number of studies have examined the possible relationship between amphetamines and adverse foetal outcomes. There is no evidence that use of either amphetamines or ecstasy has a direct affect on the foetus or the outcomes of the pregnancy and there are no reports of withdrawal symptoms.

It is often with that knowledge that newly pregnant mothers have a strong incentive to make positive changes to their lifestyles and either reduce or desist from using drugs and or alcohol. *The National Service Framework for Children, Young people and Maternity Services* states that women who misuse substances are at greater risk of a problem pregnancy and it recommends that their care is provided by integrated teams. There is a particular issue where pregnant mothers wish to withdraw from their addiction.

However, methods to help with withdrawal of opiates are not without risks. Methadone, which is often used as an opioid substitute, has a longer lasting effect and can stabilise the levels in the blood, which allows withdrawal to be less severe. There is less of a risk of a premature birth but its use may cause a reduced birthweight in the infant. It may allow the mother and her pregnancy to be monitored and lessen the risks but there is no firm evidence that it benefits the pregnancy overall.

Pregnant women who misuse substances and who are prescribed methadone should be encouraged to breast-feed, providing their drug use is stable and the baby is weaned gradually. The continuation of breast-feeding and engagement with the infant often helps the mother to stabilise her use of drugs.

The delivery of maternity care to women who misuse substances requires a specialist approach and the inclusion of multidisciplinary teams is essential to ensure effective collaboration between agencies and services. This should include maternity and neonatal services, primary care, social services and specialists in drug and alcohol agencies. There needs to be a protocol for the assessment and care management of pregnant women who misuse drugs and/or alcohol.

As in the case of other substance misuse the poor outcomes probably reflect several other factors which exacerbate the conditions, which may include multiple drug use, lifestyle and poor maternal health.

Pregnant teenagers

Whether it is because of their biological and emotional immaturity or other factors, it is clear that there are significant outcomes associated with teenage pregnancy. Low birthweight infants, small for dates, increased neonatal mortality and premature births are some of the obstetric implications (Olausson *et al.*, 1999; 2001; Scholl *et al.*, 1987; Smith & Pell, 2001). There is also some evidence to suggest that teenage mothers are more likely to suffer from postnatal depression than older mothers (Deal & Holt 1998).

Medication during the antenatal period

A meta-analysis by Kirsch *et al.* (2002) and Moncrieff & Kirsch (2005) has shown that placebos are as effective in treating depression as antidepressants. However, the use of antidepressants during pregnancy is as equally concerning as the depression itself. Active treatment for depressive states is usually a selective serotonin reuptake inhibitor (SSRI) but studies are increasingly cautioning clinicians about the uncertainty of the safety of antidepressants and in particular the SSRIs. It is thought that the drug fluoxetine is generally one of the more dependable medications (Nonacs & Cohen, 2003). It is expected that pregnant mothers and/or women treated with antidepressants would have better outcomes than those who have not had the same management. There is, however, no definitive proof that antidepressants improve either maternal or child health outcomes during pregnancy.

In depressed mothers the levels of the chemical messengers serotonin and norepinephrine are reportedly lower than in non-depressed individuals. SSRIs act by increasing the levels of serotonin in the brain. Tricyclic medication (TCA) acts by increasing the cerebral levels of serotonin and norepinephrine. Tricyclics tend to have a shorter metabolite and half-life and are the preferred medication when mothers are breast-feeding (Duncan & Taylor, 1995).

Both types of antidepressants are effective in the treatment of severe depression, but studies have reported different adverse effects. Although there is limited evidence on the toxicity of TCAs some have been noted in the use of doxepin. There have been no reports of teratogenic effects and no long-term effects have been noted.

It is advisable that the use of SSRIs are kept to a minimum effective dosage to avoid the possibility of a premature birth and any adverse drug effects in the new born (Hallberg & Sjoblom, 2005).

In a meta-analysis Hemels *et al.* (2005) found that the use of antidepressants in pregnancy has been associated with increased rates of spontaneous abortions and Alwan *et al.* (2005) and Kallen (2004) have noted an increase in birth and congenital defects.

Levison-Castiel *et al.* (2007) studied 60 infants who had been exposed to SSRIs and found that 30% had neonatal abstinence syndrome, eight of which were severe. The most common symptoms found were tremor, gastrointestinal problems, an abnormal increase in muscle tone, sleep disturbances and high-pitched cries. None of the infants with symptoms required treatment. The infants of mothers who were depressed in the antenatal period, but did not take any SSRI medication, had lower incidences of minor physical abnormalities and fewer neurological abnormalities.

Alwan *et al.* (2007) and Louik *et al.* (2007) described how mothers who took SSRI antidepressant medication in the first trimester of their pregnancy have been shown to have previously unidentified links to three birth defects. The first, craniosynostosis, a condition that varies in severity, is the premature closing of one or more sutures or fibrous joints knitting together the bones of the infant's skull. It can be secondary to an underdeveloped brain. This condition was two and a half times more prevalent in infants who were exposed *in utero* to SSRIs. Another defect, which was noted, was omphalocele. This is where the infant's main organs are on the outside of the body. The condition may be represented by the less catastrophic umbilical hernia but nevertheless was found to be more likely to affect the infants of mothers taking SSRIs.

Alwan *et al.* (2007) also found that babies of obese mothers who took SSRIs during their pregnancy had a greater risk of developing neonatal heart defects. A further study suggested that exposure to SSRIs in the third trimester of the pregnancy is associated with a small risk of developing pulmonary hypertension in the newborn (Oberlander *et al.*, 2006).

It is known that all the SSRIs are excreted into breast milk. No serious adverse effects have been reported in the infants of mothers who were taking SSRI during breast-feeding. Hallberg & Sjoblom (2005) in a review found that use of SSRIs during breast-feeding, suggests that exposure for the nursing child is lowest with sertraline and fluvoxamine and higher with paroxetine. Citalopram and fluoxetine were recorded as the highest. With the lack of available current data it is difficult to recommend the safest SSRI to prescribe for breast-feeding mothers.

Mothers who experienced depression in the first and second trimester had less in-clination to breast-feed and mothers who had depression later in the pregnancy were more likely to discontinue breast-feeding earlier.

Discontinuation of medication in the antenatal period

Women who already have a mental health mood disorder that is controlled by medica-tion may prefer to discontinue taking that medication. There is sufficient information on adverse drug reactions during pregnancy to deter some women from taking the risk, particularly if the baby is a much wanted one. One study showed that over half of the women who discontinued their antidepressant medication because they had conceived had a relapse of their condition, whereas those who continued did not.

A further study found that two-thirds of the women with a history of major de-pression who stopped taking SSRIs during pregnancy relapsed into serious depression, compared with one in four women who kept taking the drugs. Over three-quarters of mothers who have been diagnosed with recurrent depression prior to conceiving, end in relapse. This occurs most frequently during the first trimester (Cohen *et al.*, 2006).

These factors should alert the practitioner and clinician that the newly born infant should be kept under surveillance if the mother has been treated with an SSRI or TCA in late pregnancy. Withdrawal symptoms are rare and mostly self-limiting, but obvious signs of neonatal toxicity or withdrawal can be recognised and treated early.

This highlights the fact that being pregnant does not protect mothers from episodes of depression and pregnancy has the tendency to make mothers just as vulnerable to poor mental health as well as physical health.

There is evidence to suggest that screening for disorders of women's mental health during pregnancy does not always occur (Tully *et al.*, 2002) and the reasons for this are obvious when it can be argued that midwives already feel overburdened with their increasing caseloads and lack of resources. The addition of the time to screen and then to decide the most appropriate pathway of care are both time consuming and may be laborious. Often it is the case that, unlike health visitors, a pregnant woman is rarely looked after by just one midwife and it is more likley to be several in a managed caseload. Nevertheless, the evidence clearly points to the importance of recognising and managing depression during this period, particularly as this is probably the one time when the woman has extensive contacts with the health service.

It must be recognised that the majority of expectant women do not succumb to any form of mental disorder and quite probably psychologists and personality theorists will be able to explain why this occurs. The women might have other forms of support or personal reserves that give them the ability to face the problem. It is even possible that they really want to become mothers. There remain those who do not have these reserves and do not know where to look for support, and if there is an explanation of where feelings of loneliness or isolation begin, surely it is here,

Immediately following the birth of her baby Jill Tweedy (1980) recounted how she felt little for her own child:

The nurse gave me a booklet, ornamented with sketches of flowers and baby birds. There were poems inside about little strangers and violets and pink and blue and above all, about love. They bore no relation to what I was feeling because I was feeling nothing. A vacuum of immense proportions had replaced the foetus, my bruised womb was distended with it. Numb, anaesthetised, I stared over vast distances at this small creature lying on my pillow and I could not think that it belonged to me.

(p. 34)

Postnatal depression and bipolar disorder

During 2006 there were 669,531 live births in England and Wales; this was an increase of 3.7% on 2005. There were more first-time mothers in the 30–34 age group than in the 25–29 age group and the average age of a mother giving birth was just over 29 years of age. There was a 50% increase from the previous ten years in the number of women over forty who were having babies (ONS). Teenage pregnancies in the UK are one of the highest in Europe, with 7% of girls giving birth.

The number of mothers who were married or living with their partner was estimated at over 85% and 15% of mothers claimed to be lone parents. Sixteen percent of the mothers were in the lower socio-economic groups, where the household income was less than £18,000. Approximately 3.2 million people in the UK or 7% of the population, are clinically depressed and the number is increasing. More than ten million prescriptions were made out for antidepressant drugs in the ten years from 1990 to the year 2000. It is estimated that approximately 75,000 women within the United Kingdom are affected by postnatal depression.

It is well documented that social factors play an important part in both the aetiology and maintenance of mental disorders. The statistics demonstrate that a significant number of mothers are the sole providers for their infant and their vulnerability is emphasised by their circumstances, which may not be conducive to their children's welfare.

Around forty years ago, Pitt (1968) described unfamiliar and prolonged depressive symptoms, commencing with the mother's return home from hospital, which caused distress to both mother and family. Cox *et al.* (1987) suggested that the diagnosis should be restricted to mothers with a depressive illness who do not usually display delusion or hallucinations or do not usually require immediate treatment in a psychiatric hospital. It is often found that in conditions like postnatal depression the mother's behaviour is not obviously abnormal, while some others do not appear to have any life stresses at all. It is only the careful questioning about the presence or absence of particular depressive symptoms which enables the disorder to be recognised.

Postnatal depression was once a little understood illness, but over the past 30 years it has increased in both recognition and attention. The reasons for this are unclear, but during the past 20 years there appears to have been an upsurge in the debate about perinatal mental health and an increase in medically defined cases of postnatal depression.

The term perinatal mental health disorder describes a very common group of depressive illnesses, which occur in mothers following the birth of their child. Brockington (1998) suggested that the symptoms vary only in quantity from those that are part of the normal reactions to stress and unhappiness and are usually demonstrated by the spectrum of affective disorders following childbirth.

Historically, they were commonly divided into three categories, concentrating on 'postnatal depression', which, it has been argued, is a diagnosis which has the potential to be misused. Often the term is applied to include any mental illness in the postnatal period. This may have serious consequences as there is a danger that the condition the mother is experiencing is given an equal weighting to that of postnatal depression, which ultimately means that a more serious mental illness may be minimised.

However, this distinction is becoming more obvious and it is suggested in later works by Brockington (2006) that there are more likely to be over 30 perinatal disorders, which fall into six groups. These include puerperal psychosis, postnatal depression, the psychopathology of parturition, puerperal and menstrual bipolar disorder, mother-infant relationship disorders, anxiety, obsessional and stress-related disorders. Whatever label or diagnosis is given to these conditions it should be recognised that poor mental health has a significant impact on the mother's life and the lives of her infant, family, friends and the community at large.

It is commonly accepted that perinatal mental illness occurs during the first year following childbirth, though some of the diagnoses may also be applicable to mothers with young children over one year old.

The baby blues

The first experience of any mood disorder a mother is likely to have following the birth of her infant is termed the 'baby blues' or 'post-partum blues'. This is generally regarded as a fleeting phenomenon, anticipated by mothers in the very early days, probably within three to four days, following childbirth. It is familiar to most mothers; they may not have been able to function as normal and have felt weepy, oversensitive, lost the ability to concentrate or had a tendency to forget important issues. These changes in mood state are not uncommon and should be are regarded as part of the natural process whereby the mother may suffer from the withdrawal from the high pregnancy levels of oestrogen, progesterone and endorphins (Clay & ~~~4. Henshaw, 2003,).

However, it must be remembered it is not always possible for mot at this time and despite assurances, it is possible the mother is lik own capabilities and be overwhelmed by her inadequacies, togethe demands of her infant.

The careful management of this is important. It requires patience and understanding and the symptoms should be allowed to subside naturally and gradually. There is a danger the feelings may linger and prevent any pleasure or enjoyment being derived from having the child (Kelly, 1994) and it may have an adverse effect on emotional feelings.

In some case the feelings towards the partner are particularly compromised and issues around libido and sex become over stressed. This is an area that is rarely addressed but is probably one of the most sensitive subjects. It is frequently mentioned in the literature as a symptom, but there is a paucity of information on solid research which discusses the actual impact this has on the relationship between the mother and her partner. Anecdotal evidence suggests that this is a time when men feel at their most vulnerable, having the added pressure of caring not only for themselves and the mother of their child, but also the infant. The emotional needs of the father may be ignored in the midst of other emotional events and this may lead to further complications in their relationship (Buist *et al.*, 2003; Condon *et al.*, 2004). Emotional support is paramount for the mother but also the needs of the father must be recognised. Any practical intervention which is required to help new mothers cope and care for their infants would be welcome in this situation.

Historically in the UK, it was the norm to share childcare, and mothers often relied on others to help with their children's upbringing (Gotts, 1988). The lying-in period, which mothers enjoyed and was traditionally forty days has now, in many cases, been reduced to 24 hours. The philosophy to encourage mothers to be discharged from hospital as soon as possible is based on the fact that pregnancy is a natural phenomenon. Unless there are medical concerns around the mother or the baby's health, both mother and baby are better suited at home in familiar surroundings, where they can receive the support and attention of family and friends. For the most part mothers are happy to accept this decision, but for the few the ideal of familiar surroundings is a myth and they may often have to cope alone with inexperience and a certain lack of knowledge.

The lying-in period is still upheld by some cultures and religions and is a salient reminder of what the West has sacrificed in terms of motherhood. In the UK the custom was to remain in bed for at least nine days, during which time lactation could be established. It also allowed mothers 'time' to rest and bond with their infant. It was expected that there would be at least the opportunity to have six hours of rest at night, including a nap in the afternoon. The mother was afforded the highest quality foods designed to nourish both her and her infant and these conditions were expected to last for about forty days.

In today's climate in the UK, following the initial few weeks postpartum, the mother is encouraged to exercise, diet and continue with the myriad household chores that have awaited her return from the hospital. The care of her other children may be compromised and grandmothers or statutory agencies might fill the gap. A 24-hour or two-day stay in hospital is the most UK mothers can expect.

Successive studies over the years (Bonnar, 1981; Toglia & Weg, 1996) determined that there were more life-threatening complications associated with the lying-in practice compared with the benefits of rest. The main problem was deep vein thrombosis, which occurred in a significant amount of cases and was often fatal. A less serious complaint was the discomfort of constipation, which necessitated castor oil and other purgatives to provide relief, which proved both unpleasant and untimely (Nusche, 2002).

Legislation has determined that fathers may have paternity leave to support the mother during this time. Many mothers report this as a wonderful experience and for the couple it is a precious time to consolidate their parenting skills. However, it might be postulated that it is the mother's mother or similar female relative who may be the more appropriate to fulfil this role and the possibility of 'grandmother leave' might be more suitable. This would enable the father to have his precious paternity leave later on in the post-partum period, thus mirroring the added advantage of traditional cultures where the mother is not pressurised into conjugal rites with her husband until six weeks have elapsed.

In the UK, the emphasis is on pain-free labour and the need to recreate the size 10, pre-pregnancy figure. However, it may be argued that the ambiguity of the mother's role is questionable when the same society, which sanctions this care, may not ultimately acknowledge the importance of women, giving more credence and influence to its male members. In the UK the mother battles with feminist ideals and macho aspirations. All these determinants conspire against new mothers, so it is little wonder that with sufficient support, understanding and patience throughout the postnatal period, the symptoms of the blues should gradually subside (Cox *et al.*, 1987).

Postnatal depression/post-partum depression

This is the most common postnatal mental disorder and can vary in severity from major acute psychotic postnatal depression to minor chronic postnatal depression. In general, only 3% of women will suffer severe depression, and 7% will tend towards a minor form of the illness.

In one-third of cases, the baby blues become progressively worse, and the mother is unable to recapture the feeling of wellness. Periods of feeling 'normal' are outweighed by the often constant feelings of tiredness and lethargy. They may complain that they have insufficient sleep or what sleep they have is erratic and unsatisfying. Everyday chores become unmanageable and there is conflict where the needs of the infant combat the needs of the house. It is difficult enough to cope with housework, but when the mother is expected to manage when feeling exhausted it becomes an almost impossible task. The mother who worked prior to her pregnancy may demand the same high standard as she achieved prior to the birth of her infant. Her expectations are high. She demands a well maintained home, meals prepared on time, shopping completed, a healthy partner, and a smiling baby. When the reality is different this can compound her feelings of failure, frustration and deflation as she struggles against tiredness, and a domestic timetable that bulges at the seams.

Often, mothers fear their inadequacy and failure to cope may have a detrimental effect on their baby's well-being and general health. This constant worry may add to the burden that she already carries (Cox *et al.*, 1987). Some mothers may become preoccupied with thoughts of self-reproach and incompetence (Pitts, 1999). They are to be blamed for every eventuality and the guilt they endure as they feel themselves to be a bad mother is overwhelming. Little wonder that the mother is reluctant to seek help or admit to her feelings.

Classical physical, biological and psychological symptoms

It is not uncommon to exhibit feelings of anxiousness which may simply manifest as anxiety and may result in palpitations, shakiness or nervousness.

One of the most distressing symptoms for the family is the subtle change in personality, where the mother may exhibit more than the usual signs of sensitivity. Careless remarks about her overall appearance and changes in her post-pregnancy body image all have a more heightened effect than in normal circumstances (Boscalgia *et al.*, 2003).

There are significant changes to body shape, which are not always obvious. Parts of the body, which were previously associated with sex and pleasure, are now programmed for the baby. Breasts provide the infant's first source of nutrition. Some women find it difficult to reconcile the changes and there has been much debate about the importance of breast-feeding, but little research into the reluctance of mothers to breast-feed because of the objection or jealousy of their husbands.

Variations in mood and mood changes can often confuse not only mothers, but also those around them. They may be familiar to the mother who has experienced pre-menstrual tension, but there is little evidence to suggest that they are one and the same. There is the added discomfort to those who were assured that once the menstrual cycle commenced they would be afforded some respite and their mood would return to normal. In postnatal depression this is not the case and they discover that there is little if any resolution in their condition.

One mother described it as:

The feelings are similar sometimes, but no, not really. I feel differently now. It is not as if I know these feelings will go away after a week. I'm sensitive, but I wouldn't say I was irritable, at least not with everyone. I feel as if I don't care, and that no one really understands how I feel anyway – not like PMT when everyone seems to have it – even my best friend. You are on your own with this.

At one time the nutrition of the mother was assured by the attention of her helpers and the support she received in the early days following the birth of her child. A mother who was fortunate to have the support of her family, and in particular her mother, could be assured of a reasonable if not normal diet. However, many studies have shown that the mood of depression suppresses the appetite. Studies have found that anorexia nervosa is less common in pregnant women. Although the cause of anorexia nervosa is unclear, it tends to occur in young people. Severe dieting and weight loss is often associated with the preoccupation of food and weight in an effort to avoid the perceived psychological and social escalation of the demands of adolescence. Prolonged severe dieting and weight loss themselves are firmly entrenched behaviours which perpetuate the distorted beliefs around eating, food and body image that are common to anorexia nervosa.

The treatment is limited and it is difficult to ascertain whether treatment should focus on the anxieties which surround the adolescent period or tackle the habitual dieting and weight loss.

One survey has revealed that one in every fifty women develops an eating disorder during their pregnancy but there are no reliable statistics to prove there has been an increase in the numbers in recent years. There is a populist view, nurtured by the media and celebrities, that mother are expected to return to their pre-pregnancy weight, which may lead to an increased risk.

One study examined the relationship between low-income, depressed mothers who suffered from obesity and their children. It was found that the children were more likely to stay indoors and watch at least three hours of television a day, and an average of sixty minutes more television than the children of non-depressed mothers. The theory suggested was that depressed mothers are less likely to plan activities for their children and find it difficult to interact in play. The mothers also watched a significant amount of television and the children tended to emulate this behaviour (Burdette *et al.*, 2003).

Postnatal depression (major)

A third of postnatal women who subsequently develop depression may present with signs and symptoms within the first four weeks of the birth of their baby and two-thirds between ten and fourteen weeks. Women who present early tend to have the most profound and obvious illness, whilst those who present later are often misdiagnosed, or sometimes missed altogether (Gerrard *et al.*, 1993).

Occasionally, the condition becomes more severe and debilitating, and those with the most profound symptoms usually present their symptom early, particularly if the signs and symptoms are neglected or the mother chooses to avoid talking about, or conceals, her condition. Symptoms exhibited in major forms of postnatal depression are usually more extensive than in the milder form of the condition.

Major postnatal depression involves profound and consistent lowering of the state of mood. An alteration in clear thinking is evident, with a slowing down of psychomotor functions, and all the clinical symptoms of a severe depression. Thoughts are often sluggish and at times there may be 'thought blocking', where the mother is unable to release her thought processes and may often stop in mid-sentence or 'forget' what she wanted to say next. She may even find it difficult to speak in response to questions, not because she does not know the answer, but because she is unable to formulate it into one that is comprehensive. It may be difficult or sometimes impossible to initiate conversations with adults, let alone engage in baby talk with her infant.

Some mothers will admit they feel guilty about how they felt and how it must have affected their families:

> *I was tired all of the time, I could not summon up the energy to play with my children. I got angry and felt it was the baby's fault for me feeling this way. I could manage to cope with everything when there was just my husband and me.*

Another said:

> *Looking back on my illness I realise how much they must have been affected by my actions, though I was not aware of it at the time. I was irritable and cried at the least thing. I thought I hid it well, but I don't think I did as my son makes reference to the time that 'Mummy cried all the time'.*

The quick responses that are often required when considering the needs of the inf
may be absent. This is not because the mother does not care or know how to re?

the enormity of the task may not be mentally possible for her to achieve. The mother may not be able to rationalise why her child is screaming, either because the infant is hungry or requires attention. It is possible that in the depths of her depression she may interpret the infant's screaming as the denunciation of her as a bad mother, who is unable to predict and respond to the infant's needs.

Nappies may be left unchanged, as that chore would not only necessitate the ritualised performance of getting the necessary equipment ready, but it would incur more work as the clothes will require laundering, and the mother may have to go out to purchase more nappies. In this instance it is easier to let the infant cry.

The mother may be incapable of foreseeing her own dietary needs, and getting up from the bed to walk to the kitchen to prepare a meal may be an enormous effort. Perhaps more strenuous would be the decision of what to prepare. It would be less demanding to eat a tin of cold soup or grab a biscuit. Once the hunger is satisfied this method of eating may be preferable in the future. A vigilant family may notice that the mother is becoming anorexic but there might also be an increase in the mother's weight as she feasts on foods with high calorific values, to obtain the sugar rush as an antidote to her depression. Her infant may be bottle fed, but the undertaking involved to organise the warm bottles of the correct quantity of milk, may also require more effort than she is capable of. Babies may suffer the indignity of cold milk or insufficient nutrients.

Delusions are also a concern and may form part of the symptomatic range. A delusion is commonly known as a 'false belief', something that the mother holds to be true and certain even if someone demonstrates evidence to the contrary. One of the main features is that the mother is convinced that she is being lied to and that what she believes is real. This perception is regardless of the mother's level of intelligence, cultural or her religious background. Sometimes it may be difficult to differentiate between what is an unreasonable idea and what is abnormal in her thought processes.

A delusion of jealousy may have serious repercussions for both her infant and her partner. Here, the mother may believe that her partner is having an affair and will become obsessed with gathering information that may incriminate him. Despite evidence to the contrary she may confront her partner, which may have devastating results. Likewise, she may feel that her infant is receiving more affection than she is and may harbour thoughts of malignant jealousy. This also has the propensity to conclude in a grave outcome. Equally, the mother may be deluded about the fact that someone famous or of a higher status is in love with her. This irrational belief may cause her to respond and thus make her stalk the unsuspecting 'lover'.

In very rare cases the depression can be so debilitating and the symptoms so exacerbated that it is possible for the mother to suffer from catatonia. This is characterised by an interruption of her normal psychomotor movements and thought processes. She is in a 'catatonic state', which is disconcerting and similar to a deep trance-like state. Other symptoms may include a total lack of response when being spoken to, either because she is unwilling or unable to speak. However, if she does make any sounds it may be in the form of echolalia, which is repeating a phrase or word which is spoken to her in a parrot like fashion. The mother appears to be unable to respond to any external stimuli, including being shaken or shouted at. Conversely, there may be excessive and random motor activity that appears to have no purpose; this may accompanied by inappropriate gestures and grimacing. As in the case of echolalia, the mother may mimic the movements of another person. Sometimes, but very rarely, catalepsy may be present and the limbs are so rigid they remain in whatever position they are placed by another person. It is possible for her hand to be held above her head until she tires. One of the distressing features of this condition is that it appears as if the mother is totally out of control – of both her thoughts and locomotion. If the mother is not treated, then deterioration is caused by pure exhaustion, accompanied by malnutrition. In some cases the mother may have sufficient insight into her condition to self-harm.

One psychiatric nurse told of her experience in the West Indies during the late 1970s, when a mother was brought into the ward in a catatonic state:

> *She just sat there not saying a thing. We couldn't seem to reach her at all, so she just sat in the corner staring into space. We later found out that she was depressed following the birth of her twin sons. She was so ill she could not feed or care for them. No one knew about it so no one helped. The twins starved to death and she was found in her house just sitting next to them, not responding, saying nothing.*

In some instances it is common for the mother to suffer from mild auditory or visual hallucinations. A hallucination is defined as abnormal sensory perception that occurs while the mother is both awake and fully conscious. What she sees or hears is totally unrelated to anything that is around her. She may believe she sees a black cat running through her kitchen or see a stranger standing in her lounge. She may be so convinced she has seen the images that they may cause extreme agitation, anxiety or even cause her to react to them. As they are invisible to the onlooker, who will deny the existence, this causes further distress and will confirm the mother's intuition that tells her that she is going 'mad'. In some instances the images are innocuous and the mother, although she still sees them, may choose not to draw attention to them. It has been reported that some mothers repeatedly have mild hallucinations and accept them as part of their everyday life.

Whether postnatal depression is caused by bio-physical or societal problems it is nevertheless a debilitating condition. The period following the birth of a child brings many transitions into a woman's life that affect major psychological and social changes. Mental health problems following pregnancy are more distressing and have even greater impact than the same problems at other times in a woman's life. Some of the signs are obvious and some, as have been discussed, are confused with normality. Sharing experiences and understanding why it happens can go halfway to managing the condition and helping mothers to make sense of their own well-being.

Some of the problems seem to stem from societal perceptions of psychiatric disorder that do not appear to be helpful to mothers of young children and there does appear to be a reluctance to think about perinatal mental health in such terms. This is compounded by a general ignorance about the condition and a fairly common notion that 'baby blues' is just something that comes and goes. Even when there is an awareness of the problem there will be denial, because admitting to the condition somehow reflects badly upon the woman's ability to cope. It is possibly true that belief about psychiatric illness has not progressed greatly in the last few decades. However, there is some awareness of the condition, if only because it has afflicted celebrity mothers. The paradox is that their conditions are often treated with derision, as the media tend to over emphasis their hopeless plight and suggest that their madness prohibits them from remaining the 'stars' they were and they then become figures of pity and scorn.

In the main there is an awareness that seems to be limited to it being 'something that happens to somebody else'.

Bipolar disorder

The more common name for bipolar disorder is manic-depression. Until recently little was known about this condition, which primarily affects the brain and causes severe shifts in mood function. When at its most severe, bipolar disorder can cause episodes of extreme mania, which may predispose the mother to high energy levels. The moods may swing dramatically and it is equally possible for the mother to suffer from a debilitating depression, with feelings of sadness and despair. There are often periods of normal mood in between. This paradoxical mix of moods has baffled doctors for centuries. In 1854, Falret and Baillarger were the first psychiatrists to describe the symptoms of 'circular insanity' and hypothesised that patients with depression in the community who experienced moments of elation following their depressive episodes would be found to have a circular illness. This theory was regarded as the precursor of the current concept of bipolar II disorder (Akiskal, 2006) but it was Kraepelin, a German psychiatrist, who finally outlined manic depressive illness. It develops in late adolescence or early adulthood, but some women may have their first symptoms during childhood, and some develop them later in life. It affects around 2.6% of the population aged 18 and over. When Judd *et al.* (2002) followed people with bipolar disorder over twelve years they found that depressive symptoms ruled over half of their lives.

The signs of mania are the opposite of those experienced during a depressive phase. The mother's mood may be excessively euphoric. Thoughts are rapid and the ideas expressed are disjointed and superficial. Her speech may be verbose and sometimes incoherent. She is unable to concentrate for long and is easily distracted. One mother described the feeling as *'about to go over the top of a roller coaster – only the feeling is with you all the time'*.

Sometimes the inability to communicate effectively causes the mother to become irritated, irritable or aggressive. It is thought to affect a high proportion of intelligent people and those who have been gifted with creativity and talent and this often makes diagnosis difficult. Often famous personalities make surprise revelations about their health and when Stephen Fry admitted to his bipolar disorder it conjured up multiplex interest within the media and heightened the awareness of the illness in a way that no other health education campaign had managed. He described the massive highs and miserable lows that dominated his life, which prompted others in the media to describe the surges of exhilaration which led to debt and drug abuse and the deep depression which alienated family and friends.

The increased energy levels cause the mother to be constantly active, with periods where she feels incapable of resting. It is not unusual for the mother to be overtly provocatively sexual in her behaviour and have increased libido. This can provoke a great strain on relationships and has been described as *'a stain on a relationship which sometimes proves almost unbearable when your partner is subjected to this kind of behaviour day in and day out'*.

The mother may be deluded and believe that she is capable of anything, however unrealistic. In an effort to enjoy or enhance the experience there may be a tendency to abuse alcohol, or illicit drugs. Often mothers who experience the milder manic phases will confess that the feeling of euphoria is wonderful and when they feel at their most creative. The most distressing feature of the condition is that the mother may have glimpses of insight into the behaviour they are unable to control. The majority of mothers tend to have little or no insight into their condition: '*I just felt invincible all the time and when I saw expensive baby clothes I needed to buy them, even though I had the insight to know I really wasn't able to afford it.*'

When first seen by a GP, mothers with the condition are often misdiagnosed as having a personality disorder or overreacting to some situational or environmental disturbance and it is only with the benefit of hindsight that the real condition becomes obvious. In reality diagnosis is only really reliable following a clear cut episode of mania. Equally, other causes of mania should not be ruled out. Illicit stimulant drugs may induce manic symptoms and any drug-induced psychosis usually diminishes once the drug is stopped. The misuse of drugs and alcohol may also include mood altering drugs and coexist with manic episodes. L-dopa and corticosteriods are also the most commonly prescribed drugs which are associated with mania.

There is also the possibility that mania may be caused by organic conditions. The most common is thyroid disease, but likewise multiple sclerosis or any lesions which involve right sided sub-cortical or cortical areas may be associated with secondary mania and it is important that these are considered before a diagnosis is decided upon.

As it is possible for a mother to present to her GP during the depressive episode so it should be equally important to ascertain whether the woman has recently had an elevated mood which has caused her to be unusually excited or irritable for an extended period. It is also important to ascertain whether she intends to or has any ideas about harming herself, and if so what does she intend to do about this, and to what extent is she prepared to carry it out.

Once mania is diagnosed admission to hospital should always be considered, though in some areas it may be possible to offer intensive and specialist management within the community.

There is compelling evidence to suggest that women with bipolar disorder are at high risk of developing puerperal psychosis. The episodes occur following 25–50% of deliveries (Jones & Craddock, 2001). The high rate of illness represents a several hundred-fold increase from the base rate of approximately 1 in 1000 deliveries. There is also the problem that if a mother has suffered from a previous incident of puerperal psychosis then the chances of a repeat of the condition are significantly increased.

One mother volunteered:

I developed bipolar disorder when I had my first child. I would dearly like another one but I could not put my family through it again. I was fine, on top of the world, everything was wonderful, but then I realised what a nightmare I was during that time and how my husband was at his wits' end wondering where I was and what I was spending his money on. I want to cry at the thought of if but I just cannot consider another pregnancy.

There is growing evidence to suggest that bipolar disorder has a familial trait and the risks are heightened if a close family member has a history of bipolar disorder, puerperal psychosis or both. There is a plethora of social and environmental factors which may predispose the majority of mothers to bipolar disorder but there is almost certainly a genetic factor and it is postulated by Jones & Craddock (2001) that one inherited gene may be responsible for the condition. This opens up interesting terrain and suggests that in the future it may be possible to screen a foetus for the gene. This naturally is not without its own ethical dilemmas and some mothers affected with bipolar disorder may resent the inference that this is a condition that needs to be exterminated, particularly when they may find their own mood state liberating.

However, there are lessons to be learned about the future treatment and management of the condition and perhaps the most important is the early identification of mothers who may be at risk of developing or who have developed the condition. It is clear that the condition requires careful management, probably more meticulous than other screening, as one of the features of bipolar disorder is that it may lie dormant and the mother may feel well for long periods and not have the need to be in contact with mental health services. It is during these periods of stability that a mother may try to conceive another baby.

It is suggested that all pregnant mothers should be screened for the risk of bipolar disorder in the antenatal period. Pregnant mothers with a history of either bipolar disorder or puerperal psychosis are particularly at risk.

This raises the problem of a more specialised approach by midwives and the need for more input from specialist perinatal teams. This has been recognised in several Government papers and protocols and the indication is that in the future this should be part of the antenatal care, but in the meantime the fact that awareness of the condition is raised may be sufficient in itself (National Institute for Clinical Excellence, 2003; RCOG, 2007; Royal College of Psychiatrists, 2000; Scottish Intercollegiate Guidelines Network, 2002).

There would need to be debate and discussion over the most appropriate screening methods, quantitative measuring tools or whether simple qualitative questionnaires would suffice. There may be a predicament if the mother refuses to acknowledge she has bipolar disorder and indeed if she presents with the condition in her euthymic mood she may be able to disguise her happiness as that of being elated about her early pregnancy.

Although there is a genetic predisposition to the disorder it is not necessarily the case that everyone with an inherited vulnerability develops bipolar disorder, and this is a strong indicator that other, external factors may influence behaviour.

Risk factors are likely to be a major life event, which induces severe stress. This might be bereavement, a change in social or employment circumstances. In mothers prone to bipolar disorders, this may trigger off an episode or even prolong one. Therefore it may be wise for mothers to postpone a major house move or change of job whilst pregnant or shortly after the infant is born. In the case of a bereavement or loss it would be pertinent to monitor the mother's progress and mood state if there is any indication she would be unable to cope or begins to behave irrationally.

Although substance abuse does not incite bipolar disorder it is possible that drugs like cocaine and amphetamines may overstimulate the mother's mood state and make the situation considerably worse. There is also the danger that alcohol and tranquillisers have the ability to deepen any depressive state the mother may experience.

There have been reports that the changes in mood states may reflect the changes in the seasons. More cases of mania have been reported in the spring and summer months, whereas the depressive episodes seem to be confined to the autumn and winter

(Hakkarainen *et al.*, 2003). There is no conclusive research which suggests an exact reason for this, but as with research into seasonal affective disorder (SADS) efforts are being made to identify the reasons for the effect of the intensity and length of natural light on mood.

Sleep deprivation, as with other mood disorders, appears to have a profound effect on the mothers with bipolar disorder and it is possible for the minimum amount of sleep loss to trigger an episode of mania. Of course, this creates a vicious cycle as the mother is unable to sleep because she is in a manic state, which acts as a catalyst for further mania.

Onset of the condition usually occurs in the first few weeks following childbirth and any deviation from the normal behaviour of the mother should be investigated, with careful questioning of both mother and those members of the family concerned with her care. There are no strict rules governing the management or medication of mothers, but ensuring that she receives the correct medication at the prescribed times is paramount and should ideally be the remit of the perinatal psychiatrist.

The traditional treatment for bipolar disorder is the medication lithium, though light therapy is also included in the more recent treatments (Colombo *et al.*, 2000).

Treatment for acute manic or mixed episodes

When there is a severe manic or mixed episode it is important to initiate the oral administration of an antipsychotic or valproate because of the rapid anti-manic effect. Sometime the mother is so unwell, and in an agitated state, that she is unable to give consent to any form of treatment. It is probable she will require parenteral treatment and an antipsychotic drug or benzodiazepines following established protocols. The lowest dose necessary should be given in the first instance, as it is tempting to escalate the dose of antipsychotic drug to obtain a sedative effect as soon as possible.

For mothers who are less manic, the treatment of lithium or carbamazepine may also be considered in the short term. For mothers who find it difficult to sleep because they are so agitated, then clonazepam or lorazepam should be considered. To achieve the best results for the mother it is important that she has control over her own medication too, and is able to negotiate a sensible dosage with her clinician. If she feels she is being over prescribed medication, does not feel comfortable within herself or feels that it interferes with her daily living then she may not comply with the dosage; this in turn will cause her condition to relapse. If the mother was previously on any antidepressant these should, ideally be tapered and discontinued.

Long-term treatment

For some mothers there may not be a long-term cure for their condition and they are reliant on medication to stabilise their mood to enable them to live productive lives. For these mothers the long-term treatment is usually lithium, carbamazepine or valproate. Blood is regularly taken to check the lithuim serum levels to establish tolerable levels, which means that if a mother is not responding to her dosage of medication then it may be increased or decreased. Once again this regime relies on the compliance of the mother and her family to ensure it is possible to lead a comfortable, functional life.

If symptoms are inadequately controlled and the mother is severely ill then electroconvulsive therapy (ECT) may be considered. For some women this is often a preferred option as it offers a more rapid solution and enables them to function more quickly. It is sometimes the preferred option for women who are pregnant and severely manic.

Once the initial symptoms of psychosis and sleeplessness have elapsed then it is pertinent to discontinue any medication used to control them. In short-term treatments, once the symptoms have subsided, the dosage of medication used for acute treatments may be reduced over a few weeks until all the drugs are eventually discontinued. It is possible for the episode to last for about three months.

It is known that there is a 1% risk of having bipolar disorder. When one parent has bipolar disorder, the risk to each child is 15–30%. When both parents have bipolar disorder, the risk increases to 50–75%. The risk to siblings and fraternal twins is 15–25%. The risk in identical twins is approximately 70%.

It has been suggested that symptoms can begin in early childhood, but more typically emerge in adolescence or adulthood. Research by the American Academy of Child and Adolescent Psychiatry shows that up to one-third of 3.4 million children and adolescents with depression in the USA may actually be experiencing the early onset of bipolar disorder.

The symptoms are similar to those experienced by adults, with the moods alternating between highs and lows. However, instead of elation or euphoria the children's manic outburst may present as irrational behaviour or destructive outbursts. During the depressive phase they may complain of the physical symptoms of headaches, stomach pains or lethargy. Parents have described the behaviour of their children as 'silly' one minute and withdrawn the next. The timing of their moods is unpredictable. It has also been suggested that children affected this way are at greater risk of anxiety disorders and attention deficit hyperactivity disorder (ADHD) and whether the two conditions are related is debatable.

There is increasing debate about the diagnosis of bipolar disorder in children but this remains controversial. It is compounded by the fact that bipolar disorder is difficult to recognise and diagnose in children because they do not have exactly the same established symptoms as adults, and because the symptoms can resemble those of other common childhood mental disorders. In the USA the incidence of the condition is reported to be significantly higher than the rest of the world.

Acute depressive episode

The treatment with selective serotonin reuptake inhibitors (SSRIs), an anti-manic drug, such as lithium or valproate, and an antipsychotic drug is recommended for mothers with a history of mania. Antidepressants alone are not advised (Goodwin, 2003). Once again, if there is a high suicidal risk then it is recommended that ECT is considered.

Antidepressants

There is insufficient evidence to suggest how effective SSRIs are as therapy, and there is always the possibility that the mother's mood may change from the depressive phase and more to mania during the treatment. However, this can be counteracted by adding either lithium, valproate or an antipsychotic drug. Tricyclic antidepressants, on the other hand, are more likely to alter the mood state more rapidly.

There is little more than anecdotal evidence to suggest that long-term combination treatment is superior to single therapy. Recent studies have shown that the strongest evidence is that lithium is the most effective treatment. It certainly prevents manic relapse and probably depressive relapse too.

Adverse effects of long term medication

One of the unwanted effects of long-term medication is the propensity to put on weight. And this is a major problem for women in particular. The reality is that for many women it is a struggle to lose the weight gained in pregnancy and because the weight loss is not instantaneous many may be discouraged from attempting to continue on a diet regime. A further dilemma is that once the medication is discontinued, either voluntarily or because the condition has subsided some mothers expect weight loss to be instantaneous, but this is not the case. They may receive little sympathy from clinicians as the argument is often that it is preferable to be overweight than suffer the surge of depression. However, the side effects of the weight gain are also debilitating. Blood pressure may be higher and cholesterol levels may increase, which may involve additional medication to control both of these risk factors. Of course it is important to stress that once the weight gain is under control the other risk factors diminish. This is a long-term problem with long-term solutions and mothers have to adapt to a new lifestyle in more ways than one.

Discontinuation of medication

Whatever the drug of choice it is only capable of stabilising the mother's mood to enable her to function normally. What they are unable to do is cure the condition, so the danger remains that if the mother chooses to discontinue her medication there is always the risk of relapse, even if she has been taking the drugs for many years. Should there be a need to discontinue the medication this is a considered risk and it is advised that the dosage is tapered over a minimum of two weeks. Scott & Colom (2005) found that between 20–50% of patients do not adhere to or receive mood stabilising medication. Neglect of the mother during this time is also a consideration as she may withdraw from the services completely and believe that no further intervention is necessary. Therefore, continuation of psychological interventions can reduce the risk of relapse. The form of cognitive behavioural therapy specifically designed for bipolar disorder should also be offered.

Cognitive behavioural therapy (CBT)

While bipolar mothers share many of the common cognitive distortions described in depressive illnesses, a cognitive model is not convincing as a complete theory of the illness. However, cognitive theories can address some of the specific problems of bipolar disorder. CBT can produce a reduction in symptoms compared with women who are treated with drug therapy (Lam *et al.*, 2003). The therapy includes education of the condition, enhancing the motivation to comply with taking medication, self-monitoring, identifying and preventing any deterioration in the overall mood state, recognising how to solve problems which may lead to relapse and how to recognise signs of impending relapse. However, the action plans and modification of behaviour do not depend on the mother to recognise her own abnormal mood state. This is where the involvement of family is important and the implementation of family focused psycho-educational sessions can have a significant effect on maintaining the good mental health of the mother.

Six sessions of CBT, compared to outpatient follow-up, were more successful in improving the mother's ability to adhere to her drug regime. However, Scott *et al.* (2006) found that the most practical amount of CBT session offered by the NHS schemes was 20 sessions of CBT with two follow-up sessions. This may not be effective for most patients but for those with an early history of bipolar disorder it may be very helpful. It is important that CBT is considered as an adjunctive treatment option to help to stabilise moods more quickly. However, in reality it was found that the average attendance for CBT sessions amounted to 14.

In extreme cases it is vital that the appropriate use of legal powers is initiated and employed to detain mothers in a place of safety. This is usually a psychiatric hospital, psychiatric unit within a general hospital, or, ideally, a mother and baby unit.

Recovery

It is unusual for the mother to make a full recovery in less than three months following remission of her symptoms; this is important to understand if the mother is working and needs to have time off work. It should also be stressed that any life-changing decisions should not be made during this period.

Currently, interventions that have been offered are in response to the presenting clinical symptoms and do not depend on specific models of psychopathology.

There should be consistent outpatient follow up and information on the mother's care and progress should be shared with other professionals in the multidisciplinary team. Ideally, if the mother is in danger of relapsing she and other professionals should know how to access early interventions within the community. Arrangements should be in place to ensure the mother has the option of having a hospital admission if that is necessary.

There is also a need for education of health professionals and there is merit here in the use of clinical supervision as each individual may bring their own different experiences and beliefs to the therapeutic relationship. There may be value in discussion about how mothers may be reluctant to forgo their manic phase, when they may feel at their happiest or most creative, for the undetermined phase of stability or depression.

The importance of regular patterns of daily activities should be emphasised. The mother and her family could be taught to identify the habitual and very irregular patterns of behaviours, which are common to bipolar patients and attempt to try to modify them. The use of diaries for recording and monitoring moods or activities may be very useful. Recognising the inconsistencies in behaviour may help to identify the onset of mania and being aware of the signs and symptoms of manic behaviour may indicate early signs of relapse and the need for early intervention. There is no doubt it is necessary to have a sound long-term relationship amongst the physician, the mother and the family to ensure continuity of care.

Puerperal psychosis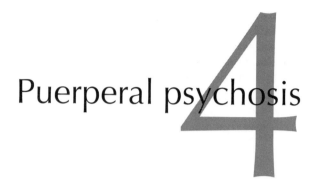

Psychosis

One or two in a thousand new mothers may require hospital admission to an acute unit or mother and baby unit following an episode of puerperal psychosis or a recurrence of affective psychosis disorder. Puerperal psychosis is a severe mental illness and is regarded as an emergency situation. It usually occurs a few days following childbirth and often where there is a family history of mental illness. It is more common in the first-time mother and the risk to women with bipolar disorder is much greater. There is the added risk that about one-quarter of mothers will suffer from a recurrence in subsequent pregnancies. Should it be left untreated it is possible it will last for more than six to eight months, but with early intervention the mother may feel completely well within one to three months. However, it is possible there will be relapses and the sad fact is that some mothers may never completely recover.

Some research has found that it may be more common in mothers who have been treated with some steroids, or bromocriptine in particular. The drug bromocriptine, Parlodel, is a dopamine antagonist and it works by stimulating dopamine receptors in the brain. Bromocriptine is mainly used to treat disorders that result from high levels of the hormone prolactin in the blood. Bromocriptine decreases the production of prolactin from the pituitary gland by stimulating dopamine receptors. High levels of prolactin are associated with several conditions. Over-production of this hormone can cause abnormal production of breast milk in women (galactorrhoea) and infertility. High prolactin levels are also associated with some breast and menstrual disorders. Reducing prolactin levels with bromocriptine can improve these conditions. Bromocriptine is also sometimes used to prevent or stop milk production for medical reasons following childbirth, miscarriage or abortion. Prolactin is the hormone that stimulates the production of breast milk, hence decreasing the production of prolactin with bromocriptine stops milk production. It is also used to treat hypogonadism, acromegaly and Parkinson's disease. It has been reported that rarely, amongst the adverse effects of hypertension, stroke and seizures, there is a possibility of a psychiatric disorder, which may include confusion, hallucinations, increased libido, hyper-sexuality and an uncontrollable urge to gamble. For these reasons its use is not recommended in women who have a history of a serious psychiatric illness.

Causes

The wealth of evidence suggests that the triggers for the condition are pregnancy related. It may occur following a miscarriage or termination of a trophoblastic tumour. The hypothesis that hormonal changes may cause puerperal psychosis was supported by Abdullah *et al.* (2006) when they reviewed the association between surgical procedures and psychosis. It was found that there was an episode of puerperal psychosis in a woman when a trophoblastic tumour was removed. These findings prompt a need for awareness, ability to diagnose and an understanding of the cause of psychotic symptoms following surgical procedures, which will ultimately provide better care and more effective treatment.

The pregnancy itself makes vulnerable women more susceptible to episodes that may occur during the third trimester of the pregnancy. However, the most powerful determinant appears to be during the first ten days following delivery. In some cases some mothers have been known to relapse once menstruation recommences and there is evidence which points at a strong link between the menstrual cycle and psychosis. A review of world literature by Brockington (2006) discusses the association between the onset of psychosis and the menses and documents case reports of childbirth, which concentrate on the menarche.

There is some limited evidence that the psychosis may occur when the baby has been weaned from the mother's breast and a proposal that breast-feeding may have had a protective effect against the development of schizophrenia; however, this was not supported in a study by Leask *et al.* (2000).

The first indication that the mother is unwell is usually signalled by her bizarre behaviour, but this is not always the case and sometimes the odd way in which the mother behaves is associated with the normality of childbirth and is often overlooked. Mothers with some insight may conceal the way they feel for fear of the reality of going 'mad' and as a result having their infant removed from their care. In this respect their fears are correct, as often infants may need to be placed in a place of safety, until the mother is well enough to look after the infant herself.

The mother, too, requires a place of safety and specialist help where she may be nursed in a protective environment to help her recover more quickly. Her medication should be closely monitored, as there is a tendency for it to have a both a sedative and tranquillising effect, which might render the mother incapable of rational thought.

Delusional states

In puerperal psychosis delusions are often present but they are more florid and more frightening than those experienced in major postnatal depression. Some delusions may be described as bizarre and these are fairly easily distinguishable from the non-bizarre types. A bizarre belief is totally implausible and opposed to the mother's normal behaviour and thought processes. A common example is that the mother believes she has been abducted by aliens and her brain used in experiments. The mother may openly admit that she feels an external force controlling her, which she is unable to resist, such as a perpetrator may have instruments that they have inserted into the mother's body or brain, which send electric impulses making her react uncontrollably to situations. She may fling out her arms or lift the infant repeatedly out of the crib. The instrument may even drain her thoughts from her head making her not responsible for her actions. This may account for the way she moves, speaks or, indeed, thinks.

The mother may experience a nihilistic delusion where she is fixed in the belief that the world is about to end and to prevent her infant or her from suffering a terrible fate she may make the decision to end her own life and that of her infant. Further negative thoughts may centre on guilt and shame, where the mother may be convinced she is wholly responsible for a natural or accidental disaster. For example she may think that the plane crashing was her fault as she cleaned her windows with the wrong type of chemical or the typhoon occurred because she was unable to control the heating in her house. Once she is convinced that she is not to blame the mother may invent further occurrences to maintain her feelings of guilt.

The mother may experience 'delusions of grandeur' where she may firmly believe that she is born of royalty or a 'super mother' and the way in which she nurtures her infant has been ordained by God. She may feel that this talent has previously gone unrecognised and the birth of her infant is an opportune moment to proclaim this to the world. These types of belief may permeate the mother's thoughts and result in distorted thinking. The more prevalent and eccentric the belief then the more likely the mother is to enact them, perhaps by refusing support and assistance with her infant from family and friends or counteracting the delusions by defending her infant, secreting it away from any destruction or hurt. This has serious repercussions for the welfare of the infant, particularly if the mother feels she has a need to protect the infant from harm, while in the process she may indeed harm the infant herself. These thoughts and actions are more likely to occur in puerperal psychosis but should not be discounted in a mother who may otherwise behave 'normally'.

Some delusions may have a somatic component and the mother may feel that her body has become distorted or diseased. The symptoms are extraordinary in that she may feel she is infested with worms or that her breast milk consists of pus and blood. Any attempt to help her to understand this is not true will be met with derision.

A non-bizarre delusion is where it may be possible but highly improbable that the mother experienced the event. This type of delusion is more prevalent in severe postnatal depression. The most common type is where the mother feels she is being persecuted. She may feel, though not reveal, that her care of her infant may be scrutinised by social services, or that the midwife is using microphones in the home to record her conversations with her partner. She might believe that the health visitor is following her when she is out walking with her baby. Additionally, she may feel that these agencies are responsible for controlling her thoughts and, as a result, her actions. Some of her thought processes may be simple and just involve one set of circumstances, but often she may construct a more complex set of scenarios which may alienate her from the services and justify her reticence or refusal to allow any statutory interventions. From a professional perspective it may be difficult to decipher whether this is a voluntary action or whether the mother is actually suffering from paranoid delusions.

Auditory hallucinations

As with all hallucinations, only the mother is privy to hearing the auditory hallucinations. Sometimes she may recognise voices which are not her own. Sometimes they are completely coherent and at others times they may be distorted, so that the mother is aware of voices or noises in her head but is unable to interpret them. Often the language is offensive, but gestures such as covering the ears to block out the sounds helps to obscure full impact of the noise; nevertheless it is difficult to control them. The voices may also be loud, sometimes shouting or screaming at the mother. They occur unpredictably, too, and this is equally distressing as it may be impossible to distinguish what is actually being said to the mother and what is actually a hallucination.

When she is able to interpret them the mother may be highly disturbed by the array of voices in her head telling her she is being watched and that her every move is being scrutinised to determine whether she is capable of being a good mother. The voices may offer suggestions about what to do next and guide the mother in her parenting of the infant. However, they are more likely to be abrupt, aggressive, controlling, negative and confirm that the mother is indeed a bad person who is obviously incapable of caring for her own child. The bombardment of sounds often allows little space for rational thought and she may feel reluctant to comply with these, but as they are, she believes, coming from a greater authority she is bound to act upon them. She feels that she is to blame for her infant's distress and it is reasonable to expect her husband to be violent towards her. It is her fault that her vacuum cleaner stopped working and she is responsible for the groceries not being delivered. These words are often repeated until they become almost unbearable. Her every effort may be thwarted and she may feel that family and friends are constantly judging her. It would be feasible, then, to suggest that she may succumb to the voices and either plunge into despair or react against them by attacking what she sees as her assailants.

Visual hallucinations

The voices are often accompanied by visions, which create a more vivid, violent scene and where the mother is surrounded by sights of terrifying evil and disaster. The image of her infant may be seen as the devil incarnate and she may feel that it is her duty to rid the world of this corrupt and depraved being. This may account for some of the known cases of infanticide. Conversely, the mother may believe that she has borne the infant Jesus. It is important to her that people believe she has given birth to the Son of God. Sinners must listen to what she has to say and there is need to preach the word of God. She might be there to protect her infant and the constant need to watch over him/her may reflect this.

One mother described her psychotic experiences as:

I could see God rising in front of me in all his glory. He blessed me and was telling me it was my duty to help him to save the world. I must preach to my family and get them to tell everyone that Jesus had come into the world and I was his helper.

In more lucid moments the mother may recognise this as abnormal and seek help, but the stark reality is that sometimes the voices can be overwhelming and it is difficult to distinguish between reality and fantasy. The words may confirm the mother's perception of herself and although she may have some insight into her condition, she may sometimes feel that her internal world is more 'real' than the external world. This state causes women to be profoundly ill, and, as a result, significantly disabled by the illness. What is equally distressing to the mother is that it may be impossible to distinguish what is actually being said to her and what is actually a hallucination.

Schizophrenia

Schizophrenia was first described by Emil Kraepelin, a psychiatrist, who thought its origins were an organic dysfunction of the brain which eventually led to its premature deterioration. He gave it the title of 'dementia praecox'. However, this was disputed by Eugene Bleuler, who noted that it affected older as well as young patients, and that the progression of the condition normally stabilised and then plateaued for the duration of their lives. The patient got neither better nor worse but learned to accept and live with the condition. The name schizophrenia is translated from Greek meaning 'split' and 'mind'. This has been misinterpreted to mean that the person is in two minds and acts as separate people, but Bleuler's intention was to emphasis the differentials in the cognitive and the affective functioning of the patient.

Schizophrenia is defined as a group of mental disorders which are at psychotic level. It is estimated that over 1% of the population suffer from it. The condition is characterised by marked disturbances in the thought processes and of the mother's perception of life. The prime symptoms are her bizarre behaviour, which is usually generated by a distortion of reality manifested in hallucinations and delusions. Sometimes the mother is apathetic and may withdraw from what she sees as reality. It used to be possible to catergorise it into several types which included hebephrenic, catatonic, paranoid and schizoaffective disorder, but these have been superseded by Type 1 which is an acute schizophrenic episode and Type II which is a process schizophrenia. It is probably the most serious and debilitating of all mental disorders. Its complexity sometimes defies diagnosis and the causes of the condition remain unclear.

Type I refers to a reactive schizophrenia, the onset of which is sudden and usually precipitated by a life crisis, which might be closely related to the infant's birth or an unresolved relationship problem. As the presentation is so acute it is often easily recognised and treated in the early stages of its development. As a result, the mother is able to respond more rapidly to the medication and therapy, whereas Type II tends to have its roots in a more protracted onset. If a history is taken it becomes obvious that the mother has been 'ill' for a longer period of time, and has a history of being withdrawn and socially inept, amongst other signs. Often this behaviour has been recognised in the past and there is usually involvement with the Child and Adult Mental Health Service (CAMHS).

The mood is affected and there is an excessive lack of correlation between what the mother is saying and the emotion she is expressing. The example often used is when she is describing a sad or distressing event yet is genuinely laughing at the thought. Often when they lose touch with reality they become preoccupied with themselves. This has serious implications for their baby as they may unintentionally 'forget' or not notice that their baby has needs and as a result these may be neglected.

There are positive and negative symptoms. The positive usually occur during the initial phase of the condition but can present at any time. They include delusions, hallucinations and/or thought disturbances. The negative symptoms consist of the more chronic loss of normal function which presents as lethargy, lack of concentration and withdrawal.

Schizophrenia has been further classified into paranoid schizophrenia, undifferentiated schizophrenia, residual schizophrenia and schizophreniform disorder. Paranoid schizophrenia relates to a mother who displays psychotic symptoms which include being paranoid about the intentions of people and objects. Undifferentiated schizophrenia is where the symptoms are of a schizophrenic nature but include other types of mental disorder. The residual schizophrenic is a mother who, during a six-month period, has suffered from at least one episode of schizophrenia which has been treated and from which she has recovered. Schizophreniform disorder is probably the less serious form of the condition, where the mother has had an episode, which has lasted for more than two weeks but has subsided after six months. She is then able to return to resume her lifestyle and has no further events.

As in psychosis, a diagnosis of schizophrenia is rare before the age of 15 years. Usually the onset occurs between the ages of 15 and 35 years and affects men and women equally. It affects one in a hundred people. Despite several reviews there appears to be little difference in the way in which both genders experience hallucinations. Hallucinations, which are the core symptoms in schizophrenia, have been described as a sensory perception in the absence of external stimuli.

There has often been debate about the causation and whether the symptoms are induced by socio-environmental issues or whether it is caused by pathological origins. In a study by Silberweig *et al.* (1995) of patients with auditory, verbal hallucinations it was possible to detect changes in thalamic, hippocampus and paralimbic (which included the orbito-frontal cortex) regions of the brain. Activity was also found in the cortical and subcortical network of the brain in a patient suffering from visual and auditory hallucinations. It was postulated that the interaction of the distributed neural systems provided a form of biological basis for the causation or effect of hallucinations in schizophrenic patients. Further research is continuing in this area.

The onset of the condition is often insidious and it is not immediately obvious that a mother may be suffering from it. Often schizophrenia is diagnosed prior to the pregnancy and community mental health teams and other agencies and health professionals are alerted to the fact. However, in a small minority of cases the condition may not be so apparent and it is only when more bizarre behaviour is detected that schizophrenia is diagnosed. Families might notice that the mother is becoming remote and isolating herself from family and friends. She may refuse help of any kind and assure others that she is self-possessed and able to manage. However, this is not evident, as there are indicators that she is obviously not coping, as indicated by failing to do the housework or the appearance of an overflowing laundry basket. She may indicate that she is not sleeping at night but spends most of the day dozing. As a result she is unable to manage everyday tasks and again the care of her infant is compromised. She may neglect her personal hygiene and be neglectful of her infant's care.

Further unusual behaviour may indicate that she finds it increasingly difficult to converse and will resort to monotone answers, which are sometimes incoherent because they are whispered or muffled. There may be a refusal to talk altogether. Eye contact can sometimes be avoided and the mother may appear as if she is listening to someone or something else. She may turn to look or search for the sounds in response to the hallucinations. Often she may respond inadvertently, and not appear embarrassed that she has done so. She may appear preoccupied with a visual or olfactory hallucination or in a minority of cases may flinch as she responds to a particular sensation. She may discuss her delusional ideas which might sound foolish or odd, but sometimes they sound so florid that they sound insane.

Causes

Some studies have shown that in one in ten cases schizophrenia is familial. For those mothers with no family history of schizophrenia the chances of developing the condition are one in a hundred, those with a parent diagnosed with the condition may have a one in ten chance, whereas an identical twin may have a 50% chance of having it as well. The genetic make-up is known to account of approximately half of the cases, but as yet, the actual genes have not been isolated. When Slater & Shields (1953) studied twins it was found that if one twin had schizophrenia the prevalence of schizophrenia in the other twin was similar. Later studies also suggested some genetic relationship. However, current theories suggest that this cannot be wholly linked to genetic make-up, but if a mother does have some component that makes up a schizophrenic gene then this may make her more susceptible to the condition if environmental factors should become a trigger.

Buka *et al.* (2001) found that the children of mothers who had elevated levels of immunoglobulins and antibodies to the herpes simplex virus were at an increased risk of developing schizophrenia later in life.

Examination of the brain has demonstrated that there are significant differences in brain development, which may be attributable to anoxia at birth, or it has been postulated that it may be due to a viral infection during the first trimester of the pregnancy. Recent studies have suggested that if a mother suffers from influenza during the second trimester of pregnancy the risk of the foetus suffering from schizophrenia increases. The statistics suggest the risk is three to seven times higher and it has been suggested that over 20% of known cases of schizophrenia have been triggered by a viral infection whilst they were in the womb. These observations have led to a resurgence of interest in this hypothesis, particularly with regard to prenatal and perinatal infection.

In a study with mice, Limosin *et al.* (2003) found that a maternal viral infection of influenza had a significant effect on the behaviour of the offspring of adult mice. It has been postulated that this was probably caused by the effect of the mother's immune response on the foetus. An innate immune response is driven by proteins called cytokines, which are produced by the body in response to infection. The researchers speculated that something was being transmitted to the foetus by one or more of the cytokines, which were produced by the mother in response to her infection. Schizophrenia is apparently more evident among people born in the winter and spring months, as well as those born following an influenza epidemic.

There is also the suggestion that infection from the *Toxoplasma gondii* parasite (toxoplasmosis) which is found in cats' and farm animals' faeces may also increase the risk of infection. In a large study Niebuhr *et al.* (2008) found that a small percentage of schizophrenics had been infected with the parasite prior to having the diagnosis of schizophrenia. However, most people who are infected with toxoplasmosis will never develop schizophrenia, but it is suggested that the parasite might be a trigger in those who are genetically predisposed to the disorder.

These studies are inconclusive as there have been several failures to replicate the findings, but although not definitive, they have demonstrated that exposure to infections, including influenza and toxoplasmosis are associated with an increase in the risk of schizophrenia. There are, however, effective antibiotic treatments for toxoplasmosis and an immunisation against the influenza virus, but it is unlikely that these alone are the cause and that lifestyle factors may also have a significant impact. If it can be clearly proven by more rigorous and extensive research that infection during the prenatal period is responsible for schizophrenia this will have clear implications for treatment to prevent the disorder.

There have been recorded incidents where the ingestion of illicit drugs, in particular ecstasy, amphetamines and LSD has induced schizophrenic episodes though it is unclear whether this causes long-term problems. Cannabis is a drug that is well known for having the potential to double the risk of developing schizophrenia, particularly if it is smoked excessively during the teenage years. The frequency of inhalation is also indicative, as the more it has been smoked the greater the risk. There is now converging evidence to suggest that the use of cannabis is a risk factor for schizophrenia. In a Danish study, Arendt *et al.* (2005) found that cannabis-induced psychotic disorders were diagnosed in just under half of the sample population. Three-quarters had a new psychotic episode and episodes were prevalent in younger men. There was a delay in receiving a diagnosis and it was often over a year later that treatment was sought for the psychosis. Frequent and extreme consumers of cannabis were over 600% more likely to be diagnosed with schizophrenia over the following 15 years than those who abstained. It has been estimated that between 8% and 13% of cases of schizophrenia are linked to marijuana use during adolescence. In a systematic review by Semple *et al.* (2005) it was found that the early use of cannabis did not appear to increase the risk of psychosis. However, all of the evidence pointed to the fact that cannabis is an independent risk factor both for psychosis and the development of psychosis.

In studies around the world it has been estimated that cannabis may double the risk of schizophrenia and that this risk increases in proportion to the drug used. The theory that self-medicating increases the use of cannabis is discounted. However, continuing research is necessary to understand the mechanisms by which cannabis causes psychosis.

Stress is often associated with deterioration in symptoms and a psychotic episode is often precipitated by a life crisis. However, the process by which stress can affect schizophrenia is unclear. It is often described in terms of the impact of life events and expressed emotions. Despite medication to control symptoms it is not always possible to reduce the mother's reaction to stress and even relatively minor stress may invoke a crisis. This raises the possibility that schizophrenic mothers have an altered sensitivity to stress and it is probable that they are unable to adapt to their environment as easily as others. This might be acute difficulty in a relationship, moving home or an accident. Long-term stress may also generate an episode; over exertion when studying for exams, great expectations to perform or emotional difficulties. It would appear important, therefore, that there is consideration for any reduction of stress-related factors. As in other forms of stress, the release of corticosteroids plays an essential role. The biological response to stress is impaired in schizophrenic mothers as their cortisol response to stress is blunted.

It was once thought that schizophrenia was caused by a dysfunctional family where there was a failure to communicate successfully with family members. However, studies have shown that there is little evidence to support this hypothesis.

Schizophrenia has been recorded in cases of women who have been abused in childhood.

Care of the infant

There is evidence that schizophrenic mothers have poorer interaction with their infant, particularly for the duration of their illness as they are often preoccupied with their own thoughts and feelings and are unable to manage themselves, let alone the needs of an infant. Unfortunately, even when they have recovered clinically they remain vulnerable to continuing a stable relationship with their offspring. This area is still under investigated but preliminary findings suggest there is a subtle difference in the way in which these mothers speak and behave with their infants. One study suggests that the symptoms specific to schizophrenia may be particularly harmful for interaction and that parenting interventions need to be developed specially for these mothers to improve their interactions with their infants (Wan *et al.*, 2007).

Management

In most instances it is necessary to consult a psychiatrist and then be assessed by the mental health team. Sometimes hospital admission is necessary, but often the mother's care can be managed in the home. Drug therapy in the form of antipsychotics is probably the first treatment as it is important to stabilise mood and counteract, or at least reduce, the severity of hallucinations, which will help the mother to increase motivation and self-esteem. These help to reduce dopamine in the brain.

There are two groups of antipsychotics, first and second generation. The first generation consist of the familiar Largactil, trifluoperazine and haloperidol. The Depot injection is designed for those who are unable or reluctant to take oral medication. Frequency varies and it is possible to have the injection, which is given by the community psychiatric nurse, every week, fortnight or month as is necessary. There is a newer atypical antipsychotic called risperidone which is currently in use.

Unfortunately, these have the distressing side effects of Parkinsonian-like symptoms of uncontrollable tremors and stiffness in joints and muscles. Akathisia, a feeling of restlessness, may also be present. The additional drug Artane is given to control this. The mother's libido is often affected. One of the problems with long-term medication is that some patients may develop tardive dyskinesia, which affects the tongue, and mouth and may cause persistent movement of both areas.

Over the past ten years there has been a significant improvement in drug therapies. This has produced a group of drugs known as the 'second generation' or 'atypical medication'. These have the familiar names of clozapine (the generic name is Clozaril) and quetiapine (generic name is Seroquel). Clozapine is found to be one of the more effective treatments and the incidence of suicide is considerably lower when this drug is used. Studies have found that the drug can affect the bone marrow, and the drop in white corpuscles lowers any resistance to infection. As a result, levels of the drug in the blood are monitored carefully.

The drugs interact specifically with the serotonin in the brain. The side effects are less likely to cause Parkinsonian side effects, such as tardive dyskinesia, but still cause problems with the woman's libido. The drugs have the added unwelcome side effect of causing weight gain. It is recommended that all of the drug treatments continue for at least six months as it has been shown that if the treatment is terminated before then there is probability of relapse. Gradual reduction of the drug is recommended and it is important that no drug is stopped without consultation with a psychiatrist.

In addition to drug therapy, other forms of behavioural therapies are recommended and encouraged. Research is currently looking at the efficacy of CBT in the early stages of schizophrenia.

The severity of the condition often necessitates admission to a psychiatric unit. However, because the mother is unaware of her bizarre behaviour or how fixated or fanatical her actions are she may refuse to be admitted. The legislation in the Mental Health Act (England and Wales) (2003) ensures that procedures are in place to compulsorily detain the mother in a place of safety, which is the unit, even if it is against her will. Criteria have to be addressed and these include the agreement of three professionals that the mother's health is at risk, she is a danger to herself or a danger to other people. The professionals are usually the family general practitioner, who is familiar with the mother's condition, a doctor with specialist mental health training, usually a psychiatrist, and an 'approved social worker' with specialist training in mental health.

Recovery

Statistics are more positive than in previous years and it is estimated that one in five will improve within five years of the first episode of schizophrenia. Three in five will improve but will not be asymptomatic and sometimes their condition may deteriorate, leaving one in five with persistent and debilitating symptoms.

Suicide attempts and suicide is more prevalent in mothers with schizophrenia. This is usually due to untreated symptoms or mothers who refuse to engage with prescribed treatments. Suicide has consistently been the most common cause of premature death in schizophrenia. A number of risk factors have been identified and some studies have identified females as being substantially at greater risk than males and they are invariably under the age of 35 years (Appleby, 2000). This probably reflects a more complex concept encompassing the stage and severity of the illness (Raymont, 2001). Heila *et al.* (1997) found that one-third of all patients who committed suicide were non-compliant with their medication and over half were prescribed insufficient medication. A large proportion of the suicides occurred during the active phase of the illness.

Early intervention, as in psychosis, has a greater success rate and hospital admissions are lower, less intensive treatment is necessary and there is a quicker recovery rate.

Community day centres

Sometimes, particularly where the mother has been severely ill, it is important to integrate her back into the community slowly. Day centres offer this resource. The mother is contained in a safe, comfortable environment with trained specialist workers in mental health. There is the opportunity to socialise with others, participate in a range of activities, which may include exercise classes, or the creative arts, where she is allowed to express herself in the form of painting or pottery. The support of the community mental health team (CMHT) is important and is able to act as a facilitator for the 'care approach programme' and provide information and advice on treatment.

The support of family and friends is vital, and a support network is often provided for them. As in all cases, early detection and treatment is the preferable course of action. It is important that not only the immediate family is familiar with signs of relapse but that the mother is also aware of and recognises impending signs. These may include an unusual loss of appetite, difficulty in sleeping and often suffering from sleep deprivation. This will be particularly important if her infant is experiencing problems at night and demands her attention, so that she is unable to extradite herself from the responsibilities. She may experience feelings of anxiety or distress that are often precipitated by misinterpreting the actions of others. This may lead to feelings of mild paranoia, such as thinking that people are questioning her ability as a mother, or people are discussing her in the street, or behind her back. There may be the insidious return of the controlling angry voices or sounds which make it difficult to concentrate.

The mother may not be as particular in her hygiene and there may be a noticeable and sometimes alarming lack of care, both of herself and of the infant. This may include leaving soiled nappies unattended or failing to bathe the infant.

It is important that the mother should not to attempt to counteract or diminish these symptoms by resorting to alcohol or illicit drugs. Situations that are likely to be stressful should be avoided, but should this be inevitable then it is important that the family are aware of the potential difficulties that the mother may experience.

Performing the relaxation techniques that have been learnt during therapy will be helpful to the mother, as will using avoidance methods to alleviate or at least reduce the input of the voices. These might include listening to the radio, television or personal stereo, or chatting with other people. Convincing herself that the voices are unreal and not allowing them to control her are equally important.

Menstrual psychosis

One neglected issue in the psychoses is 'premenstrual psychosis', which is not to be confused with premenstrual tension or premenstrual depression (Deuchar & Brockington, 1998). This has the characteristics of a brief, but acute, onset, with a brief duration followed by a complete recovery. The symptoms include confusion, delusions, hallucinations or mania and are synonymous with the mother's menstrual cycle. Its prominence is rare, primarily because so little is known about it and it tends not to be diagnosed. The similarities in the symptoms indicate that menstrual and puerperal psychoses are related and it is possible for women to suffer from both at different times in their lives.

Mother and baby units

Where the mother should be cared for is subject to debate. There are the practicalities that mothers who are severely ill and are admitted to hospital are unable to engage with their newborn infant. There is little possibility of building a relationship and being allowed to continue breast-feeding. These are all associated with mother-child interaction, which is discussed in another chapter. The mother is often isolated from her family, albeit for a short period of time, but nevertheless it fractures her role as a mother, partner and homemaker, with all the obvious consequences, not only for herself but also for her family as a whole. Therefore the most obvious form of treatment is at home, in the community. The reality is that this must be effective and vigilant and in partnership with the primary care team.

There is always the danger and indeed the risk that a mother with a florid psychosis may harm herself, her family or her partner. The twenty-four hour observation that can be effectively provided by a hospital admission is not always possible and more likely impossible. It also relies heavily on the support of the extended family that must also take responsibility for the infant and all the care that entails. This may be too heavy a burden for some, particularly if the mother is unsupported by her partner or is a teenager who relies on her own family for support. The primary pharmaceutical need is for powerful sedation and in particular the neuroleptics, but these are not without the debilitating side effects of drowsiness and apathy, which when the needs of a newborn are considered are probably not the most welcome of treatments.

The most obvious solution is to admit the mother and infant together into a mother and baby unit. However, the reality of this is that these are scarce and whereas some parts of the country are well served by these, in others there are none. In total there are eight units in the UK. Although clinical need for a mother and baby hospital is likely to exist in many parts of the country it is postulated that it is only feasible to establish a separate service in locations where the population density provides sufficient and ongoing demand. Hospitals located in rural settings may not have adequate clinical demand to warrant development of a specialised mother and baby unit (Howard *et al.*, 2006).

The idea of mother and baby units was conceived at the Cassel Hospital over fifty years ago. They are designed to enable the mother to feel relaxed and well supported with supervision to whatever degree is appropriate. Some amenities will include arrangements for relaxing, a private room for feeding and for receiving visitors, a nursery and sometimes en suite facilities are available. The aim is to maintain the mother baby relationship. The average stay at a unit is six weeks. Staff at the units are constantly vigilant of the need to re-integrate the mother back into the community. Regular liaison with the community services is important to ensure there is a seamless transition from the unit back to the mother's home.

However, the positive outcomes of a mother and baby unit may be over estimated as it may not be in either the mother's or the infant's best interest to be exposed to multiple caretakers. Lovestone & Kumar (1993) also found that men whose partners and infants were admitted to psychiatric hospitals were subject to high rates of depression. It is possible that they were reacting to their inability to provide a suitable and conducive environment that would allow their partner to recover, as well as being confronted with the severity and devastation that comes with enforced separation. Conversely, they may also reflect the mental state of other men whose partners remain at home.

There are few studies which validate the use of mother and baby units, and it may be argued that there is a lack of rigorous systematic analysis to either justify or argue against the existence of them in the treatment of puerperal psychosis (Cawley *et al.*, 1999). More research is needed to compare the overall costing of the different models of care, and to measure both the long and short-term outcomes.

Early interventions in psychosis (EIP)

An early intervention in the treatment of psychosis is a new preventive paradigm, which has been borne out of a general deep dissatisfaction with the traditional services. Its aim is to reduce the duration of untreated psychosis and provide optimal psychosocial treatment, where the focus is on social as well as clinical outcomes. This ensures that the mother is able to return to work or resume her college course. It is now well accepted that the most effective and critical period to treat this is during the early years. If treatment is offered for a period of two to three years it is predicted that the outcomes are better 15 to 30 years later. The focus on the duration of treatment is from one to two years and should be 'phase sensitive'.

Girls who later develop a psychosis are known to present with the first episode of illness at around 14 years of age. The diagnosis of any mental disorder is distressing but for girls and parents alike, the discovery of a psychosis must be particularly devastating, particularly as there is no known cure and the consequences remain for a lifetime. There is a need to cope with the initial grief and loss over what might have been.

The idea of EIP is to improve the girl's mental state and ultimately reduce the time she may stay in hospital. In some instances it is postulated that the full blown psychotic episode may be prevented or at the very least delayed. It would also allow the identification of women who might be at ultra high risk of relapse. There is evidence to show that there is less reluctance to disengage from the services and serious attempts at suicide were reduced from 18% to 10%.

Personality disorders

Personality disorder has been defined by the *International Classification of Mental and Behavioural Disorders* (ICD-10) (World Health Organisation, 1992) as:

A severe disturbance in the character, logical condition and behavioural tendencies of the individual, usually involving several areas of the personality, and nearly always associated with considerable personal and social disruption.

In the fourth edition of the *Diagnostic and Statistical Manual of Mental Disorders* (DSM-IV) (American Psychiatric Association, 1994) a personality disorder has been defined as:

> *An enduring pattern of inner experience and behaviour that deviates markedly from the expectations of the individual's culture, is pervasive and inflexible, has an onset in adolescence or early adulthood, is stable over time, and leads to distress or impairment.*

There are nine categories of ICD-10 personality disorder and ten categories of DSM-IV personality disorder. The classification scheme is unwieldy, as personality disordered patients rarely belong to just one category of personality disorder. However, the DSM clustering system provides a useful solution to this problem by grouping the subcategories of DSM-IV personality disorder into three broad 'clusters': A, B and C.

It is generally believed that borderline personality disorder is a gendered diagnosis whose construction and patterns of diagnosis are based on the assumptions of how people should behave. It is believed that one of the main predispositions to personality disorder is caused by traumatic events – and more commonly sexual abuse and it is probable that the disproportionate number of women who are diagnosed with this disorder reflects the high numbers of women who are distressed because they have experienced such trauma.

Studies have indicated that over 70% women diagnosed with the disorder have experienced some form of childhood sexual abuse. This is supported by Goodwin *et al.* (1990) who argue that borderline personality disorder may be conceptualised as a complicated post-traumatic syndrome caused by childhood trauma. The national website 'Personality plus' argues that from their research it is unhelpful to label distressed and traumatised people as having borderline personality disorder as it is stigmatising, victim blaming, obscures the impact and extent of childhood sexual abuse and does not offer a useful model for treatment. They recommend a psychosocial approach to the management and treatment of the condition.

Distinctive personalities have usually developed by the early twenties, with recognised and acceptable ways of thinking and behaving. This equips individuals with the ability to interact with other members of society in a meaningful way. However, for those with personality disorder this is not an easy option and it is often difficult for them to relate to other members of society. It is often difficult to sustain relationships and they feel unable to adapt to strange situations. This can cause anxiety and frustration that can lead to irritability or irrational behaviour, which is often difficult to control. This often has the propensity to cause upset or harm to other people, which in turn may or may not result in affecting the mood and may compound other mental health disorders like stress or depression.

The concept of describing what is a normal personality is difficult in itself as there is no clear-cut set of rules, and the variants are substantial. Describing the signs and symptoms of schizophrenia or psychosis are less fraught with controversy. The label 'personality disorder' seems to be a panacea for all irrational and unsociable behaviour, some of which may be part of the 'normal' traits in any personality.

What does make recognition and diagnosis easier is the common patterns of behaviour that appear to be similar in some sectors of the population. It is the identification of these patterns that enable effective strategies and treatments of personality disorder to be implemented.

There is little doubt that the condition has, in the past, lacked the attention and recognition of other psychiatric disorders. Emerging research has indicated that there is a clear argument for managing people affected with the disorder to enable them to sustain a place in the society in which they live. In order to make a clearer diagnosis and therefore direct patients to an appropriate source of help, personality disorder has been categorised into three types, or clusters. It is possible to feature only one cluster but it is not unusual for people to experience more than one type.

The first is labelled cluster A. Although some of the traits are familiar to most people, those with personality disorder will experience this type of behaviour in the extreme. The first group is 'paranoid'. This describes feelings of unfounded suspicion, where there is a true belief that everyone despises the person and they only have malicious intent. These ideas generate feelings of rejection and ultimately of retribution. People in this group may not act upon the feelings of revenge but there is a propensity to hold a grudge, which can be damaging not only to the person but to the person who allegedly hates them. Those who present as 'schizoid personality' may best be described as emotionally cold, lacking in any real warmth or love. They find it difficult to interact with other people and prefer their own company. In order to sustain their isolation from society they tend to create a fantasy world where life may be full of wonderful events. They may have false beliefs about their level of status in life and elevate themselves to important positions. Their behaviour may reflect this and they may enjoy acting out the eccentricities of their life, such as dressing in vivid, bizarre colours or flaunting luxurious clothing. Gestures may be over exaggerated and they may express peculiar ideas, sometimes in response to the voices they hear or the people they see in their head, commonly known as auditory and visual hallucinations. There may be thought blocking or difficulty in judgement which may make them reluctant to make decisions or, in extreme cases, they absolve themselves from any responsibilities. This is known as a schizotypal personality as it is closely linked to the condition of schizophrenia.

Cluster B encapsulates all that is concerned with emotion and impulse. This tends towards antisocial or dissocial behaviour. Society feels aggrieved when one of it citizens revolts against the common good and acts in an antisocial manner. People with personality disorder care little for the feelings of others and do not feel guilt if they have been offensive or have committed a crime. Neither do they learn from their mistakes and will often repeatedly commit the same or similar actions. There is a tendency to be aggressive and they are easily frustrated. The behaviour tends to be impulsive and often misdemeanours happen on the spur of the moment with little forethought about the consequences for either themselves or the people it may affect. This group of people often end up in the judicial system, with many of the inmates of prison being affected or labelled with personality disorder.

The third type, cluster C, is associated with a type of anxiety disorder. Characteristics tend towards the mother feeling anxious or fearful for most of the time. Her personality dictates how she tends to behave. This borders on obsessive compulsive disorder, which although similar, is not quite the same. She lives her life in a controlled, methodical and orderly way. Generally, she is submissive to other people's requests, with an inclination to be overly dependent on them, constantly seeking their reassurance. She may be plagued by this lack of confidence and low self-esteem, which prevents her from successfully interacting on a social level. This lack of social skills often isolates her from others and she is often described as a 'loner', although this is not from choice but dictated by her feelings of inadequacy and fear of ridicule.

The 'borderline' or 'emotionally unstable personality disorder' usually presents with feelings of self-loathing which are hard to control. They, too, find it difficult to sustain any form of relationship and suffer from delusions or paranoia. The most prominent part of their lives is the propensity for self-harm, either in serious suicide attempts or non-fatal, self-inflicted injuries. There is a tendency to have excessively strong emotional reactions and they have extreme difficulty in controlling those emotions. Self-harm may include cutting, which involves drawing a blade across the skin, or a limb, or the abdomen, until it bleeds. The instruments used may range from paper clips to kitchen knives and razors. This behaviour serves as a distraction from their emotions as it is easier to cope with the physical pain than the mental anguish they feel they are suffering. It is well known that people with the condition are at risk for later suicide and indeed there is evidence of very high suicide rate amongst these people. It is also understood that self-harming behaviour affects females far more often than it does males. This begs the need for more studies on the progression of self-harm attempts.

Obsessive-compulsive disorder (OCD)

This is a potentially life-long debilitating disorder, which often emerges during teenage years and can affect as many as 1 in every 50 people. Mothers who suffer from OCD will probably experience recurrent obsessions or compulsions which are so distressing that they interfere with family relationships, social life, relationships and careers.

There is much evidence to support the fact that the perinatal period is a precipitating factor in obsessive-compulsive disorder (Abramowitz *et al.*, 2003). Symptoms are usually in the form of obsessional and compulsive behaviour which severely restricts everyday life. Pervading obsessional thoughts are a feature. They usually focus on the foetus itself and of any contamination of it or flaw that may be present.

In a study by Williams & Koran (1997) it was found that pregnancy was associated with the onset of the disorder and in over half of the cases it occurred during the first pregnancy. It has been proposed that OCD is caused by the adverse affect of serotonergic functions which occur because of the rapid withdrawal of progesterone and oestrogen following delivery. However, Kalra *et al.* (2005) proposed that it is considered as an equivalent to the lesser known chorea gravidarum which is described as the onset of involuntary movements during pregnancy which are so severe they inhibit sleeping and eating (Brockington, 2006). Once the infant is delivered all of the symptoms are completely resolved. Oestrogen is thought to be the agent, which increases the activity of dopamine.

Obsessions are described as recurrent, intrusive and often persistent thoughts which in themselves cause anxiety and distress. The mother may attempt to suppress such thoughts but is unsuccessful. As she has the insight to understand they are formed in her own mind and are not external thoughts, as in the case of psychosis, she is even more disturbed by them.

Her compulsive behaviour presents as repetitive and sometimes excessive actions, which must be performed a ritualised number of times in order to prevent any dreadful events occurring. If she goes in to check her infant is sleeping she must do this at least a specified amount of times otherwise something untoward might happen. She may have to count the number of stairs, touch the banister, open the nursery door a specified number of inches or touch the infant a pre-determined number of times. Once the task is completed she is able to relax and often does not feel any further anxiety until it has to be performed again. If the mother is hindered or stopped from her ritual this may cause even further distress and this will continue until she is allowed to finalise it. These acts are not connected in any realistic way with what they are meant to counteract or prevent.

The obsessive fear of contamination is common and this can result in her washing or scrubbing her own hands several times an hour, particularly if she is feeding or changing her infant's nappies. She may feel the need to change her baby's clothing frequently even if there is no evidence of dirt or stains.

There may be a need for complete symmetry in her everyday life. This will require ensuring that household furniture is in the correct position. Cutlery is arranged in order, tins of food are placed in alphabetical or content order, the infant's clothes are not just colour coordinated in the wardrobe but are put in order of length, type of material and price.

The mother may experience some unwanted sexual thought or feelings and may counteract this by seeking assurance that they are not as bizarre as she feels they are, or continually praying to her God for forgiveness. Repeatedly checking that the iron is not left turned on or the car door is locked helps to correct any obsessional doubts she may experience. There may be an obsession with losing or unintentionally throwing something valuable away. This will result in her hoarding possessions, which in extreme cases can cause so much clutter it is virtually impossible to gain access to any further storage space.

Mothers treated with fluoxetine have responded well and recovered.

Obsessive compulsive disorder should not be confused with obsessive-compulsive personality disorder (OCPD). The diagnosis of OCPD, as described in the *Diagnostic and Statistical Manual of Mental Disorders* (American Psychiatric Association, 2000) is given to a woman who has:

> *A pervasive pattern of preoccupation with orderliness, perfectionism, and mental and interpersonal control, at the expense of flexibility, openness, and efficiency, beginning by early adulthood.*

She strives for perfection, has an excessive devotion to her infant, home and family and is rigid in her behaviour and thinking. Relatively few women with OCD also meet criteria for OCPD, and the converse is also true.

Problems associated with perinatal mental health 5

Sleep

One of the most common problems during the perinatal period is sleep or the lack of it. Women usually suffer from diurnal variation, where they spend most of the night awake and although tired, are unable to sleep during the day. What sleep they have is fitful, perhaps waking every hour or falling asleep for a few moments, but they find that when they finally awake in the morning they do not feel refreshed and are unfulfilled. Some would describe it as similar to feeling woozy or drunk when they are not in complete control of their actions. Studies have highlighted the failure of sleep-deprived subjects to perform basic tasks at the same level as those who are well-rested. One such study demonstrated that the temporal lobe in those who were deprived of sleep was not activated, whereas there was more activity in the parietal lobe. It appeared this was to compensate for the shut down in the temporal lobe (Drummond *et al.*, 2000).

Some mothers may present with these symptoms at the general practitioner's surgery and as a result only the symptoms may be addressed and not necessarily the cause. A course of sedatives or minor tranquillisers may be prescribed to help to enhance sleep. However, this therapy merely tackles the immediate problem of impaired sleep and not the overall reasons as to why this disorder occurs. The inability to have a satisfying night's sleep is traumatic enough, but when this is compounded with the feeding and demands of an infant that make it impossible to have a fulfilling sleep, then the effects of sleep deficit are more severe.

In the first few months of life, because of their nutritional needs and immature sleep cycle, infants are unable to distinguish night from day. Studies report that sleep deprivation in the short term may have an adverse effect on maternal mood and motor functions. Ultimately, the cumulative effects of long-term patterns of interrupted sleep, as experienced by new mothers, may have a detrimental effect on their mental and physical health (Dement & Vaughan, 1999; Reimann *et al.*, 2001). It is likely therefore, that if the mother has no respite from this pattern she will suffer from the depressive symptoms commonly associated with sleep deprivation.

Adjusting to the changes in lifestyle and relationships following the birth can create physical and emotional strains on everyone, yet for the mother the added responsibility of being expected to modify and adjust to the demands of a new infant can have untold effects. Most people will be familiar with temporary sleep deprivation, brought about by an all night vigil or festivities, but to have sleep restricted and then to have little or no control on the amount of sleep that is necessary to feel replete must be tantamount to a form of punishment. Indeed, prisoners of torture have described sleep deprivation as having one of the more tenacious effects on the body and soul.

One of the most dominant and well documented facts, which is probably a universal experience for all new mothers, is the lack of a decent night's sleep. Babies normally need around 15–18 hours sleep a day but the immaturity and size of their stomachs also means that they have to feed every four to six hours. A feed at eight o'clock has to be repeated at twelve, four and eight. A mother who may already be exhausted by the day's events has also to adapt to the prospect of waking at least twice during the night. Hunger is not the only factor, as the room temperature, amount of light entering the room and level of noise or disturbance may also be of importance. Mothers are usually resigned to the fact that their sleep pattern will be sacrificed but it is only when the lack of sleep lasts for protracted periods that it becomes impossible for them to function as they did prior to the birth.

It is probable that this short-term sleep deprivation will have an adverse effect on the mother's mood, cognitive and motor functions (Dement & Vaughan, 1999). However, the effect of frequently disturbed sleep on mood is even more profound (Riemann *et al.*, 2001), and it is possible that the cumulative effect of sleep deprivation will have some impact on her mental as well as physical capabilities. Whether the lack of sleep during the postnatal period is a significant prelude or a cause of poor perinatal mental health is debateable. Research is continuing to emerge which sheds light on the risks of sleep deprivation.

At least 80% of depressed people experience insomnia, which is characterised by having difficulty falling asleep and/or staying asleep. Early morning awakening is one of the most positive symptoms of depression. In a critical review by Ross *et al.* (2005) both the quality and quantity of sleep were implicated as a causal factor in post-partum depression and it was found that maternal sleep changes in the post-partum period related to mental health outcomes.

Hildebrandt *et al.* (2007) reported that mothers whose infants developed a pattern for waking frequently and for prolonged periods throughout the night had a greater risk of having depressive symptoms. Some research has outlined how an improvement in the infant's sleep pattern has significantly decreased the mother's symptoms. However, there is limited research which concentrates on the effects of infant's improved sleeping habits on maternal mood.

It would appear that sleep deprivation has a significant effect on the deterioration of mood state and general well-being. Mothers who have been deprived of sleep are generally very tired, less happy and less sociable than those who are well rested and it is possible that they can become increasingly irritable. This also has implications for personal relationships, not necessarily for her infant, as the mother probably cannot blame them for what is usually regarded as normal phenomena, but for the partner, who may refuse to get up in the night to assist with the feeds or even take over the care of the infant. The mother may resent the lack of commitment in what she may see as a role that should be shared. Yet it is well established that the level of support a mother receives, particularly from her partner, can affect the amount of restful sleep she has.

Once again, the disintegration of the role of the extended family has not helped the situation. Previously it would have been acceptable for families, the second generation in particular, to have the space and energy to accommodate the infant at night to allow the mother some respite. She would be confident that the child was being well cared for and with this assurance would be able to benefit from a sound night's sleep. As grandmothers are often working it is not feasible to offer the support the mother so often needs, but there is the added factor that the mother may, because of pressure exerted on her to care for her own child, feel that she is unable to ask for help and will struggle on alone. The lack of family support networks and the effort the mother feels she must make only exacerbate and compound the situation, making it more difficult for her to extract herself from the enormity of the situation (Thomas *et al.*, 2000).

Findings by Skouteris *et al.* (2008) revealed that the poor quality of a mother's sleep earlier in pregnancy predicted higher levels of depressive symptoms at later stages in pregnancy. However, there was no evidence to suggest that depressive symptoms earlier in pregnancy impacted on sleep quality later on. The study concluded that there was merit in enquiring about any evidence of a problem with sleeping during the pregnancy.

One of the criteria for sleep disturbance to be classified as a sleep disorder is that it has to last longer than a month (American Psychiatric Association, 1994). In many instances mothers with infants will meet this condition. There are also similarities with this type of sleep pattern and the criteria for Circadian Rhythm Sleep Disorder (American Psychiatric Association, 1994), where the essential factor is a recurring pattern of sleep disturbance which is caused by external factors that affect the timing and duration of sleep. The diagnosis of this disorder concentrates on daytime sleepiness and the resulting functional impairment or significant distressed mood (American Psychiatric Association, 1994). This broad criteria can be open to interpretation, but the evidence suggests that mothers in the postnatal period often experience impaired functional ability, episodes of fatigue accompanied by low mood, which in some cases are linked to sleep deficiency (Dennis & Ross, 2005; Swain *et al.*, 1997). It may be argued that some mothers meet the third criterion of daytime dysfunction and distressed mood required for a diagnosis of Circadian Rhythm Sleep Disorder (American Psychiatric Association, 1994), which classifies sleep disorders as severe enough to constitute a mental health problem, indicating the severity of the potential risk which sleep deprivation has on maternal mental health.

The fact that there is a paucity of knowledge surrounding sleep deprivation as a contributing factor to poor perinatal mental health is probably because it has not been given sufficient credence by health professionals and families alike. It is anticipated that sleep patterns will be affected when the infant is very young, but although there is some understanding of the effects of sleep deprivation in its purest terms, little is known about fragmented and fitful sleep patterns and why diurnal variation should be a problem.

Sleep deprivation and insomnia

Sleep is a restorative process which relies on two types of eye movement. One of these induces the process of deep sleep: 'non-rapid eye movement' (NREM). This helps to repair and renovate of the body. There is also the lighter type of sleep, 'rapid eye movement' (REM), which serves to repair and restore cerebral function. Although the amount of sleep required for individuals varies, the normal recommended amount of sleep is on average eight hours a night. Although there is no definitive evidence about the consequences of sleep deprivation many studies have determined that if the individual's requirement for sleep is not fulfilled then there may be impaired functioning in the daytime, coupled with deterioration in mood.

Normal sleep has a well-defined architecture. Four or five times during the night there is a cycle of deepening, relaxing sleep, marked by slow waves of energy; this is followed by dream sleep which is marked by dramatic brain activity and rapid eye movements. It has been noted that depressed mothers will often lapse very quickly into REM sleep, which induces an almost immediate dream-state, which Perlis *et al.* (2005) describe as unusual in both the duration and intensity. It is further commented that this form of sleep pattern is abnormal and the way in which the depressed dream and the function of dreaming is undermined.

One of the functions of sleep is to consolidate memory and REM sleep is involved with emotional memory. This intense activation of REM sleep may invoke negative memories which are not allowed to dissipate over time and are continually repeated as the dream sequence occurs. Disordered REM sleep is usually a sound indication of depression.

The majority of research focuses on male subjects and there is no substantiating evidence that this may be applied to females. Some sleep disorders are linked to the hormonal changes experienced during menstruation or the dramatic changes which occur during pregnancy, childbirth and the postnatal period.

Swain *et al.* (1997) suggested that mothers have to make important adjustments in their sleep pattern if they are not to succumb to negative mood states. However, it is usually around the time when her infant is weaned that mothers tend to experience less interrupted sleep (Nishihara *et al.*, 2002).

Recent evidence has suggested that many mothers only averaged a total of four to six hour's sleep a night for the first three months of motherhood. This was fragmented and fitful because of the demands of the infant (St James-Roberts *et al.*, 2001). How bedtime is managed in the early days is of prime importance and the knowledge that there is a definitive time when broken nights will cease is often sufficient to allow the mother time to accept the situation. However, there are exceptions to the rule and infants waking during the night when they have been weaned onto solids is also common.

One solution to the problem is to focus on a sleep behavioural programme, which will enable both the mother and the infant to have more rest, if not more sleep. There is still little scientific evidence to suggest that an improvement in the infant's sleeping pattern improves the mother's well-being but Hiscock & Wake's (2002) use of a community based sleep intervention programme, which concentrated on teaching a controlled crying method, was shown to decrease the infant's sleep problems and the symptoms of depressed mothers.

This behavioural programme was designed to manage the way in which the parents responded to their infant's crying pattern (Hiscock & Wake, 2002). The idea was to increase the time intervals between attending to the infant. At the same time they were given information about normal and abnormal sleeping patterns and mothers were asked to maintain a diary recording the infant's sleep. The study concluded that by aiming to control the infant's crying they reduced infant sleep disorders. This opportunity to have increased periods of respite appeared to benefit the mothers and in particular those who were most seriously depressed.

Similar programmes have achieved positive results but when mothers were questioned in more depth they admitted that they were not truthful about the outcomes. They regarded the failure of their infants to conform to a sleeping schedule as a failure in themselves. There was no doubt they benefited from the interest that the interventions generated, but rather than admit defeat the mothers chose to say what they believed the researchers wanted to hear.

There are also the personal and cultural factors to be considered when thinking about an infant's sleep and determining any form of intervention. There is the belief that it is wrong to pick up a child who is constantly crying and that if left unattended they will eventually cry themselves to sleep. Presumably it is only if this is successful in the first instance that the 'leaving alone' system can be repeated. Even then there is little guarantee that the infant will cease crying every time he/she is ignored.

In some instances this may be impractical as it may disturb others in the household or neighbouring houses. Judgements will be made against the mother, as often crying infants and screaming toddlers are viewed as a child rebelling against pitiable parenting. The intensity of the cries might make it impossible to ignore and not being allowed to comfort their infant often causes mothers further anxiety and distress. For the mother who is depressed this may further confirm her poor parenting skills and the fact that her infant will cry despite her best efforts.

If the infant is left to cry for too long a period there are also impractical repercussions. Infants may become so distressed they are unable to be soothed quickly. They can become fretful, breathless, perspire and their skin becomes florid. Sometimes the distress caused will ensure the mother will not let her infant endure that state again.

Newborn infants usually sleep in close proximity to the mother, either in a crib or Moses basket, which reassures both parties that they are safe. The mother, in particular, can be reassured if she can hear her infant's breaths. Some mothers may feel more secure if their infant remains in the bed with her and some reportedly sleep more soundly. However, this has the drawback of the mother suffering from such fatigue she falls into a deep sleep and inadvertently lies on the child and in extreme cases there have been reports of the child being suffocated.

If the practice has been bed sharing then a gradual process of moving the infant from the bed to the crib is suggested. The time during which the parents are present while the infant is falling asleep is also reduced until the infant is able to go to sleep independently of the parents' company. Other methods include adjusting the infant's sleep pattern by regulating the time they are put in their cot and attempting to keep the infant awake during some part of the day. There is no recorded evidence to suggest that behavioural interventions per se are harmful and if the intervention includes health professionals who show concern and have an interest in the welfare of the mother and infant, this in itself must be therapeutic.

It has been suggested that the interpretation of sleep intervention programmes is complex, with multiple variables that requires careful consideration. Strategies used for newborn babies and infants may not be applicable for the older child. The success of the programme will depend on the mother's ability and motivation to pursue it and in the case of a depressed mother this may not always be as relevant.

Appetite

The mother that believed that any excess weight she gained during the pregnancy would be shed in the postnatal period may find it even more difficult to lose weight. Often her appetite is impaired, with episodes of overeating to compensate for her feelings of sadness and distress. More common is eating the minimal amount of food, which may ultimately result in serious anorexia. The lack of a substantial diet can lead to feelings of listlessness and fatigue, though it may also be argued that the mother's mood state controls the appetite (Cox *et al.*, 1987) and she may only desire simple sweet foods or indeed no foods at all. Another commonly experienced situation is that the appetite may be threatened because the infant's demands often coincide with the mother's own routine. The mother will usually forfeit her own nutritional needs at mealtimes and depend on eating on an ad hoc basis (Charles, 1993).

Libido

The self-limiting nature of pregnancy and the hormonal changes that occur often have a disruptive impact on the sexual desires of the partner. Sometimes, however, there can be a mismatch of communication and for some couples the woman's complete preoccupation with the pregnancy or the loss of the woman's desire to sustain the intimacy of the relationship may be misinterpreted as an alienation of the relationship.

As the pregnancy progresses, the woman whose feminine security and self-esteem hinges on a waif like figure becomes increasingly concerned over the distortion of her body image and is more needful of reassurance and in particular sexual reassurance. The lonely and dejected woman who feels that her recalcitrant partner can be erotically recaptured is often further dejected when she is unable to resolve her problems. Some women may exploit the emotional sensitivity of their pregnancy by responding to any sexual provocation with tears and distress whilst in other circumstances she may be overtly sensual. Paradoxically, the woman's urge for a loving, assuring relationship to stabilise the emotions she obviously craves, in some instances, makes it almost impossible for the relationship to survive the intensity of her demands.

For some mothers though there is the genuine feeling that their partners were un-concerned about their well-being:

> *I'm tired all the time, but he does not seem to understand. He will not put the kids to bed or do any little jobs around the house. What he is good at is complaining – the house isn't tidy enough, I haven't got his food ready, I spend too much time visiting*

friends. What he doesn't realise is that I can't stand being at home all day with just the kids and me – it drives me insane.

One woman's depression was precipitated by her partner's affair:

When I found out about the affair I was devastated. We decided to stay together for the sake of the children, but then I got pregnant, and a friend told me he was still seeing her. We haven't been right since. I don't feel that I can trust him anymore.

Conversely, some sexual urges are not affected at all and one study found that because intimacy made depressed mothers feel better, they actively initiated and participated in sexual relations. There is little evidence throughout the literature to help understand this enigma but earlier works by Kleinke *et al.* (1982), Neziek (1995) and Smith (1999), go some way to explain how women construct their sexuality to cope with their own distress. It is suggested this might be the subject of further research.

There are obvious external physical changes that occur in pregnancy, which continue to increase in size as the pregnancy advances and remain until the termination of the pregnancy. There are changes in the contours of the abdomen and the breasts, and the bulk and height of the fundus often make it difficult for the mother to find a sufficiently comfortable posture to be able to relax, let alone be able to indulge in sexual practices.

Approximately two-thirds of women experience nausea or vomiting (hyperemesis) during the first trimester of pregnancy. Hook (1978) and Profet (1995) have suggested that morning sickness serves as an adaptive and prophylactic function. It protects the embryo by causing the women to physically expel and subsequently avoid foods that contain teratogenic and abortifacient chemicals. These may be found in alcohol, caffeine and vegetables with a strong taste. Ptyalism is often confused with hyperemesis and commences soon after the onset of pregnancy and persists until the end. It is characterised by a copious increase in the production of saliva that can exceed one litre per day. There appears to be no change in the chemical constitution and it is of undetermined aetiology. When an attempt is made to swallow the secretions it is often regurgitated and it is often followed by frequent episodes of nausea and vomiting. Sexual malaise often accompanies the condition. Nevertheless, this debilitating, albeit natural, complaint may have an impact on the sexual desires of the partner, too, as he struggles with the perpetual morning or evening ritual at a time when he may feel at his most amorous.

The onset of a bleed may occur at any time during the pregnancy but is most prevalent during the first and third trimester. Often bleeding in the first trimester is frequently followed by a spontaneous abortion, while in the third trimester there is the risk of bleeding because of placenta praevia or abruption of the placenta. All of these cases are viewed as obstetric emergencies and either require complete rest or hospitalisation. In all cases, sexual activity is often discouraged and if possible avoided to prevent further complications.

There are several physical changes in the third trimester which make expressions of sexuality more difficult. Often orgasms may cause painful, prolonged uterine contractions. In preparation for labour and in response to the hormone relaxin, the supporting ligaments of the bony pelvis and symphysis pubis slacken. When this occurs there is severe pain on pelvic motion, which makes any locomotor or sexual activity very uncomfortable.

These changes to sexual intimacies may occur in a normal pregnancy that was planned and where conception occurred quickly. The more arduous the processes of getting pregnant the more sexual difficulties seem to be encountered. Studies have recorded the difficulties infertility causes as the male feels bound to conform to the successive masturbatory demands for him to produce sperm samples (Read, 1999). The couple's sexual life becomes prescriptive, with ritualistic sexual activities designed for the positive outcome of a pregnancy. Should conception prove successful, but the foetus is aborted, the resulting frustration and despair may cause the woman to blame the man for his reproductive ineptitude. This recrimination or disaffection may to some degree disrupt the normal affiliate sexual relationship, which may take the form of punitive abstention or the male partner may contentiously desensualise sex by dispensing with the usual comforts and foreplay and the woman may respond accordingly.

The women who experience multiple pregnancies and births may also regard the sexual act as something that becomes an anticipatory dread rather than a participatory pleasure. If sterilisation is indicated, with no opportunity for future pregnancies, there have been reports of mothers feeling emancipated and viewing their partners in a more positive light. However, many feel there is no change in their sexual responsiveness and some complain of an even greater degree of decreased libido.

The personality and predisposition of the woman and her partner, the desire for the pregnancy, financial circumstances, family sizes, material and non-material aspirations and unforeseen situations may impose sexually cordant or discordant patterns on the pregnancy. When the pregnancy is mutually desired and there are no medical complications sexuality is usually unaffected.

In one study the majority of women felt they had a good relationship with their partners, but not all. For those mothers fortunate enough to enjoy a sound relationship with their partner, the comments were: '*Wonderful, I don't know what I would have done without him. He is so patient he allows me to be me.*' Another felt her partner, although he had his own problems, was willing to tolerate hers:

I try so hard to disguise how I feel but somehow he seems to understand. He has never complained about the way I behave. He takes care of our son and will get up with him in the night, even though he is tired himself.

Some of them could not understand why their partners should be so tolerant and when reasons were sought were told: '*It's because I love you.*'

There is little guarantee that the climax of the pregnancy, which results in a healthy infant, will be either a festive end or an auspicious beginning for the couple's sexual relationship.

Some mothers often neglected to talk to their partners in the way they had before the baby was born and often it was only following therapy sessions that they learnt to trust their partner with their more intimate feelings:

It's funny, but we have learnt to talk again about what and how we feel about each other. I think I was so wrapped up in the baby, I forgot about how he must feel.

I just assumed he was getting on with it, I didn't realise he was really worried about me. Men don't show their feelings so much, do they?

Management of sexual issues

As depression has a debilitating effect on all of the body's systems it is not unusual to find that libido is similarly affected. The diminished activity in the brain tends to be associated with lack of interest in sex and difficulty in reaching orgasm.

Highlighting the commonality of the symptoms and the effect they have on relationships can be useful, particularly if the mother becomes withdrawn, does not pursue her normal routine and does not appreciate when her partner is attentive, which can lead to frustration for him.

As in the case of the depressive illness, there are often times when the loss of libido is not limited and there may be occasions when the mother feels aroused. The difficulty is this may not occur at mutual times with her partner. Often penetrative sex is unwelcome but cuddling or hugging may help to affirm that she is still loved. Often sexual expression is not as important to the father as it is to the mother.

Exercise can be therapeutic and just taking a walk will release endorphins, which are known to elevate the mood. This feeling may stimulate the mother to feel more receptive to suggestions of sexual activity.

Antidepressant medication has been found to interfere with sexual functions. It has been reported that between 30% and 60% of the women who took the antidepressants Prozac or Zoloft experienced some degree of sexual dysfunction. For some women lubrication is also diminished. The commonest side effect is the interference with the process of orgasm; this is sometimes delayed or does not occur at all. An option is to add the drug, amantadine, which may help to counteract orgasmic failure induced by the antidepressant.

There is the option of altering the medication to one which is known to have fewer sexual side effects and these include Wellbutrin, Serzone (nefazodone), Remeron (mirtazapine) or Zyban (bupropion). However, a different medication may not necessarily alleviate the depression. A reduction in the dosage may help, but will also reduce the therapeutic benefit. The older antidepressant tricyclic drugs that include Elavil or imipramine, or one of the MAO inhibitors, like Nardil or Parnate may be useful in reducing the amount of sexual dysfunction, but there is the risk of further debilitating side effects with this type of medication. Some women can be successfully treated for sexual dysfunction with small doses of testosterone, which increases libido and arousal. There have been reports of a decrease in sexual side effects by taking the herbal remedy ginkgo biloba.

A recent approach is to take the medication throughout the week and discontinue it during the weekends. This enables sexual function to improve or return temporarily, though this should not be attempted without medical supervision.

When offered the choice, most mothers would prefer to have the benefit of short-term antidepressant medication and forgo sexual relations. Once the medication is discontinued the libido gradually returns, but it is often with this knowledge that the mother may decide to stop taking the antidepressants and that may precipitate a relapse to the depressive symptoms.

Discouraging the partner from being paternalistic or patronising the mother will help. It is possible he may understand how she feels but it is unlikely he will understand completely. To put the condition into perspective it is compared with having sexual relations after the mother has had major heart or abdominal surgery. It is important that the partner does not become consumed by the depression too, and securing and continuing a social life is equally important.

Huang & Mathers (2006) found that there was a strong association between a poor relationship with the mother and her partner and the incidence of her suffering from postnatal depression, and those mothers with sexual worries after birth were more likely to have the symptoms of postnatal depression. The loss of libido is a salient point. Pitt (1993) suggests that it is the first emotion to disappear at the beginning of depression but it is also the first emotion to return as the mother gets well. Often men may see this lack of interest in them as a threat to their partnership and exacerbate the situation by blaming the overindulgence of the child's needs over theirs. Partners may feel neglected and unhappy with the situation. In the short term they may be prepared to accept it but if the depression is left untreated and allowed to progress, or the severity of the illness is not explained, then the loss of feelings may result in marital disharmony and the subsequent breakdown of relationships. Sometimes mothers try to explain the intricacies of their sex life but often do not understand the reasons themselves.

Following the intervention of therapeutic sessions many women find they are able to reinvent the way they communicate with their partners:

We just talked and talked. I don't feel we have to do that anymore, as now we both understand.

Once I had discussed some of the more intimate aspects of my life with a relative stranger, it was somehow easier to discuss them with my partner.

Sex lives appeared to improve too, something that is not frequently talked about, if at all, but some of the women had to make a conscious effort to partake in sexual activity:

Initially I really did not feel like sex but did it out of duty as I knew that's what my husband wanted, but then as I began to feel better, little by little the old feelings started to return. Eventually it was me who wanted the sex, not him!

I felt nothing at first, I knew that was wrong and I so wanted it to be different, but I just couldn't make anything happen for me. Then I was told to relax, not make it such a big deal, and let it happen naturally. I was on the antidepressants for several weeks before I noticed a difference and then gradually it was fine.

Sexual issues, as well as thoughts about suicide, are often a neglected subject and health professionals will admit that they sometimes feel uncomfortable discussing it with mothers. Some health professionals, with the exception of the general practitioner, may not feel sufficiently qualified to discuss intimate relations. Midwives might be concerned by the chosen form of contraception and this is reiterated by the health visitor during the birth visit. 'Are you using any form of contraception?' is a likely question at the birth visit, not 'How tired do you really feel?' or rather more blatantly 'How is your sex life?' Should the mother admit that she has experienced sexual difficulties, albeit at an early stage following the birth, the question may be posed 'How do you see yourself with this man in ten years time'? Such pertinent questions might open up a constructive dialogue and help form the sentient relationship that is often so necessary.

Society may be very liberal and accept sexual practices with the young, but there is rarely a mention about how sex or the absence of sexual contact affects young mothers. Perhaps the lying-in period, where mothers were kept in bed for ten days following the birth protected mothers from the threat of intercourse, and their reluctance to respond to any sexual advances would have been seen as natural. With this safeguard no longer in place and the neglect of health professionals to address it there is the danger that partnerships which might have relied on the support of the father are suffering as a result.

Peindle (1995) discovered that some women were so traumatised by the events of postnatal depression that it had a significant impact on future family planning. Mothers fearing a recurrence of the illness and the prescribed medication, worried about the effects on the family, but also were concerned about the severity of the episode, manifested by suicide or infanticide attempts.

Studies have found patterns of physical and emotional distress, lack of confidence and dissatisfaction with family support among depressed mothers. Hall *et al.* (1996) studied the role of self-esteem as a mediator of the effects of stressors and social resources on mothers with postnatal depression. The data collected suggested that 42% of women have high depressive symptoms. Self-esteem mediated the effects of everyday stresses and intimate personal relationships. Mothers with low esteem were 39 times more likely to manifest depressive symptoms than those with high self-esteem. This finding suggests that interventions to decrease depressive symptoms and improve the quality of intimate relationships may enhance self-esteem and this may, in turn, decrease depression.

Mothers who have *in vitro* fertilisation

In one study which looked at the medical records of women who had treatment for postnatal depression it was found that 6% of the group had conceived by IVF compared with 1.5% in the general population. The women from the study, however, were more likely to be older, have multiple births and have a Caesarean section, all of which are linked to an increase in the risk for postnatal depression. The researchers speculated that when there was a history of difficulty with fertility, assisted conception may also heighten the risk of postnatal mood disturbance (Fisher *et al.*, 2005).

Self-harm

One of the major factors which causes a mother to self-harm is her depressive condition. The cultural norms, which protect mothers against suicide, may not protect her against self-harm. She is unlikely to die but she may gain some satisfaction or relief from the impact of the pain she inflicts on herself. However, the risk of the repetition of self-harm and later suicide is high. Studies have shown that more than 5% of those who have been hospitalised will commit suicide within ten years. Its occurrence is probably more common than is recognised by most health professionals and it is only when there is a serious attempt to self-harm that this behaviour may gain empathy and some form of understanding. Those who may have intentionally harmed themselves but have survived are often described as 'deliberate self-harmers'.

Self-mutilation is the deliberate, direct destruction or alteration of body tissues without conscious suicidal intent. Self-harm, however, will include drug overdose and gestures of suicide. In one study the patients described feeling numb, empty and devoid of emotion prior to the actual act of self-harm and then during and after it had an overwhelming feeling of relief and satisfaction. In some cases they even felt elated and fascinated by the sight of their own blood. Wiessman (1975) suggested it was a way of combating their feelings of unreality and emptiness. This compares with the mother who attempts suicide in an effort to end her life and in turn all the emotions that make her feel the way she does. Self-mutilation is an instant solution to take away the negative emotions and replace them with feelings of elation. There is always the danger that the mother may be unable to manage the control she has over the way she inflicts the hurt and often there is a high risk of unintentional suicide.

There are varying degrees of self-harm, which range from the superficial to more severe. Superficial self-harm is probably the more prevalent in the population and includes pulling out tufts of hair, severe nail biting, picking at the skin, causing a sore and then picking at the sore, or scratching the skin until it bleeds. Often the mother is unaware of what she is doing and it tends to be associated with unconscious intent. The more severe form of self-mutilation may involve using tools such as knives or needles to carve, bore or stick into limbs or digits or using matches or cigarette lighters to burn into the skin (Tantam & Whittaker, 1992).

Some people are unable to explain why they self-harm or may offer some idiosyncratic reason for their behaviour. In the more severe cases this may depend on their religious beliefs and/or be influenced by the need to offer spiritual atonement, purification or respond to iniquitous demonic commands. There may be sexual connotations where a woman may feel embarrassed or uncomfortable with her female body and the paradox of becoming pregnant may have momentous significance as it confirms her status as a woman.

Research had suggested that people who self-harm often have a history of childhood sexual abuse and the earlier the age when the abuse occurred the more likely it was there would be cutting behaviour. However, Klonsky & Moyer (2008) found that this did not explain the variance in the behaviour and compared with other risk factors the relationship was minimal.

It was accepted that childhood sexual abuse might be a proxy risk factor for the behaviour and might be a causation factor for the feelings of anxiety, depression and low self-esteem.

One of the important considerations in managing the condition is to determine why the mother intended to harm herself and what her beliefs were about the methods she would employ to carry it out. It is more likely that the mother with superficial self-harm will present in primary care, as those with the more severe types will probably have been recognised and treated previously. Often scars and open sores are only visible during the summer months when the mother may have no alternative but to wear short sleeves and light clothing. It may be difficult not to make reference to them and enquire why they are there, but then the health professional has to deal with the reasons they hear. It may be difficult for the health professional to understand and make sense of the condition as they may initially view it with disgust or see it as attention seeking in its more bizarre form. Understanding the aetiology of the condition and recognising the structured pathways for dealing with the condition may lessen the difficulties and complications of discussing self-harm with the mother.

Earlier treatments suggested that the use of high doses of selective serotonin reuptake inhibitors was an effective way of treating self-harm by cutting. It is, however, becoming more obvious that these drugs have the potential to cause suicidal tendencies; they are no longer recommended unless the mother is psychotic or out of control with her behaviour. If there is a need for a pharmacological approach then minor tranquillisers and mood stabilisers are usually the preferred choice. It appears that no single treatment is effective and there is uncertainty about which forms of psychological and physical treatments are the most effective (Hawton *et al.*, 1998).

The NICE guidelines (2005) on the short-term treatments for self-harm recommend that a full assessment of the physical, emotional and social needs is performed by a specialist. There is modest evidence to suggest that the use of a psychodynamic approach has helped to reduce the repetition of self-harm. Therapists who have experience of clients who self-harm are probably the most appropriate to be involved. Clients may be asked to keep a 'thought diary', recording where events which precipitate self-harm occur, the feelings they engender and how they are dealt with. This is particularly important when thinking about issues that initiated anger or hurt. Working through and analysing these emotions helps the therapist to help the client to manage the anger and if necessary transfer it to something which is less tangible. This in turn helps to build up self-esteem and confidence. The accounts of why they deliberately self-harm are important. In a study by Sinclair & Green (2005) on adolescents who self-harmed they discussed the unpredictability and chaos of family life where there was a failure to provide validation of their experiences at the time. They gave specific accounts of sexual abuse or physical violence within the home. There were also more general memories of confusion or feeling unsupported. Sinclair & Green offered the following account to elaborate on what the adolescents felt:

> *I mean we had the slipper and we had the belt and when we did get a smack it was a smack, and occasionally you know I'd be on the brunt of someone losing their rag and I'd get a, I wouldn't call it a beating[e] ... just a good hiding, which I still, I think was too much[e] ... My mum's overdoses get talked about, about the fact that she slit her wrists and she was in [hospital], mine don't get spoken about at all.*
>
> (participant 2, female, aged 20 in 1997)

Family and friends may have been aware of the condition but found that the mother denied it or allayed their suspicion by giving spurious accounts of the cause of the injuries. Often it may have been easier to ignore the symptoms and hope that over time it would resolve itself (Oldershaw *et al.*, 2008). Once it has been recognised as an 'illness' and the process of recovery is initiated then they will need help to come to terms with what it means for both themselves and the mother and infant. There are few studies to establish whether mothers who harm themselves inflict the same harm to their infants.

Suicide

Along with cardiac disease and infections, psychiatric morbidity is the leading cause of maternal death. As the cards stack up against the mother she becomes increasingly burdened, not only with her own feelings, but those of her infant, partner, family and others (Cox, 1986). There is evidence to suggest that even mothers who are receiving treatment either as inpatients or from their general practitioner, have been unable to release themselves from this state. The mother feels her only recourse is to plummet ever downwards until she becomes so overwhelmed by her feelings of unhappiness that she decides her own fate and attempts to extricate herself from it, often permanently (Cox *et al.*, 1987; Kumar & Robson, 1984).

Even seriously depressed mothers who do not self-harm, are said to think about the act of suicide a great deal, and often contemplate it. Thoughts are said to range from dreading facing the day ahead and not wanting to get out of bed; thoughts that the world would be better off without them, to planning in detail the best way to die (Appleby, 1991; Holden, 1991). In the majority of cases it is said to be the thought of their baby, and its dependence on them, that prevents them from carrying out the act (Marzuk *et al.*, 1997; Pitt, 1993,). The exception is in bipolar disorder, where thoughts of suicidal intent may emerge as the pregnancy progresses, as part of the reactivation of the disorder.

The fifth report on the Confidential Enquiries into Maternal Deaths in the United Kingdom (1997–1999), named *Why Mothers Die*, concluded that more new mothers are dying as direct result of psychiatric disorders, with suicide being the leading cause of death. The mothers' deaths were violent. They threw themselves in front of fast moving vehicles, jumped off bridges, hanged themselves or drowned. There are several events recorded in the daily newspapers which confirm the types of deaths mothers choose and there is little sign of them diminishing.

The report is confident that the mothers were not attention seeking or seeking help but were calculating and intentionally took their lives. The psychiatric history of the mothers who committed suicide suggested they were severely depressed or suffering from puerperal psychosis. Fifty cases of reported death were due to a mother's suicide during the first year of her infant's life, making it one in eight deaths. Forty six percent of them were known to the psychiatric services and half had a previous admission to a psychiatric unit following childbirth and of the half in contact with psychiatric services none had any detailed management plan or close surveillance.

Pregnancy itself has been associated with a lower risk of suicide (Marzuk *et al.*, 1997). Studies have found that suicide during pregnancy is very low and that teenagers have a slightly higher risk of committing suicide than older women (Appleby, 1991; and Marzuk *et al.*, 1997). There is overwhelming evidence to suggest that an unplanned pregnancy is a major risk factor for suicide and this was found to be particularly so in teenagers. Deliberate self-harm appears to have a similar prevalence in both pregnant and non-pregnant women.

Suicide may occur during pregnancy, but there is little indication that the pregnancy itself is the main motivation. If has been suggested that conditions that may have an impact on the woman's life may give reason to self-harm during the pregnancy. These may be an unwanted pregnancy which can have a devastating impact on the mother's mental health, particularly if the option to terminate the pregnancy is not viable. Women trying to kill themselves by a drug overdose before or during pregnancy appear to have the need to provoke a miscarriage and this in turn may increase the efforts of the woman.

It would appear that women see their doctor if they are planning a pregnancy and require maintenance therapy, feel depressed during the pregnancy or if they get pregnant when taking antidepressant therapy (Wisner *et al.*, 1999). However, a mother may find it difficult to confide about how she really feels because of the social taboo of not wanting to sustain her life or that of the foetus.

There may be relationship difficulties or her partner may be unaware that he is not the father of the baby. She may feel unprepared for the pregnancy both physically and emotionally and recognise the difference a new infant will make to her lifestyle. She may of course be pregnant very soon after the birth of her last child and may feel unable to cope with another so soon.

A family history of suicide is also an indicator, as there is an increased risk of suicide in mothers whose mothers were suicidal; it appears to run in families and is independent of depression or other mental health disorders. Deliberate self-harm has the same prevalence in pregnant and non-pregnant women and the characteristics have been reviewed.

It has been suggested that talking about the act of suicide may be used as a threat to abandon or manipulate their children. There is evidence of this, and mothers may say that they are going to kill their children if they do not behave or do as they want them to.

Management

The management of mothers is complex and poses the dilemma of whether to discontinue the antipsychotic medication, should she already be pregnant, as this will expose her to a greater risk of suicide. There is evidence to suggest that some antipsychotics, such as clozapine, can reduce the suicidal tendencies of patients with schizophrenia. However, there is limited research on the management.

There is great merit in screening mothers before and after the pregnancy to elicit whether there are any risk factors for suicide and if the mother has harboured any thoughts about harming herself. The Edinburgh Postnatal Depression Scale (Cox *et al.*, 1987) or any recommended screening tool can be applied to help identify the mother's innermost thoughts and open up discussions. This should lead to solutions which would enable her to manage her life more effectively.

Many commentators suggest it is difficult to differentiate the variety of signs and symptoms of postnatal depression from the signs of a classical depression (Cox *et al.*, 1987; Kelly, 1994). However, very few women of childbearing age present with such feelings of unhappiness outside their childbirth experience (Cox *et al.*, 1987.) The insidious way in which symptoms appear and progress, mimics the onset of any type of depression. However, unlike the traumatic events that may trigger a 'normal' depression, it is a 'joyous' event that predisposes the woman towards postnatal depression. However, if the cause of the trauma is a young baby, extrication of the offending child is not only impractical but, in some cases, impossible. Thus it may be perceived that the main difference between classical depression and postnatal depression is the addition of a child and all the responsibilities that this incurs (Cox *et al.*, 1982; Kumar, 1994,). The birth of a baby is a cause for celebration, and should have the opposite effect. This realisation raises the question of why post-partum women become depressed, sometimes so profoundly that they have been known to attempt suicide.

Possible causes of postnatal depression 6

It has been argued that the definitions and treatment of postnatal depression are, to a great extent, in the hands of the medical profession, an area dominated by men, where postnatal depression is usually perceived as an individual illness. The extensive studies made into this condition by the medical profession bear this out. Initially, male psychiatrists, who sought to examine why women became depressed following childbirth, researched postnatal depression. This was perceived as a relatively new phenomenon in women. Indeed, it was men who first brought postnatal depression to the attention of health professionals and then to the public. However, over the past 40 years female researchers have taken on the mantle and also carry out significant research into the cause of postnatal depression, amongst other perinatal mental disorders (Dalton, 1985; Glover, 1992; Henshaw, 2003).

It would appear that there is sufficient evidence to suggest that there is a sound component for social factors, which would predispose mothers to depression in the ante and postnatal period. Epidemiological studies demonstrate that twice as many women suffer depression than do men and that childbearing years are a time of increased risk for the onset of depression in women. Pregnancy, miscarriage, abortion, therapeutic or otherwise, infertility and the post-partum period all challenge a woman's mental health. There is possibly no life event that rivals the neuro-endocrine and psychological changes associated with pregnancy and childbirth. In 1984 Kumar & Robson reached the logical conclusion that the chemical constituents of the human female body play a very large part in determining predisposition to postnatal depression.

In recent years a wide variety of research has been undertaken to establish the causes for postnatal depression other than psychological ones. This may be related to the fact that mothers would rather admit that a chemical imbalance is responsible for their mood state, than a more taboo psychiatric disorder. It also enables mothers to have more control over themselves and their bodies, and dismisses the need for intervention from the psychiatric services.

Oestrogen and progesterone

During pregnancy there is a rise in the levels of plasma, oestrogen and progesterone. There is also a large increase in cortisol and corticotropin releasing hormone (CRH). Once the baby is delivered, all of these levels drop rapidly. Ovarian hormones are known to enter the brain easily and act as external modulators of neural activity. Receptors for ovarian hormones have been found not only in brain areas that control reproductive functions, but also in locations that are involved in the regulation of mood and higher mental functions. Hamilton (1962) and Wieck *et al.* (1991) demonstrated that an overdose of steroid hormones was surprisingly difficult, even in great quantities.

The hypothalamic-pituitary-adrenal axis (HPA)

The hypothalamic-pituitary-adrenal axis (HPA axis) is one of the key systems involved in the human stress response. It is a complex set of interactions between the hypothalamus, pituitary gland and the adrenal glands. This is a major part of the neuro-endocrine system which is responsible for the regulation of the immune and digestive system but primarily controls reactions to stress, for 'flight or fight' and is of particular interest to scientists as it also regulates mood, emotions and sexuality.

The HPA axis is governed by the secretion of corticotropin releasing hormone (CRH) from the hypothalamus. CRH activates the secretion of adrenocorticotropic hormone (ACTH) from the pituitary. ACTH then stimulates the secretion of cortisol from the adrenal glands. The cortisol interacts with the receptors – the corticosteroid receptors throughout the body. The binding of the cortisol to the corticosteroid receptors in the brain inhibits the further secretion of CRH from the hypothalamus and ACTH from the pituitary (Pariante *et al.*, 2004). Several monoamine neurotransmitters regulate the HPA axis. These are dopamine, serotonin, and noradrenaline. In animal experiments it has been found that there are two different types of stress – physical and social. Both these types activate the HPA axis through different pathways.

The function of the HPA axis changes considerably during pregnancy and the postnatal period (Wadha *et al.*, 1996). The hormone of the HPA axis, which is normally released from the hypothalamus into the blood circulation, is produced from the placenta as the pregnancy progresses. Halfway through the pregnancy CRH levels are detectable and continue to rise until the birth, until it is almost one hundred times the normal range. It has also been noted that there was a significant association with the low mood and the concentration of ACTH, six days after the birth of the infant. This suggests that hypothalamic CRH secretion is 'kick started following delivery'.

Kammerer *et al.* (2006) have suggested that the symptoms of antenatal and postnatal depression may be significantly different and those differences in part are linked with the function of the HPA axis. One group, the melancholic-type depression, is more likely to be connected with antenatal depression, where the cortisol levels are raised. The 'atypical' or postnatal depression is affected by the withdrawal of cortisol and is associated with the reduced cortisol levels. This may explain why mothers might experience either mild bipolar depression or post-traumatic stress disorder following the birth. They also argue that mothers may have a genetic predisposition to either melancholic or atypical depression.

It has also been proposed that the rapid fall of oestrogen in the postnatal period can be a contributing factor to postnatal depression (Bloch *et al.*, 2003; Sichel & Driscoll, 2000). Fink *et al.* (1996) state that oestrogen exerts profound effects on mood, mental state and memory by acting on both, 'classical' monoamine and neuropeptide transmitter mechanisms in the brain. The researchers reviewed an example of each type of action and found that low levels of oestrogen in women are associated with premenstrual tension, postnatal depression and post-menopausal depression. Fink's study was the first to demonstrate that oestrogen also stimulates a significant increase in the density of chemicals in areas of the brain concerned with the control of mood, mental state, cognition, emotion and behaviour. These findings explain the efficacy of oestrogen therapy or 5-HT uptake blockers such as fluoxetine (SSRIs). Other research findings demonstrated that the mood of depressed postnatal women receiving oestrogen supplements improved at a significantly faster rate than the control group (Gregoire *et al.*, 1996). It was also noted that there is preliminary evidence that natural oestrodial has a significant effect in the treatment of postnatal depression (Ahokas *et al.*, 2001), and another study suggested that oestrodial in physiological doses may have a mood elevating effect.

Neuro-endocrine data in women predisposed to postnatal manic-depressive illness suggested that the interaction of oestrodial with hypothalmic D2 dopamine receptors might be abnormal. Various effects of female sex steroids on aspects of serotonin function have been described in animals. In healthy women, recent studies suggest that ovarian hormones influence serotoneurogenic function in a way that is consistent with an antidepressant action.

Progesterone and some of its metabolites have a powerful effect and may be responsible for some symptoms associated with mood disorders such as changes in sleep, alertness, concentration or anxiety. The development of increased sensitivity of hypothalamic dopamine D2 receptors in the post-partum period appears to predict the onset of depressive and anxiety disorders. Harris *et al.* (1994) found that mothers who suffered from minor depression had a greater drop in progesterone, but other studies failed to find any difference between mothers who were depressed, and those who were not (Bloch *et al.*, 2003). Although progesterone has been advocated as a useful treatment in postnatal depression, as yet this has not been rigorously tested.

It has been suggested by Bloch *et al.* (2003) that women who are vulnerable have a different sensitivity to the increase and, or decrease in the hormones rather than the different levels of hormones themselves. Cortisol levels rise considerably during the pregnancy and reach their maximum levels during delivery. The levels drop gradually over time, usually over weeks. It has been suggested that these raised levels predispose a mother to feelings of anxiety during the pregnancy and the withdrawal of cortisol once the infant is born causes the mother to feel depressed.

Electrolytes

Work was done to attempt to identify if there were any biological changes in puerperal disorders. These studies concentrated on changes in blood plasma and urine. Some of the studies indicated that changes in mood might correlate with changes in blood sodium concentration, but not with urinary vasopressin output. Reid *et al.* (1977) recorded many cases of thirst abatement, coinciding with depressive symptoms, on days three and four post-partum. They felt this might coincide with a reduction in renin secretion. In a further study, Stein *et al.* (1984) demonstrated that a peak period for mild change in the puerperium occurred between the second and seventh days post-partum. This also correlated with a significant weight loss and increase in thirst, as well as a rise in urinary sodium excretion. However, the peak mood change did not correlate with any change in vasopressin concentration.

It was suggested that increased plasma calcium is important in determining the onset of puerperal mental disorders in women who have no genetic background of mental illness. Raised levels of calcium plasma have been noted in relation to mood change.

Vitamins

It was postulated that vitamin B6 was responsible for mood changes in the premenstrual period. Livingstone *et al.* (1978) in their studies found no evidence for vitamin B6 (pyridoxine) deficiency in women suffering from post-partum depression. Some success has been claimed in alleviating puerperal depression with pyridoxine administration. Mothers were treated with a daily administration of 100 mg of pyridoxine, for 30 days post-partum, which was found to cause a statistically significant decrease in depressive mood scores in women suffering from the 'blues'. Its use in the treatment of premenstrual tension is well documented. Perhaps this is an area that requires more research, but the application of pyridoxine may be too simplistic a measure to invite investigation.

Thyroid

Harris *et al.* (1992) acknowledged that post-partum thyroid dysfunction, usually of mild severity, has been known to occur for the past 50 years, yet it is only in the past 30 years that a link has been established between this dysfunction and auto-immune thyroid antibody status. Following the description, by Hamilton (1977), of a number of such cases and in view of the fact that mood disorder was known to occur in patients with primary thyroid disorder, a hypothesis emerged suggesting a link between post-partum auto-immune bipolar and post-partum depression. A weak link was confirmed when a large sample of thyroid antibody positive women was compared with antibody negative women, at several points in the six months post-partum period. An increase in depression (but not major cases of depression) occurred in thyroid antibody positive women, whether or not actual thyroid dysfunction was determined in terms of plasma thyroid hormone levels. Possible explanations were that either rapid fluctuations in plasma thyroid hormones have been missed, or that the depressive symptomatology was a reflection of the general malaise in thyroid positive women. When this hypothesis was tested the negative result suggested that an alternative explanation should be sought for post-partum depression in thyroid antibody women.

Vitamin C

There has been significant research on ascorbic acid (vitamin C) which is essential for normal brain function. A deficiency in ascorbate during pregnancy increases the risk of adverse birth outcomes. However, little has been investigated into the impact of ascorbic acid in pregnant mothers and how this may affect their mood state. Work by Bodnar *et al.* (2006) found that women who had low mood also had low levels of vitamin C. As this was one of the few studies in this area it is worth noting that further research is necessary in order to establish the facts.

Genetics

The way in which a mother manages the changes following childbirth may, to a certain extent, be dictated by her genetic make-up and a history of depression is a strong indicator of a propensity to postnatal depression. The French psychiatrist Jean-Étienne Esquirol (1772–1840) first noted the tendency for puerperal psychosis to run in families (Goldstein, 1987). Several family studies have focused on puerperal psychosis and have consistently demonstrated familial aggregation of bipolar disorder, raising the possibility of one or more recessive genes contributing to susceptibility (Jones & Craddock, 2001).

It is evident that the biological explanations need to be better understood. The mechanisms of resilience and protective prenatal and postnatal environments, coupled with the efficacy of interventions, are worthy of further investigation, which will help to reduce maternal stress.

Feminist views

The feminist movement has been critical of this intrusion of professional knowledge into women's lives. They have drawn attention to the sexist nature of scientific definitions of human nature and in particular scientific definitions of health and illness in women's lives. Since these definitions are based on 'science' it is said they have been projected as women's biological destiny rather than any form of social oppression. Yet many researchers believe that masculine definitions of women's circumstances or experiences, couched in scientific terms, predominate (Orr & Luker, 1985). This hard held view maintains that women, who are acting out overall dissatisfaction with experiences of motherhood, are diagnosed as having a depressive illness.

Anxiety

Anxiety is a powerful force in the coping process; it may be present both as an antecedent factor, in the form of a personality trait, and as a contributory factor, in the form of state of anxiety in response to stress. Kumar & Robson (1984) found the relationship between anxiety traits and emotional distress reduced with the passage of time. Anxiety during pregnancy also appears to be a risk factor for postnatal depression (Heron *et al.*, 2004). It is probable that the high levels of cortisol during the pregnancy stimulate feelings of anxiety and when they decline following the birth it fosters depression. This indicates that anxious women need a longer time to adapt to motherhood than women who are less anxious. The interactive relationship between anxiety trait and emotional well-being is indicated in a study by Ball & All (1987). There is no doubt that personality is a powerful influence upon the way women cope with the demands of motherhood and that anxious mothers are more vulnerable to emotional distress.

Anxiety and class is another indication of the complexity of the situation surrounding the vulnerability to depression (Brown & Harris, 1978.). Anxious women found it difficult to relax and 'feel at home' whilst in the maternity ward. Their anxiety was manifested in physical as well as emotional symptoms. There was no evidence to suggest that anxious mothers received less efficient care than other mothers in the same ward, but their natural anxiety did not enable them to cope with the unfamiliar ward environment. Anxious people find it difficult to relax, take in information and learn new skills. It is unrealistic, therefore, to expect anxious mothers to learn how to care for their new babies, and cope with carrying out that care, as rapidly as less anxious mothers. These mothers need more time to become confident and may need to have the same information constantly repeated before they can fully absorb it. Anxious people become more anxious when they feel that they are not conforming to other people's expectations.

It may be argued that the symptoms are very distressing, but, as women have successfully reared babies for generations, the question raised is whether postnatal depression is a cultural phenomenon of modern times. Are today's women different in any way from their forebears?

Risk factors

The childbearing years are a time of increased risk for the onset of depression in women. Pregnancy, miscarriage, abortion, therapeutic or otherwise, infertility and the post-partum period all challenge a woman's mental health. There is possibly no life event that rivals the neuro-endocrine and psychological changes associated with pregnancy and childbirth.

Epidemiological studies and meta-analyses conclude that no one particular factor is responsible for causing perinatal mental health disorders but it is becoming increasingly clear in recent studies that depressed mood or anxiety during pregnancy are the strongest factors. Work by Beck (2001), O'Hara & Swain (1996) and Robertson *et al.* (2004) conclude that this depressive episode is by far the most compelling evidence.

Other risk factors include the lack of social support both in the antenatal and postnatal period. This may involve the intimate support received from the father of the baby as well as financial and emotional support. Teenage mothers are particularly vulnerable because of the fragility of their relationships with their partner. This may be based on the superficiality that having a baby is the prime reason for having a baby. Girls have complained of being 'dumped' or deserted when they became pregnant and of the boyfriend terminating all ties and refusing to acknowledge he has any genetic attachment. Popular television shows often encourage fathers to establish the DNA results of an infant to establish whether they are the biological parents. Often the mother will claim to have had postnatal depression following the birth of the infant and will attribute this primarily to the lack of social and emotional support from her partner but also the neglect of his financial duties. This may often be compounded by an estranged boyfriend demanding visiting rights to his child, whether they are negotiable or not.

There are many recorded cases of teenagers' mothers refusing to take any responsibility for their own daughter and her child, or offer them emotional and social support. Often there is a lack of financial support too. The prejudices of 'you made your bed so lie in it' are often applied and it is then the remit of social services to provide the necessary care for the girl and her child. Occasionally there might be the luxury of lodging with relatives, but this is often a temporary measure and the girl may find she has to make provision for herself.

Even in the more wholesome households the support from the woman's own mother is not always as steadfast as it used to be. Now they are encouraged to go out to work and may not be able to provide the practical support they would wish. This may be particularly pertinent at night when mothers are deprived of sleep but are fearful of asking their own mothers to care for the infant to allow them to sleep, as they are aware of the burden they are incurring (Hanley & Long, 2006).

The closeness of friendships may also affect how the mother is feeling. Many mothers in a full-time occupation continue to work into the last two weeks of pregnancy, leaving little time or space to acquaint themselves with their immediate neighbours or friends. Some have complained that they are unfamiliar with the area and do not feel comfortable requesting help from 'strangers'.

Although there are significant numbers of mothers with postnatal depression across all sectors of society, those on lower incomes appear to be at greater risk, with over a third of mothers with postnatal depression living on annual incomes of under £10,000. This is compared with under a quarter of mothers whose annual household income exceeds £50,000. It was suggested that over half of mothers found that financial worries were the main cause of stress (Netmums, 2004). Other figures suggest that one in three working class mothers develop postnatal depression as opposed to one in twelve in the middle classes (Littlewood & McHugh, 1997).

There is a growing body of evidence to suggest that there would be great merit in assessing the emotional well-being of the woman prior to her pregnancy, and to take great heed of the added emotional stresses that may be encountered during and after the pregnancy. Often if there is no supportive social framework, in the words of one woman 'you just have to get on with it'.

An awareness of postnatal depression

Postnatal depression is emerging as one of the 'trendy' illnesses and public acceptability and empathy towards this hitherto much maligned illness has increased greatly. Over the past ten years there has been an increase in the number of newspaper articles, popular women's magazines, television chat shows and radio interviews which have highlighted the plight of women following childbirth.

Emphasis has been placed on the symptoms experienced by depressed mothers and the cause of their condition. Often there is criticism of the care they have received, which mostly focuses around the fact that the recognition was not early enough or the necessary support networks were not offered or accessible to help the mother through this time. Often the mothers will concede that with the help of the GP or another health professional they gradually understood their condition and made a slow but sure recovery. Though some mothers will confess that they are still recovering, others felt they would not be able to recover.

There is little reason why the modern day mother should not have learnt something about postnatal depression from the media, though for most mothers the advent of the condition comes as somewhat of a surprise. Studies confirm that most women still appear to have little knowledge of it, unless they have either suffered from it, or know someone who has had the condition. It would appear that little knowledge is absorbed unless the problem is personally encountered and only then does it become a major issue.

When one woman was asked about her previous knowledge of the condition she said: 'I knew it existed but I can't say I knew much about it.' Another claimed that although she had vaguely remembered someone on the radio discussing it, she was not really aware of the condition and had little knowledge of it: 'No I didn't really think much about it.'

Some may be aware that there is a possibility that they may experience feeling weepy a few days after the birth of the infant, and are able to describe the symptoms of the 'baby blues'. This information is sometimes part of the programme in antenatal classes and designed to warn mothers of any impending or intrusive feelings. It is understandable that pregnant mothers do not retain the information as there are copious amounts of information that need to be learnt about the imminent birth. It is more likely for the woman to take on the practical aspects of her pregnancy, such as a description of the birth itself: is it going to be painful, how long is labour likely to last and what is the correct way to bathe the infant? Matters of mental health may have little relevance and it is unlikely that the woman will want detailed information or want to research into the area to be better informed.

Even for some mothers with experience of a family member suffering there is un-likely to be a great understanding of the condition or motivation to gain a greater understanding. She may have been involved with the childcare or even had to support

LIVERPOOL JOHN MOORES UNIVERSITY
LEARNING SERVICES

someone through their 'black hole' (Hackney & Sherlock, 2006). On one television programme a mother who had experienced severe puerperal psychosis admitted to not having any knowledge about the effects of any perinatal mental health issues.

Some have reflected on their mothers' experiences and recollect that they must have been suffering from depression but could not remember it being discussed in the home:

She was a very quiet woman, cheerless[e] ... She still is. I felt unloved as a child. My mother was very strict with me, always chastising me or being cruel. She used to beat my legs with a stick if I misbehaved, for even the slightest thing. I was the only surviving child of twins. My older sister, on the other hand was spoilt; she could have anything or do anything she wanted. My mother had been pregnant once before and miscarried that child too. I believe my mother never got over the death of her stillborn children and in some way blamed me, I always seemed to have the brunt of her anger.

It is probably those mothers who have a history of a mental disorder who are the most informed and aware of the implications and devastation the condition can cause. It is most likely that the majority of the women feel that postnatal depression or a perinatal mental disorder is something that happens to others, but would probably admit that it neither alarmed nor interested them.

Studies have shown that women have little, or in some cases poor, prior knowledge of what postnatal depression, in particular, entails. It was only if they or someone close to them had experienced it that they were aware of it. Knowledge of the 'baby blues', however, seemed far more widespread. This raises the question of whether mothers are really prepared for any mental health issues which may occur. There is no doubt mothers have access to exceptional physical care from the maternal services but often the fact that postnatal depression is not detected by a health professional in the postnatal period is testimony to the lack of the awareness of the condition by the mother herself.

Self-awareness of health status

Several studies have indicated that women who have suffered from premenstrual tension may be prone to postnatal depression (Garcia-Esteve *et al.*, 2008; Sugawara *et al.*, 1997). One mother recorded her history of premenstrual tension from onset of her first menses at the age of 12 years. Six years later she became depressed with anxiety overlay; she felt the feelings of anxiety were more debilitating than the depression itself. She felt irritable, sensitive and cried most of the time for at least one week a month prior to her menses:

I always feel I am not doing the right thing with my baby, I am always questioning what I am doing. I let my mother take over because I can't seem to do it right, she always stops the baby crying and I never can.

Was there any correlation between the way she felt having premenstrual tension and being postnatally depressed?

The feelings are similar sometimes, but no, not really. I feel differently now. It is not as if I know these feelings will go away after a week. I'm sensitive, but I wouldn't say I was irritable, at least not with everyone. I feel as if I don't care, and that no one really understands how I feel anyway – not like PMT when everyone seems to have it – even my best friend. You are on your own with this.

'*I have always been sensitive,*' recorded one mother of two children. 'My mother said I have got my bladder next to my eyeballs!'

She was depressed after the birth of the first child. The second bout of depression following the birth of her second child did not come as a shock but it was frustrating nevertheless: '*Yes I suffered from PMT for as long as I can remember, but it has not been so bad since the kids are born, but then I don't know which is the worse when it happens!*' Some mothers assume that all women suffer from premenstrual tension at any one time and that it was part of the normal pattern of life.

Premenstrual tension

Premenstrual mood change or premenstrual tension (PMT) and its relevance to maternal mental health have been discussed. Research by Sugawara *et al.* (1997) investigated the relationship between premenstrual tension and postnatal depression. Women who had PMT before their pregnancy showed significantly higher levels of depression than those who did not suffer from PMT. In addition, the research showed that women with PMT had greater anxiety about pregnancy and delivery, were more reluctant to accept maternal roles and were more likely to feel their babies were vulnerable, suggesting that PMT is correlated with unstable mental health throughout the perinatal period.

Substance misuse

There has been an increase in substance misuse over the past decade but there is no conclusive evidence that the taking of illicit substances is linked to postnatal depression. There can, however, be serious physical consequences for the mother, the foetus, her offspring and the family. Anecdotal evidence suggests that some mothers who have a history of drug misuse may also present with high EPDS scores (Appendix 2). One woman admitted to regular use of the drug ecstasy. She commenced the habit at the age of twelve years. Prior to her pregnancy she was taking one 'tab' for five consecutive days to get 'high'. She stopped taking the drug whilst she was pregnant but recommenced once the infant was eight weeks old. She described taking the drug to '*help stop feeling depressed*' but within weeks she had the same thoughts and feelings as she did prior to the pregnancy: '*All mixed up in my head, I can't get it together*'.

The increasing culture of substance misuse amongst the younger mothers raises the question whether this may predispose them to anxiety and depression or merely camouflages an existing condition.

Previous abuse as a cause of postnatal depression

Little evidence is available on the incidence of child physical abuse resulting from a mother suffering from depressive symptoms. As the condition has such a high public profile, several mothers have used it in their defence, as a reason for harming their child. There is a little evidence to suggest that mothers who have been physically abused themselves as children tend to suffer depression following childbirth.

There are few studies on the incidence of child sexual abuse in relation to postnatal depression (Buist & Janson, 2001; Raphael, 1994). The reasons for child sexual abuse are complex and evolve over a long period of time. It is possible that a depressed mother may allow the abuse to occur, being too labile to prevent it, but there have been no documented cases of this, for even if her affect is flat, judgment should be relatively unimpaired.

In studies of women who were admitted to a hospital in Melbourne with postnatal depression, Buist & Barnett (1995) hypothesised that a history of childhood abuse predisposes to a more severe prolonged postnatal depression, with increased parenting difficulties and a poor prognosis for the child's development. Mothers who have experienced sexual abuse are more likely to be single, stay in hospital longer, have fewer supports, experience lower self-esteem and increased parenting distress. Women who have experienced sexual abuse as a child may be more likely to have traumatic pregnancy, birthing and postnatal experiences. Extensive interviewing of abuse victims revealed that the experience of childbirth can have lasting negative effects on the mother, especially during her matrescence, the stage when she is becoming a mother. However, there is reasonable doubt in both cases about which is the independent variable and which is the dependent.

In a follow-up study (Buist & Janson, 2001) it was found that the same mothers had a more impaired mother interaction compared with the control group. There was some evidence of a significant difference in the child's cognitive scores and the fathers rated the children as being more disturbed. The mothers also suffered from higher anxiety and depression scores. This appears to be further confirmation of the fact that a history of sexual abuse has potentially long-term effects.

The parallel between rape and birth may be very real: being strapped down and not in control; spoken to impersonally without eye contact; having unwelcome fingers around the vagina; and the sensation of an invasive object pressing against the cervix. An abused woman may not allow the usual vaginal examination or operating room procedures. These powerful feelings may trigger memories of the abuse, memories that had been safely closeted, until that moment of crisis.

Work done with sexual offenders highlights abuse in a very different context. It is only with knowledge of the 'cycle of abuse' that the deviousness of the abuser can be understood. The abuser's ultimate goal is to perform a sexual act with his victim. If he wants the abuse to be more than a single episode he has to be skilful in his manipulation of his victim, giving her the power to control. The act, contrary to being painful, is often pleasurable. Fingers may be welcome and it is not always impersonal. The most damage is sustained when the victim falsely believes the act to have been performed under the label of 'love'. The perpetrator will often remark, '*I do this to you because I love you and you do this to me because you love me*'. Perhaps when researchers get a clearer view of the abuser's methods of targeting and grooming they will have a more passionate and less prejudiced viewpoint.

Post-traumatic stress disorder

Recent research on post-traumatic stress disorder (PTSD) suggests it may occur after a painful childbirth. The variant of this is called a traumatic birth experience (Reynolds, 1997). Whereas most women recover quickly from the event, others appear to have more difficulty. Little research has been done in this area as most of the evidence is based on qualitative research and studies of women seeking elective caesarean sections for psychological reasons. It is postulated that elective caesarean section exemplifies avoidance behaviour which is typical of PTSD, and that health professionals are in a prime position to take a woman's history to establish if she has experienced trauma that could place her at risk for a traumatic birth experience. Providing excellent pain control during childbirth and addressing feelings about the pain and birth postnatally has been seen to help. Work by Czarnocka & Slade (2000) identified the mothers' perceptions of low levels of support from her partner and the maternity staff, having someone to blame when something went wrong and having little control over what happened during labour as being likely predictive symptoms.

All, some, or even one, of the above factors, can contribute to the illness. Perhaps the most important reason given by mothers is a feeling of being 'alone', not having anyone to talk to or most importantly not having anyone to listen to them (Ball & All, 1987).

Recognition and detection of perinatal mental health disorders

7

Use of the Edinburgh Postnatal Depression Scale

One of the key factors in the prevention of postnatal depression and other mental health disorders is the early detection of the condition. In most instances the gradual onset makes it difficult not only for the mother herself, but the family, to recognise the insidious changes in behaviour and mood. Health professionals come into contact with a large number of clients where their emphasis is primarily on the physical and social health of the infant and in previous years there has been significant neglect of the emotional and mental health of the mother. There have been significant inroads into the awareness of the mother who may be susceptible to postnatal depression and other disorders, but rates of detection remain poor as this is an area which continues to cause controversy, and it may be argued that mental health issues have always been the Cinderella of medicine.

Postnatal depression may be recognised in the early stages, by sensitive and careful monitoring. In an effort to address this, the Edinburgh Postnatal Depression Scale (EPDS) was designed by Cox in 1986. This screening tool is currently the most widely recognised means of monitoring mothers in the postnatal period. This is the tool that contains a series of questions designed to examine the mother's mood. It takes the form of a self-administered questionnaire which asks mothers to choose the response which is closest to how she has felt in the last seven days. The ten questions inquire about the mental state of the mother: is she as happy as she always has been; is she able to laugh; has she still retained her sense of humour? Other questions denote her anxiety state, by questioning her behaviour: does she blame herself when things go wrong or can she cope as well now as she did prior to the birth of her child? The responses range from positive to negative answers and the mother completes the form by ticking the appropriate box. Negative answers score higher, the higher the score, the more likely the mother is to be depressed.

There are specific protocols for using the screening tool and it is suggested that it is routinely given to the mother at home, approximately six weeks following delivery. It has not been validated for use in the first week post-partum, and is not used in the hospital (Holden, 1991). In practice the health visitor is usually the first to introduce the scale. Cox (1986) recognised that mothers are capable of masking their symptoms for several months and therefore it is wise to use the EPDS several times over during the period of the first year following childbirth.

Its use is recommended particularly during the second or third month post-partum; therefore it has become normal practice to administer this screening tool at eight weeks, eight months and twelve months post-delivery. The mother must complete all ten questions, and ideally should not discuss her answers with anyone else as this could influence her own answers. Since it is a self-report scale, only the mother completes the form. It may be filled in at the clinic or at home but should always be handed back to the health professional concerned, on completion. The scoring for individual questions ranges from 0–3 according to severity and the total score is calculated by adding the scores for each of the EPDS questions. The EPDS relates to how the woman has been feeling during the previous week and a score of 12 or more indicates that the mother is probably depressed and requires further investigation (Cox, 1986). Mothers who have low scores at eight weeks may present with a higher score at eight months, although in many instances the mother will not admit to any previous feelings of low mood. If there is a high score it is pertinent to retest the score after two weeks, if only because one high score could indicate a temporary low mood. One of the great strengths of the EPDS is that it can be used as a tool to enhance discussion between the health professional and the mother about the overall condition of the mother's well-being. This can foster further discussion to allow mothers to examine their thoughts and actions more fully.

Designed as a screening instrument, the EPDS has been used in wider perspectives and its current use has been extended to include a measurement of the effectiveness of various forms of treatment within the postnatal period (NICE, 2005). The authors of the EPDS have always been very clear that the scale is meant to be used for screening purposes only, and that is was never intended as a diagnostic tool. It was developed from a positivist perspective, which, it is argued, ignored any of the social contexts in which the new mother may find herself. During recent years this lack of scientific rigour has caused significant controversy. The use of the EPDS as a diagnostic instrument has been scrutinised and critics from the National Screening Committee (NSC) (2002) outlawed the tool as not matching any of the criteria essential to diagnose illness. It was accepted that it might be conceptualised as a continuous measure of well-being but is not sufficiently robust to satisfy the concise cut-off required of a diagnostic tool.

As a result the commissioning bodies, which include the Scottish Intercollegiate Guideline Network (SIGN) (2002) and NICE Guidelines (2007), recommend that the EPDS should be used only as part of a postnatal depression screening programme, as the ability to diagnose requires sound professional judgement.

In current practice, specific difficulties were identified where mothers who recorded higher scores were referred for urgent mental health treatments without any consideration about the experiences of the mothers and the uniqueness of their situation. This prompts many critics of the EPDS to view it as more suited to the clinical aspect of the mother's care than her situation.

Other findings of Shakespeare *et al.* (2003) and Cubison & Munro (2005) suggested that mothers often feel compelled to complete the questionnaire because of pressure from health professionals and, as they were aware of the consequences of any negative responses, were prone to distort their answers to give false negatives.

Often when EPDS is given to mothers, few express concern about the outcome of the results. Some women were conscious it had something to do with the way you felt after the baby was born, but did not associate this with clinical symptoms of depression. However, when it is explained that the EPDS monitor is intended to screen for PND, this often raises anxiety and a frequent question is, 'Are you testing me to see if I am mad?' And another, 'If I had filled this in a week ago you would have certified me!' Yet relatively few ask any questions about the diagnosis or the course of postnatal depression.

Following discussion with the mother to confirm that the score on the EPDS was high (greater than 12) or if one particular question rates a high score, this often provokes discussion. It is not unusual to see the mother break into tears of relief as she explains the reasons for her distress:

> *I was frightened to tell anyone, but things have been getting on top of me. I thought it was just lack of sleep and this heavy cold. I thought that after a good night's sleep, it would get better, and I would be able to manage again.*

One mother suggested that her demanding job and the responsibilities of her domestic chores and family, compounded the feelings of tiredness and anxiety: '*I did not think for one moment I was depressed, but now you come to mention it, I believe I am.*' Mothers rarely approach the health visitor to suggest they may be suffering from postnatal depression.

The tool has been further identified as being unreliable when mothers' understanding of the questions are disadvantaged by their language, culture and literacy (Garcia-Esteve *et al.*, 2003; Gaskin & James, 2006; SIGN, 2002; Sobowale, 2003). The EPDS has currently been translated into 28 languages.

In contrast to the elaborate and detailed EPDS the NICE Guidelines have proposed the addition of the Whooley *et al.* (1997) questions (http://www.ncbi.nlm.nih.gov/pubmed/9229283). These are two brief focused questions that address both the mood and interest of the mother. Their strength is that they may be used in either in the ante or postnatal period. The first question is: '*During the last month, have you often been bothered by feeling down, depressed or hopeless?*' The second is: '*During the last month have you often been bothered by having little interest or pleasure in doing things?*' If there is a positive response to both questions then it is recommended that the third question, devised by Arroll *et al.* (2005) is asked: '*Is this something with which you would like help?*' There are three possible responses, which are 'No,' 'Yes, but not today,' or 'Yes' (Sobowale, 2003).

Concern has been voiced about the dismissal of the EPDS in preference to the three-question approach of Whooley *et al.* as there appears scant evidence for the reduction in the number of questions. It is unclear what the evidence base is for the decision, and whether these studies have been validated for use with childbearing women. The evidence for discouraging or abandoning the use of paper and pencil questionnaires is questionable.

Despite all its critics the EPDS has been and remains one of the most widely known screening tools for postnatal depression. The dismissal of the EPDS, which has been formalised, validated, widely used and accepted by practitioners as an opportunity to introduce mothers to an awareness of their emotional health, seems to have thrown some practitioners into confusion. The NSF for Mental Health (Department of Health, 1999) recognises the importance of good maternal mental health and also acknowledges that the EPDS is the most frequently used tool for the detection of postnatal depression. However, it is now clearly reluctant to advocate its use. The EPDS has an important function helping clinicians and practitioners who may be uncomfortable asking mothers about their mental health. It is currently an integral part in the facilitation in the detection of maternal mental health issues. Many practitioners will argue that the role of intuitive knowledge cannot be underestimated and that scientific practice and intuition are not mutually exclusive and both have a role to play in their professional practice (Leviston & Downs, 1999; Rowley & Dixon, 2002).

Until recently, health professionals working with non-English speaking communities had to rely on translations of link workers to translate the EPDS. Attempts to translate it to maximise sensitivity often resulted in a loss of meaning, particularly in those languages where there was no accepted term for depression. The illustrations, in poster form, depict socio-cultural expressions and physical symptoms and are available in Arabic, Bengali, Chinese and Urdu. The material is called '*How are you feeling?*' and has been produced by the Community Practitioner's and Health Visitor's Association (CPHVA). A resource and training pack has been designed to support those delivering training in implementing the information and includes a copy of *Postnatal Depression and Maternal Mental Health in a Multi-cultural Society: Challenges and Solutions.*

The Hospital Anxiety and Depression Scale (HAD)

The Hospital Anxiety and Depression Scale (HAD) was developed by Zigmond & Snaith during the early 1980s (an article on which can be found at http://www.ncbi. nlm.nih.gov/pubmed/6880820 with an updated version at http://www.ncbi.nlm.nih. gov/pubmed/118322521983). This self-assessment scale was found to be a reliable instrument for the detection of anxiety and depressive states in the general population. It has been validated for use in both hospitals and general practice. The HAD scale comprises 14 statements which relate to the experiences of the user over the past week. Seven of the statements explore feelings which would relate to a generalised anxiety state where the mother may feel she is worried (though not unnecessarily) and unable to relax. The other seven questions relate to general feelings about her appearance, ability to concentrate and general feelings of happiness. Negative responses to these questions could indicate a depressive state. The idea is not to think too deeply about the meaning of the questions, but to answer them quickly and honestly.

Each question has four responses and is scored on a scale from 3 to 0. The maximum score is 21 for depression and 21 for anxiety. A score of 8–10 generally means the mother is probably feeling down, and may require some form of intervention to help her feel back to her old self again. Scores of 11 or higher may indicate a mood disorder which requires further investigation. Following further study the HAD scale has now been divided into four ranges. Normal is a score of 0–7, mild is 8–10, moderate is 11–15 and severe is 16–21.

The HAD scale is widely used in the community and hospitals but there is usually a preference for the use of the EPDS, which, although similar, has been validated for use for women during their ante and postnatal periods.

The Patient Health Questionnaire 9

The Patient Health Questionnaire 9 (PHQ 9, http://www.pubmedcentral.nih.gov/articlerender.fcgi?artid=1495268) is based directly on the diagnostic criteria for major depressive disorder in the *Diagnostic and Statistical Manual*, fourth edition (DSM-IV). It has two components, which are to assess the symptoms and functional impairment. These ascertain whether the mother has signs of depression. It gives a baseline score on which the management and treatment may be underpinned. When it is repeated it can help to monitor the progress of the mother following the interventions.

The Patient Health Questionnaire 9 may also be used over the phone by a health professional to determine how a mother may feel, and it is proposed that instead of listing the questions it may be used as an aide-memoire to help the health professional cover all likely aspects of the mother's lifestyle. The question about appetite can generate discussion about the mother's eating habits and patterns. However, if the mother has an eating disorder the question may be ambiguous as they may not see their appetite as being particularly poor and any overeating may be compensated for by vomiting the food at a later time.

The Beck Depression Inventory for Primary Care (BDI-PC)

Aaron Beck was the first to design the scale (in 1961) and it is amongst the longer established self-reporting scales for a depressive condition. In its original form it tested for 21 items and was intended to provide a 'quantitative assessment of the intensity of depression'. It was used to detect, assess and monitor changes in the depressive symptoms of people in mental health care settings. The scale was revised in 1966 and developed to reflect the revisions in the fourth edition text revision of the *Diagnostic and Statistical Manual of Mental Disorders* (DSM-1V-TR).

More recently in 1996, the scale was revised again to the BDI II. The BDI II reflects both components of depression: the cognitive component or mood state, and the somatic component, which may reflect the changes in sleep patterns or appetite. The individual questions assess mood, feelings of pessimism, irritability, self-esteem, guilt and suicidal ideas, sadness, concentration and libido. However, it was considered that the inventory relied too greatly on the physical symptoms and as a result the scores might be inflated because of an undetected physical illness rather than depression. In response to this the Beck Depression Inventory for Primary Care (BDI-PC) was designed. The final version has a shorter form and now consists of seven questions. It is designed for use in the primary care setting. The BDI has been extensively validated for use in general practice. It normally takes a few minutes to complete, but, as with the other self-report scales, is intended to be administered by a health professional.

Limitations of self report scales

As the scales are completed by the mother there remains the problem that she might exaggerate or minimise the scores. For some mothers it might be a double check, out of curiosity to find out how they really are feeling as opposed to how they think they feel. The way in which the form is administered is also important and if the mother feels hurried, under scrutiny or overwhelmed by the questions this may affect the final score. With all the questionnaires, it is important that there is a full and detailed discussion about why the questionnaire is relevant and what will happen if the mother has a high score. The scales are not diagnostic tools but rather a measure of the presenting symptoms. It is recommended that any self-report scale is accompanied by a clinical interview. The most important thing is to reiterate that high scores do not necessarily mean she is a poor mother and to put into perspective that in some cases a significant majority of mothers will also have high scores. This will help her to have the confidence in the scale, the professional and the consequent management.

LIVERPOOL JOHN MOORES UNIVERSITY
AVRIL ROBARTS LRC
TITHEBARN STREET
LIVERPOOL L2 2ER
TEL 0151 231 4022

The effect on the family

In contrast to the plethora of information on the mother's experiences of motherhood and her perinatal mental health there has been comparatively little research which investigates the father's experience of the transition to fatherhood and how this might affect him. Furthermore, unlike mothers, there is little evidence to demonstrate how the rapidly changing cultural perspectives, changing roles and changing attitudes contribute to his experience. In a qualitative study by Draper (2002) the accounts of partners and their transition to fatherhood were explored. It was found they wanted to be included and involved with all aspects of the pregnancy and to feel a part of the bigger picture. This knowledge appeared to prepare them more fully for the advent of fatherhood and the expectations of it.

It is significant that men express concern that the arrival of a child, particularly a male child, will adversely alter their relationship with their partner (Fujita et al., 1991). Some men may feel excluded from family interactions after the birth of a child, and may feel unable to discuss this with their partner in the midst of all the attention focused on the mother and child.

Most men have the ability to deal effectively with the transition to fatherhood. However, it was noted in a study by Buist et al. (2003) that men who have the propensity to be worried by the effect of the pregnancy will continue to have problems with their role as a parent and partner.

In the main, mothers rely strongly on support from their partner rather than from family and health professionals. This is particularly pertinent when they have depressive symptoms. They rely on the stereotypical strong man to help them through their distress; however, if the partner himself becomes distressed this may have a detrimental affect and may even exacerbate her own feelings of depression. It has been estimated by Huang & Warner (2005) that up to 30% of new fathers may suffer from some form of depression, whilst a further study found that more than double the number of men suffered from depression. In the light of the findings it has been suggested that paternal postnatal depression needs to be more accurately identified and the assessment scales to include male depressive symptoms should be developed (Masden & Juhl, 2007).

A consistent association has been found between marital or relationship dysfunction and depression. The interaction of a couple where one partner is depressed shows episodes of greater conflict and tension. There is also a tendency to be negative in the way in which affections are expressed. This creates a potential 'circle of despair' and is usually exacerbated by the subtle gender differences in the conduct of relationships (Gotlib & Hammen, 1996).

In a study by Davey *et al.* (2006) the fathers reported that they were overwhelmed by their partner's postnatal depression. Some complained they felt isolated and frustrated by their inability to deal with and understand the situation. However, their stress levels were significantly reduced and they were able to cope with their partner's depression when they were allowed to share their experiences in a group situation with their peers.

There is a tendency for men to have smaller networks of individuals to whom confidences are disclosed, than do women. Social expectations of male gender often preclude men from feeling able to disclose personal concerns and this means they may experience rejection if they do attempt to admit concerns or weaknesses to others.

Indeed, it may well be that postnatal depression is a particular situation where both male and female partners, out of their own recognition of gender role expectations, feel unable to seek outside help. For mothers, there is concern that their competence in childcare may be in question, whereas men do not want to admit that they are unable to cope. The male gender role places an unrealistic social expectation on men, so that in order to be respected as a 'man' they must always be seen as being able to cope. This will be particularly pertinent when there are expectations to be providers for the vulnerable infant and mother. Most men are aware of this burden placed on them, not only by their own families, but also by the media and outside influences that perpetuate the myth. Since depression itself is purportedly incongruent with the gender role, there is a general feeling that a man cannot be a 'victim'. In the light of such studies, it is not surprising, therefore, that a collusive phenomenon occurs between the couple, to hide or deny the depression.

One study aimed to discover whether a couple-orientated approach to postnatal depression could enhance the recovery rate for mothers. It was Ryan (1995) who identified that when partners lacked a fundamental understanding of postnatal depression, they lost the ability to cope with their partner's distress. It was only when the men were offered support and counselling to explore their own relationship issues that the women showed significant improvement in their own depression (Misri *et al.*, 2000).

Deater-Deckard *et al.* (1998) also found similarities in the patterns and correlates of depression after the birth of a child, for both men and women. This points to the importance of family and partnership in the adjustment of men before and after the birth of a child. Other studies agree that postnatal depression is a significant issue for fathers as well as the mothers.

Gjerdingen & Center (2003) found that both parents experienced significant problems following the birth of the infant. Some fathers had lower energy levels but both the mother and the father experienced lower levels of good health for at least six months post-partum. Additionally, fathers reported an increase in the number of days ill and a decrease in their general health and vitality. Notably, the level of post-partum health was associated with the satisfaction of their partner.

Lovestone & Kumar (1993) found that over half the partners of mothers who had a diagnosed psychiatric illness also suffered from a psychiatric disorder, which typically followed admission of their partners to a mother and baby unit. It was also discovered that other factors prevalent for the fathers were a history of a mental health episode, social problems and, interestingly, a poor relationship with their own fathers.

It has also been found that obstetric risks during pregnancy have some effect on subsequent paternal competence. This is related to male anxiety and depression which the father may have experienced (Ferketich & Mercer, 1995).

Causes of depression in men

Whereas the mother seeks support from the father, equally the father seeks support from the mother. If the mother is herself depressed this adds to the friction within the relationship and this paradox can only lead to further disharmony within the relationship.

The inability of the father to cope with the maternal depression is also a strong factor. The unrealistic expectations of society for fathers, particularly young or inexperienced, to understand or cope with the emotional demands made upon them, not only by their partner but their new infant is understandable and many fathers feel ill equipped to deal with this (Huang & Warner, 2005). This also presupposes that that the relationship was fully functioning prior to the pregnancy and both parties felt supported and prepared for the birth. If the relationship is at all tenuous this may have future repercussions not only for the mother's but the father's mental health.

There is evidence to suggest there may be issues around the pregnancy itself, with some men not wanting the pregnancy in the first place because of the possibility of being not only financially but emotionally burdened (Matthey *et al.*, 2001).

There may be issues with drug and alcohol abuse where where they feel that their original lifestyle is disrupted with the advent of an infant and the incumbent responsibilities (Anderson *et al.*, 2005).

Having both parents depressed brings about further detrimental consequences for the family, as studies have shown that the emotional and behavioural problems in children were associated with an earlier depression in their fathers (Ramchandani *et al.*, 2005).

Nevertheless, the role of the father when mothers are suffering from perinatal mental illness cannot be underestimated. Where parent-infant bonding is an issue, it is found that the interaction of the father is crucial. Some studies have found that fathers can protect infants from the deleterious effects of their mother's condition and infants will respond favourably to their fathers when social communication and responses have been denied by their mothers (Edhborg *et al.*, 2003; Kaplan *et al.*, 2004). Retrospective studies have found that women who had depressed mothers were less likely to develop the depression themselves if they had a sound relationship with their father (Crockenberg & Leerkes, 2003; Lewis & Lamb, 2003).

It is not unusual for the needs of the partner of a depressed mother to be ignored and often the management and treatment are decided upon without referring to the father's views. Fathers often feel marginalised and prefer to avoid any confrontation with health professionals, often because they may feel they are wholly responsible or their presence might exacerbate the situation. They are equally affected by the fragmentation of society and previous family norms where the father was the mainstay and breadwinner. With the increase in divorce rates and separation men, too, have the disadvantage of their own children being brought up without a father in the household. They often do not have a role model to whom they can aspire. Current data shows that women account for the majority of teachers in both primary and secondary schools, further disadvantaging younger men who may require support and guidance on parenting.

There is growing evidence of the importance of planning and implementing future care, incorporating the perspectives of the father. A deeper understanding of the father's role, own needs and perceptions will help to coordinate and collaborate services to support the family as a whole unit.

It is obvious, in the light of research, that where relationship distress exists prior to pregnancy, it is more likely to be compounded and deteriorate even further during the pregnancy, or the birth of a child. It is worrying to know that this a particularly vulnerable time when the woman needs the support and care of her partner. Men appear to confine their confidences to a small, select number of people who will empathise with their difficulties, whilst the women, according to society, should experience few difficulties except those surrounding the birth. Depressed parents often report that high levels of conflict mark their close relationships, or that they perceived their partner to have made excessive demands on them prior to the onset of depression. Research has shown that men fail to understand the emotions expressed by the depressed mother and may view this behaviour as rejection by their partner, which may compound an already fragile situation. This evidence suggests that the quality of any relationship should be assessed as a predictor of potential vulnerability for postnatal depression.

Effect on the child

Bowlby described 'attachment' as the strong emotional link, between two people. He called it an 'affectionate bond'. Most of the close intimate relationships between individuals, throughout the life span, can be thought of in terms of attachment. When children become attached to a person they use them as a safe base to provide the comfort and encouragement which allows them to explore their environment. It has been found that a basic repertoire of attachment behaviours is instinctive in the infant and has even been found to be present at birth. Newborn babies are able to cry, make eye contact, cling, cuddle and respond to efforts at being soothed (Bowlby, 1980). This highly effective behaviour ensures that people are always on hand to care for the child.

Specific family circumstances affect the stability of the child's early relationships. The quality of the baby's temperament to the first attachment may predispose the child towards secure or insecure relationships with others. The mothers of securely attached infants have been found to be more supportive of their infant's independent play, more sensitive to their child's needs and more emotionally expressive towards their baby. In studies of infant/mother behaviour it was observed that a mother, who uses this type of interaction, naturally paces and modifies her actions, observing and allowing her infant time to respond to her (Murray *et al.*, 1996a).

The evidence that impaired maternal mental health has adverse effects on the infant, socially, emotionally, behaviourally and cognitively is extensive (Kurstjens & Wolke, 2001). It has been suggested that many depressed mothers provide distorted environments for their infants. Numerous studies have been conducted into the impact of parental depression and the possible effects of perinatal mental health disorders on infant development and children (Horowitz *et al.*, 2001; Murray, 2001; Sharp *et al.*, 1995). Often it is in the postnatal period and the ensuing months, more than at any other time, that the infant's primary environment will, in all probability, be the mother herself. Some mothers may become overwhelmed with the responsibility of care required by their infant. It is not unusual for mothers to be overindulgent to their infant's needs by overfeeding them, overprotective of the safety of their infant or even show the characteristics of compulsive obsessive disorders. These unreasonably high standards often leave them feeling guilty and inadequate. Alternatively, the mother may lack any concern for her infant but might also be feeling helpless and guilty at her lack of parenting skills. It is in these instances that she might resort to hostility.

It was during the 1970s that interest was first aroused in the possible impact of depressed mothers on infants and children. Zajiecek & de Salis (1979) and Uddenberg & Englesson (1978) found that mothers who had suffered from postnatal depression gave more negative descriptions of their children at two and four years, than did mothers who had not suffered from depression. Weissman & Paykel (1974) assessed mothers with long-standing mental health problems who had significant deficits in relation to their children, which persisted even when depressive symptoms had remitted. It was found that difficulties communicating with their children continued and the friction in the relationship between mother and child endured.

This picture of continued impairments in those with a history of postnatal depression continues, despite symptomatic improvement. It was found that the quality of the mother infant interaction continued to be dysfunctional both for mothers who were still depressed and those who had recovered. Paradoxically, follow-up of three-year old children whose mothers had had a brief postnatal depression revealed more behavioural disturbance than in children whose mothers had experienced prolonged postnatal depression, or those whose mothers had not been depressed. One explanation for the indirect effect of depression might be that women with low self-esteem and confidence in their capability to be a good parent may behave in ways that reinforce their beliefs.

According to Field *et al.* (1996), from as early as three months of age, infants of depressed mothers generalise their depressed style of interaction with their mother compared to those of non-depressed mothers. In addition, three-month-old infants of non-depressed mothers reacted vehemently when subjected to conditions of simulated maternal depression. They were wary and tended to look away to avoid any interaction. They demonstrated clear signs of protest, (Tronick *et al.*, 1992). Many researchers have suggested that mother-infant interactions following depression differ from interaction between babies and mothers who are not depressed where the behaviour of the former is more likely to be withdrawn.

The successful interaction between a mother and her infant occurs, for example, when an infant pulls at his/her mother's hair and the infant appreciates both the positive and negative responses that the mother imparts. The infant has a well-organised response of its own, and responds in a reciprocal fashion. When the mother smiles, the infant smiles in response; however, if the mother frowns unexpectedly then the infant becomes confused.

When micro-analytical studies were carried out they showed that the depressed mother showed more face-to-face sadness and this sadness was reflected in the facial expression and in the behaviour of their infants. When faced with this situation the infants exhibited more 'fuss' crying behaviour and were prone to gestures of misery. This emotional detachment of the mother has serious consequences on the process of speech and communication between the mother and child. In mothers with postnatal depression it was found that the amount of interaction and play with their infant was significantly reduced and that mothers tend to disengage from interacting with their infants and are unable to re-engage with them.

Murray *et al.* (1996a) studied the five-year-old children of mothers with postnatal depression and concluded that at 18 months the infants were insecurely detached, failed on the cognitive tasks, had problems with eating and sleeping, and the language development was poorer. Hay & Kumar (1995) found that some of the infants exhibited irregular spans of attention, impaired search abilities, lack of attention to contingencies, matching of negative affect and suffered from periods of distress that prevented active learning. This resulted in a failure to learn from non-depressed carers. The infant mimics the depressed mother and, in turn, this depresses the mother. Consequently this whole process impedes the baby's need for attention.

There is a strong belief amongst behavioural scientists that it can be catastrophic if this emotional detachment occurs at any time. If this input from the mother is missed, for example, because of a period of depression, then the child has no means of catching up and is unable to recapture what has been missed. There are, however, instances where this may be compensated for, but this relies on other members of the family. A sibling, father or grandparent may be in a position to provide the necessary stimulation, whether knowingly or not, by engaging in play or smiling spontaneously at the infant in social interaction and thus the gap is filled.

Murray *et al.* (1996b) examined subsequent infant cognitive development and attachment to explore the impact of depression in mothers and on mother-infant, face-to-face interactions at two months. Primiparous mothers, who were at low risk of depression and their infants did not exhibit the extremes of behaviour that were seen in severely depressed mothers. The depressed mothers were less sensitively attuned to their infants and were less positive and more negative about their experience of the infant. There were also difficulties in social and personal interaction. This early work discovered that these disturbances in early mother-infant interactions predicted that the infants would have poorer cognitive development at 18 months than those infants of well mothers.

Similar research was done with five-year-old children, where the cognitive functioning of the children was compared with non-depressed mothers. The infants' early experience of insensitive maternal interactions predicted the persistence of poorer cognitive functioning. Work done by Beck (1998), following similar lines to Murray *et al.*, found that postnatal depression has a small but significant effect on a child's cognitive and emotional development. A sample of primiparous women was studied from early in their pregnancy until the children were four years old (Hay & Kumar, 1995). It was found that the perceptual and performance abilities of the children were most affected. Once again, this study supported the findings that there is a significant correlation between postnatal depression and the cognitive abilities of the children. However, this study produced some important modifications as it was found that low birthweight infants and the infants of poorly educated mothers were most at risk.

Sharp *et al.* (1995) looked at the impact of postnatal depression on the intellectual development of boys. Those boys whose mothers were depressed during the first year of their life had a lower intellectual attainment than did those boys whose mothers were well. This work is supported by further studies, which report behavioural problems and impaired cognitive functioning (O'Conner *et al.*, 2002a).

Hay *et al.* (2001) found that the eleven-year old children of mothers who were depressed at three months postnatally had significantly lower IQ scores than children of non-depressed mothers. Four-year-old boys whose mothers had suffered from postnatal depression were fifteen points behind on the 'Intelligent Quotient (IQ) measurement scale' and they remained behind even at 15 years old. These boys also recognised they had attentional, emotional and behavioural problems. They also had problems with attention and difficulties in mathematical reasoning. They were more likely than other children to have special educational needs. It transpired that the boys were more severely affected than girls. At the age of eleven twice as many boys as girls were rated, by their teachers, as having significant psychological problems.

Gender differences

The difference in behaviour between both sexes has been the subject of numerous studies. Girls showed more social interaction than boys. They were more focused, but the boys were more vulnerable and were dependent on social input from their mother. Girls exhibited more joy than boys, were more able to self-comfort, displayed fewer gestures and were fussier. The boys declared their own problems earlier, their behaviour was distinctly more demanding and they had more conduct disorders. In general they emphasised their anger and irritability and were prone to be downcast. It was noted that the girls' behaviour, however, went unnoticed, until it became problematic. It therefore followed that boys should have been more affected by depressed mothers.

Rade-Yarrow *et al.* (1985) explored the impact on children of mothers who were depressed with unipolar depression (depression only) and bipolar depression. In the 15-year study it was found that the children, who were otherwise competent, became 'nagging' and 'annoying'. There was a distinct inability to interact and an inability to sustain relationships. In the unipolar group, the children had problems at all ages, whereas in the control group there was only low core morbidity. The children who were affected by bipolar mothers performed better academically than did unipolar children.

Those who were most strongly linked were the ones with the most persistent problems. Some of them also had personality disorders. This was significantly related to their behaviour. When mothers suffered from a unipolar depression the interpersonal relations showed lack of engagement with their children. This was emphasised at certain ages but was most significant when their children were toddlers. The study concluded that if good mothering were available, this would decrease the child's problems.

One Australian study found that depressed mothers with only one child reported more behavioural problems in their infants. These included poor feeding, difficulty in conforming to a sleep pattern, constant crying and 'miserable' children (Williams & Carmichael, 1985).

It is estimated that one million children suffer from mental health problems in the UK and that attention deficit hyperactivity disorder (ADHD) has increased by 850%. There is an increasing drive by the pharmaceutical companies for a quick medication fix to solve the problems, but it may be argued that children's mental health is suffering from more socio-environmental issues. The need to grow up earlier and the demands from school, family expectations and peer pressure all add to the growing burden those children have to carry. More worryingly, seven out of ten children believed that body image was important, with some on a diet all or most of the time. Sadly, in one report the Children's Society (UK) found that one-third of children had said that they felt their life did not have a sense of purpose. More than a quarter of 14 to 16-year-olds questioned said that they frequently felt depressed, though it is possible that although they feel this way they may not be suffering from a mental illness. Compared with other industrialised European countries the children in the UK were at the bottom of a league for well-being. The report claimed children were unhappy and unhealthy (UNICEF, 2008).

Other national surveys have suggested that children generally felt well and good about themselves. However, even here it has been argued that problems still exist and children have new challenges to face. Children's mental health issues have often been dismissed in the past but in view of the increasing evidence of the long-term issues, there is growing recognition of the need for early intervention and management.

The evidence for a mother's mental health affecting her infant appears strong, and it is with reluctance that this information may be imparted to mothers. It may be argued that whilst the mother is in the throes of depression she does not need to be aware also that her condition may significantly damage the well-being of her infant. Fundamentally, there is little a mother can do as she contends with her own despair.

In the field, however, this vital information is of importance to promote the cause of early intervention for postnatal depression. Despite all the years of research, it is true to say that in our society there remains some reluctance to believe in the concept of postnatal depression. As a consumer society our needs are ever growing, the social structure makes more demands on the State than ever before. It is only in recent years the media have been aware that maternal mental health disorders can have long-term consequences for the emotional, psychological and physical health of their children. There have to be premeditated decisions about the necessity for money to be spent. Social services will usually only acknowledge that a mother is depressed if there is significant and serious harm to the child. The child may be at serious risk of impaired cognitive development and may experience difficulty in sustaining future relationships, but is not in any immediate danger. Thus the dilemma, to tell and stress or not to tell, confronts many professionals who are concerned with preventative care.

Rejection of the child

In a small minority of cases there may be rejection of the child, which can be either covert or overt (Brockington, 1998). Although there has been significant work on the rejection of children there is very little research into the rejection of newborn babies. There is evidence to suggest that children who have suffered from rejection suffer from higher levels of loneliness than other children do. It is further noted that there is considerable variability in the levels of loneliness even in groups of children and it is postulated that this may be due to the amount of overt rejection they received (Leary, 2003).

The past forty years have seen the fragmentation of the nuclear and extended family and it is more probable that an emphasis is placed on securing sexual relationships with partners than forging secure relationships with siblings and parents. The word 'family' is synonymous with the image of a close knit unit, as frequently referred to in one particular television programme based on the East End of London 'cause we're family', demands loyalty, allegiance and gives license to protect, support and embrace it, no matter how great the sacrifice. The fact that 'charity begins at home' is testimony to the fact that individuals are more inclined to support the needs of their family than that of an acquaintance and as a general rule are more likely to confide in a family member than a stranger (Fitness, 2005). The phrase that 'your mother will never lie to you' is reassuring when her opinion is sought or her advice requested, and it is your mother that you should be able to rely on.

There are different responses to hurtful behaviours from family and non-family members and it is possible to tolerate extremes of damaging behaviour in order to maintain family ties. There is little known about the types of behaviour that will be tolerated without actually completely rejecting family members and what is too serious or destructive to avoid the decision to reject them. There is a paucity of studies noting the interaction within families as a whole.

In order to address this shortfall in social research, Fitness & Parker (2003) asked respondents to describe what was the 'very worst thing' that parents could do to their children and vice versa. The most remarkable finding was that just under half of them gave prominence to familial rejection and ultimately abandonment. This, they felt, was the most heinous of crimes; to desert your children implies the most profound of rejection of all social norms and duties to protect and nurture children.

Bowlby (1973) once described how children who were threatened by abandonment, which might include suicide, were highly dysfunctional and had bouts of violent disruptive anger. This was such a potent mixture and caused such insecurity within the child that sometimes it could lead to the murder of the parent, as once they were dead the parent could never threaten to leave them again.

What makes a mother reject her child is a matter of conjecture: the familiar traits of the errant father, an unwanted pregnancy, a depressive illness that flattens all emotion, whether towards infant or partner, an infant who is the reason for her suffering the depressive symptoms, an inability to 'bond' because the pressures and responses to hallucinations are too great, or simply an unexplained innate disregard for her own infant. It has been postulated that there is an relationship with the birth order. The first born tend to be regarded as sensible and accountable, the last indulged and spoilt (Herrera *et al.*, 2003; Sulloway, 1996), whereas middle children may feel marginalised and rejected. Should a child be out of favour with his/her mother, for whatever reason, including birth order, there is a likelihood they will receive less attention from their mother and as a result will probably exhibit negative behaviour towards everyone. This behaviour in turn will perpetuate their mother's lack of preference and her consequent disdain for the child.

The rejection of a mother in older children can precipitate depressive episodes but this is still an area that has been under researched and is little understood. Neither is there any firm research on the consequences of being rejected emotionally rather than physically as an infant. The rejection may not be intentional but the effect on the infant must be incalculable.

The behaviour of rejection is rarely recognised by health professionals as not only is it disturbing but also a taboo subject that is sometimes too difficult to comprehend. One noticeable feature is that the mother's depressive or anxious state is considerably improved when she is separated from the infant.

There is also emerging evidence of the rejection of babies born by *in vitro* fertilisation (IVF). This is even more difficult to comprehend when the time and effort to become pregnant is considered. A small number of studies concluded that it was found that mothers who experienced a multiple birth via IVF were more likely to express negative feelings of tiredness, feelings of stress and depression and to question their parenting abilities. Whereas mothers of singleton births felt elated and delighted at their new infant (Sheard *et al.*, 2007).

Child abuse

As the awareness of disorders of perinatal health emerges, so does the evidence that some depressed mothers may harm their child. Anger is probably one of the crucial features in the mother and child relationship. Irritation is usually expressed by the mother raising her voice to the infant should crying disturb her. The only response, from the anxious infant, is to increase the volume of noise, which may agitate the mother even further and cause her to increase her commands by shouting. This is not a new phenomenon and most mothers will be able to identify with the feelings of frustration and desperation; however, what is different and what divides the way in which mothers react is that this is where the anger subsides. The shouting helps to release the build up of pressure and some may even recognise the effect on both themselves and their infant. For some, however, the shouting may be a precursor to more serious assaults. In an effort to stop the infant from crying the mother may resort to picking up the baby, handling the body roughly and shaking it until the infant stops. This is commonly known as 'shaken baby syndrome' and is caused by an adult holding an infant by the torso, giving no head support and then violently shaking the whole body.

There are usually a group of features in 'shaken baby syndrome', which includes subdural haemorrhage; sometimes there is retinal haemorrhage and in some cases there is brain swelling and evidence of damage to the brain. What is usually conclusive is that the findings are accompanied by other injuries outside the head, marks on the sternum and fractures to the ribs caused by holding the torso tightly.

It may be argued this is a momentary loss of control, neither predetermined nor malicious. The infant is violently shaken, thrown and the mother suffers from remorse. There is no scientific evidence to support the view that any shaking causes the characteristics of those which are described in 'shaken baby syndrome' and more recent research has suggested that from a biomechanics perspective the science is fundamentally flawed. However, this assertion is premature, as there are extensive clinical reports of confessions from the perpetrators of infant brain injuries indicating that they were caused by shaking. There is also evidence to show that retinal haemorrhages are overwhelmingly more common in abuse cases than in accidental injuries.

The aggression can take many forms and may lead on to cruelty and neglect. There may be pressure bruising; cigarette burns and other intentional burns from fires, stoves, lighters; broken bones; starvation; bites; and sexual abuse.

Sudden infant death syndrome

There have been reported cases of mothers confessing to the impulse to suffocate or strangle their infant and it has been estimated that over a third of cases classed as sudden infant death syndrome (SIDS) or cot death have been caused by suffocation. SIDS is the explanation for a cause of death when no other is apparent or where the post-mortem has concluded that there is an insufficient evidence to determine the cause of death. The confidential enquiry into families with more than one unexpected infant death revealed that there was a high rate of psychiatric illness (Wolkind *et al.*, 1993).

Other risk factors have been reported and the most common are the sleeping position of the infant (which generated the back to sleep campaign) and parental smoking. The socio-economic status of the family has also been cited, with those in the lower income bracket and poorly educated more at risk. Studies have examined the possibility of an increase in the incidence of SIDS where the mother is at risk of postnatal depression (Mitchell *et al.*, 1992; Sanderson *et al.*, 2002). Both papers confirmed that there was an association between sudden unexpected death in infancy and postnatal depression. High scores on the Edinburgh Postnatal Depression Scale (EPDS, Appendix 2) were associated with SIDS. However, despite some plausible theories, the nature of the association remains unexplained. Howard & Hannam (2003) examined studies which linked SIDS to psychiatric disorders but found that at the time there was no clear evidence for an association between the two and that further research was required in this area. However, further research by Howard *et al.* (2007) found that there was some evidence, albeit limited, to suggest an independent association of SIDS with postnatal depression during the six months following birth.

It has been found that infants who die from SIDS have symptoms in the days prior to their death and it has been postulated that mothers with postnatal depression are less aware of their infant's needs and are unable to respond as readily. Conversely, it was noted in a study by Murray *et al.* (1996b) that infants aged two months who scored poorly in their muscular activity and presented with greater irritability had less face-to-face interaction with their mother. This in itself could have led to a greater degree of depression in the mother.

SIDS has prompted increasing investigation into determining how an infant died. One method being developed is a more accurate measure of blood in the lungs, although the researchers concede that blood in the lungs does not necessarily indicate smothering. Currently, lung tissue is examined under the microscope but this is a fresh method. As the death of a child is distressing in itself it is important that the evidence is 100% accurate before falsely accusing the mother. It is therefore important that a full case history is obtained from the mother prior to any further investigations. Once again there are conflicting reports about the causes of death and cot death.

The 'Back to Sleep' campaign is designed to encourage the mother to place the infant in the supine position when putting the child in the crib to sleep. This has alerted health visitors and health practitioners to the importance of preventing cot death and to heighten the awareness of the mother to the precautions she should take. Smoking in the same room as the child is also discouraged. However, anecdotal evidence has suggested that although mothers do try to adhere to that advice, sometimes, particularly when feeling the symptoms of depression, they find solace in cigarettes and therefore have more difficulty in controlling their infant's exposure to smoke (Shrivastava *et al.*, 1997).

Care of the next infant (CONI)

The death of an infant can be devastating for a mother and her family, no matter what the cause. For the depressed mother the event is even more overwhelming and the coping mechanisms that would normally help the mother to try to rebuild her life are absent. Should the mother have another baby, the anxiety and distress of the same fate occurring to this infant is greatly increased. The Foundation for Sudden Infant Death set up a programme called Care of the Next Infant, or CONI, to help and support mothers. This is a nationwide scheme and exists in both primary and secondary care, with almost 90% of the country covered by the scheme. It adopts a multidisciplinary approach, with midwives, health visitors, paediatricians and general practitioners involved.

The midwife ensures the parents are offered the programme for subsequent pregnancies and helps parents as they begin to use the support programme after the new baby is born. The programme offers weekly visits by the health visitor, but she is also supported by a specialist CONI health visitor specifically trained in the management and outcomes of mothers who have suffered from an infant's death. The mother is encouraged to keep a symptom diary which records her baby's health. This will include appetite, general behaviour or any signs of infection or distress. A room thermometer is supplied to help the mother determine the room temperature, which should be around 18°C (65°F). Advice is offered on the most suitable type of clothing and bedding. Each detail may be discussed with the health visitor, or if there is a more pressing need, the general practitioner can be contacted. The infant's growth is monitored and specifically on the 'Sheffield' centile charts completed on a weekly basis or more frequently if required. The foundation supplies apnoea monitors which are sensitive to the infant's movements and an alarm will ring if the movement stops for more than 20 seconds. This does not prevent cot death but can alert parents to any changes in the infant's condition. The parents are offered training in resuscitation and those who choose to monitor their infants at home must complete the course.

The support is often intensive and there is evidence which suggests mothers and their families welcome the extra support. The mother is given the opportunity to discuss her fears, not only about the health of the infant but those which may be more personal to her. If any problems are raised which are beyond the skills of the health visitor or midwife, then the mother and infant are referred to the general practitioner and subsequently on to the paediatrician or mental health teams for further help and support. The scheme is designed to help mothers to have the opportunity to enjoy subsequent pregnancies and have a fulfilling experience with their new infant.

The writer Mary Shelley gave birth to an unnamed daughter who died a few days later. Her *Journal* records:

Monday Mar 6th – find my baby dead. Monday March 13th, Shelley and Clare go to town. Stay at home. Wet, and think of my little dead baby. This is foolish, I suppose; yet whenever I am left alone to my thoughts I do not read to divert them, they always come back to the same point – that I was a mother. [e] ... Monday March 19th – dream that my little baby came to life again; that it had been cold, and that we rubbed it before the fire, and it lived. Awake and find no baby. I think about the little thing all day long. Not good in spirit.

(Mary Shelley 1797–1851)

Infanticide

Probably one of the most distressing and frightening consequences of postnatal depression is the possibility that the mother may injure or indeed murder her infant (Friedman *et al.*, 2005). In the early 1970s it was recognised that mothers with puerperal depression may be obsessed with the fear that they may harm or kill their children. It was recommended that these mothers should be admitted to hospital as an emergency (Resnick, 1970).

Maternal aggression towards offspring is not a new phenomenon but when she kills her infant *'belongs to the territory where the law and medicine meet and to some extent carries the difficulties which attach to both'* (Hansard, 1938). Prior to the introduction of the Infanticide Act it was the mother's conviction for murder, with the resulting execution, that made juries find the hanging of the mother abhorrent. Many courts refused to find the mother guilty and it was the first Infanticide Act in 1922 which made manslaughter a more acceptable verdict, on the basis that a mother was insane if she *'had not fully recovered from the effect of giving birth to such child, but by reason thereof the balance of her mind was then disturbed'*. This meant the incarceration of a mother rather than the mandatory death penalty which judges were obliged to pass. The verdict of manslaughter carries the maximum life sentence.

No link was made between the causation of the aggression in the postnatal period and the mother's intention to harm her infant. In 1938 the law was revised and the age of the infants was extended to 'from newly born to under the age of 12 months'. This captured the period during which a mother might breast-feed and therefore be prone to bouts of 'lactational insanity'. This was recently challenged as there appears to be no firm evidence of the link between mental illness and lactation, but was disputed in an unpublished work by Marks (1996) who found that psychotic episodes may be activated by increased dopamine sensitivity which is increased by the process of lactation. Raising the age limit to two years was also considered. This would then include all child killings committed by mothers with postnatal mental disorders. However, it was decided that *'in the light of current medical knowledge and the existence of the defence/offence of diminished responsibility the defence of infanticide was absolute'*. It was also proposed that the Infanticide Act pardoned mothers who might have killed older siblings or spouses during this period (Pearson, 1997). The possibility of expanding the scope of the offence/defence to cover '*circumstances consequent upon birth*' was debated; however, this was felt to be unsafe as it was possible this could provide persons who had criminal intent with a sound alibi.

It has been the subject of much criticism but the Infanticide Act appears to be the most '*practical legal solution to a particular set of circumstances*'. The mother is recognised as having 'diminished responsibility' which distinguishes it from other offences (Law Commissions Act, 1965) and the Act '*does not require the act or omission of killing to be causally linked to the disturbance of the mother's mind. There need only be a temporal connection*'.

The majority of infanticide cases occur within the first three months of birth and are unlikely after twelve months. After twelve months the defence is 'diminished responsibility'. Infanticide itself is very rare, with less than ten mothers being charged each year. However, that figure may be inaccurate as it is often difficult to determine the cause of death and there is often confusion with cases of Sudden Infant Death Syndrome (SIDS). It has been estimated that the incidence of infanticide is approximately 30 to 45 per year (Marks & Kumar, 1993; 1996). It is suggested that infants have a greater risk of becoming a victim of infanticide than any other age group (Craig, 2004).

Neonaticide, a term used to describe the killing of an infant less than 24 hours old, is more common amongst teenagers. Several studies have noted the risk factors inherent in cases of infanticide, which include young mothers, usually teenagers from economically deprived backgrounds, with poor educational standards, who are socially isolated and in a dysfunctional or violent relationship (Friedman & Resnick, 2007; Palmero, 2002; Siegel et al., 1996). Recent cases, however, have involved mature mothers from middle class backgrounds. Most of the mothers have a history of mental disorder, which includes psychosis, depression or attempts at suicide (Alder & Polk, 2001; Meyer & Oberman, 2001; Rouge-Maillart et al., 2005). Mothers who kill all of their infants either at the same time or over an extended period of time are usually found to have episodes of psychosis or depression (Friedman et al., 2005; Spinelli & Spinelli, 2002). There is a complexity of symptoms compounding the vulnerability of these women, which include dissociation from the event: a feeling of having no control over her actions and the feeling of depersonalisation, describing it as watching herself outside her body. Most mothers admit to being amnesic for most of the event. Some may describe additional symptoms, which may include confusion, hallucinations and a denial of pregnancy. Research which is able to compile a complete and accurate portrait of a likely perpetrator is still evolving.

In the USA the defence of infanticide does not exist and there is no legal distinction between the murder of an adult and the murder of a newborn. In many States, mothers who commit infanticide can be tried for murder and could face life prison terms or death. Here there is great controversy about the nature of postnatal depression and puerperal psychosis, primarily because the condition almost always necessitates admission to an acute psychiatric wing of a hospital. The insurance companies that pay for the hospital care refuse to acknowledge the illness and therefore refuse to pay for treatment. In the USA all past history of depression has to be declared and this is taken into account when the premiums have to be paid by the insured. As a result there appears to be a disinclination to declare knowledge of the illness.

There was the famous incident of Andrea Yates, who was convicted of the murder, by drowning, of her five children in Texas, USA. When her friends were questioned following the incident, they considered Yates as a doting mother. However, she concealed a history of postnatal psychosis and days before the murder her antipsychotic drugs were discontinued. Yates based her motive on the premise that Satan possessed her and the only way she could possibly save her children from the eternal damnation that was to befall them was to cause their deaths which would then allow them to enter the Kingdom of Heaven.

It was the influence of the evidence from a psychiatrist, who had no significant expertise in postnatal psychosis, which convinced the jury to give the verdict of guilty. Yates was sentenced to 40 years in prison. The condition of postnatal psychosis (or post-partum psychosis) appears still to be unrecognised in some parts of the States, despite being readily diagnosed.

It is well known that there is a deep-rooted preference throughout cultures for the birth of a son to a daughter. Female infanticide is not uncommon, particularly where resources are limited and a son can bring wealth and status to the family. Research has indicated that female infanticide is more common in the higher socio-economic groups, as the son has the probability of siring several children, which in turn will enhance the family's growth and future (Kauppi *et al.*, 2008; Stone *et al.*, 2005).

In order to attempt to prevent or at least avoid further infanticides it is important that the subject, albeit difficult to comprehend, is tackled in a sensitive and supportive way. Early screening and recognition of any mental health disorder within the perinatal period is essential. Midwives are in the prime position to understand and determine whether a pregnant mother harbours suicidal thoughts about herself or indeed her infant in the womb. There are some studies which recommend the use of the Edinburgh Postnatal Depression Scale (EPDS) as a screening tool in the antenatal period, and some midwives welcome this. However, as most care tends to be holistic and managed in a multidisciplinary way it is important that there are clear indicators about the way in which referral pathways are established. The NICE Guidelines have influenced the way teams should and can respond in the future.

It has been estimated by Palmero (2003) that up to 4% of mothers with untreated postnatal psychosis will commit infanticide. Mothers whose depressive symptoms have been detected, probably by the health visitor when administering the EPDS, should explore at length the question which asks if the mother has any intention of harming themselves. Asking the questions 'How do you intend to harm yourself?' and 'What will happen to your children when you are gone?' allows the mother to be more honest about her actual feelings and not feel as if she has to conceal her intentions. One clinical practice study by Cubison (2006) revealed that mothers suffering from severe postnatal depressive illness reported intrusive thoughts, with over half of them experiencing thoughts of death and dying. The thoughts they shared in the study were so graphic they had been afraid to express them to health professionals. This was partly blamed on high profile cases of infanticide, where blame was cited primarily against the mother. Mothers have often calculated the future of their children, who will either be under the care of their father or they will have plans to take the children to heaven with them (Friedman & Resnick, 2007). Threats of such a nature should be taken seriously and the mother referred to the psychiatric team for immediate assessment. If her thoughts are seriously delusional and profound, then admission to a psychiatric unit or mother and baby unit would be advisable. In some cases the child protection team is alerted and provisions made to take the infant and any other siblings into a place of safety. This might be the grandparents or foster home if they were unable to be accommodated by the father. More frequent home visits are also recommended where the mother has the opportunity to raise issues about her thoughts and fears about her parenting skills. This will allow the appropriate intervention from social, voluntary and non-government organisations, all of which are designed to support and help with her domestic and social interests. There is little written evidence to support the intervention of health visitors but experiential evidence and statistics show that in the light of few other resources available, this has the best possible outcome.

Alder & Polk (2001) found that often the infant does not die as a direct result of an aggressive act but because of systematic physical abuse, though there are few studies which support this and it is often unclear what underlying behaviour leads to infanticide. This can often lead to or be a part of a fabricated illness.

Fabricated illness or illness induced by carer

This term was preceded by the phrase '*Munchausen's by proxy*', which was created by an infamous paediatrician (Meadow, 1977). It is commonly known as a disorder of parenting and the children of parents who have this disorder have either a fabricated or induced condition which requires medical assistance. The parent will visit a health professional and claim that their child is unwell or has a serious medical condition when it is in fact fictitious. In order to convince the doctor or nurse to take them seriously the parent, usually the mother, will be highly deceptive and describe symptoms that accurately describe a condition and will even present a contaminated sample. The mother might claim the infant has copious vomiting or diarrhoea, consistently cries or has epileptic type fits, all of which is difficult to disprove unless the child is strictly observed all the time. Visits to the Well Baby Clinic may be frequent, and each time there may be a catalogue of exaggerated ailments. Each one is discounted by the nurse, health visitor or doctor. There may be obvious signs of harm, which are inflicted by the mother but explained as occurring naturally. An example is of a rash, which has been caused by the mother rubbing irritants into the infant's skin. The age of the infant makes it impossible to clarify any of the claims made by the mother and the health professional has to rely strongly on the history she provides. This is what makes the diagnosis difficult.

There is little evidence of the psychopathology underlying the intentions of the mother and with such a wide variation in presentations and symptoms it is difficult to categorise a particular type of illness or condition. However, it seems to be an effective and complex way of seeking attention for both themselves and the infant.

It has been argued that fabricated illness does not exist and because of the difficulty in detecting and recognising it as a condition, there is very little literature on the subject and the numbers of infants who are subjected to it. One study has found it is more common amongst mothers, who often have a history of a mental health disorder. There have been some suggestions that it relates to the mother being abused as a child. A national survey concluded that there are approximately fifty cases of the condition reported each year, with just under half involving infants less than one year of age (McClure *et al.*, 1996).

There has been significant controversy over the subject in recent years, in particular where there have been child protection cases. When the theory of Munchhausen syndrome by proxy was discredited it left a trail of confusion and anxiety amongst health professionals, in particular those who had experienced the damage and concern those mothers engendered. There was the danger that this label would make unwarranted assumptions about the mother's mental state and her motivations (Craft & Hall, 2004). However, the damage to mothers wrongly convicted of harming or causing serious harm to their child was equally serious. It is estimated that only a minority of parents deliberately harm their infants and the revision of the term allows the health professional to focus on the needs of the infant rather than on the mother.

Mothers who have committed infanticide in the UK

Case one

A mother in her early thirties was heavily pregnant, seriously depressed and anxious about the state of her marriage when she poisoned her young son then cut her throat with a circular power saw. Her son was found in the bedroom.

Case two

A depressed mother suffocated her two sons with a pillow after a row with her ex-boyfriend. The two children were found in the bedroom of the family flat. The mother hanged herself.

Case three

A Bangladeshi mother poisoned her daughter and then set fire to herself.

Case four

A mother suffering from postnatal depression drowned her five-week-old baby in the bath.

The incidences are not exclusive to the UK.

Mothers who have committed infanticide in Europe, Canada and the USA

Case one

A woman surrendered to police in an East German town after her newborn child was found in a blue plastic rubbish bag trapped in the reeds of a lake.

Case two

In the same week another mother was arrested on suspicion of throwing her baby out of a ten-storey apartment building, wrapped in a plastic shopping bag. She had given birth to him half an hour before, in the bath. A dog found the bag and scratched it open.

Case three

A mother in Bavaria was arrested for strangling her baby daughter and putting her in the freezer. The mother of two children aged ten and four, feared her boyfriend's disapproval. 'He threatened to throw me out if I concealed another pregnancy from him,' she told the court.

Case four

Another woman was arrested after police found two dead babies in her freezer. One baby was stillborn a year before; the other was a recent live birth. A driver pulled up at a car park and found the corpse of a young baby in a waste-paper basket. The DNA coincided with that of another baby who was fished out of a rubbish-sorting depot a year before; the mother had not been traced.

In the USA during the years 1976 to 2005, over ten thousand parents killed their children. In Canada there were 33 homicides committed against children under the age of twelve in 2003, the lowest number in over 25 years. Of these victims, 14 (or 42%) were under one year of age. Of the 27 solved homicides against children, 23 were killed by a parent: nine by a father, four by a step-father, ten by a mother and one by a step-mother (in one incident, both parents were accused).

Weissman & Paykel (1974), on the basis of clinical observations of women admitted as consecutive cases to a clinic for the treatment of acute depression, described the predicament of depressed women as experiencing feelings of inadequacy and being overwhelmed by the care required by an infant. As a result, mothers often became overindulgent, overprotective and compulsive. Their failure to achieve unreasonably high standards lowered their self-esteem and they lost faith in their ability to perform the mothering role efficiently. This inability to cope was noted as the women tended to overfeed their infants and had a real fear of harming their babies, psychologically, if not physically. The women showed an awareness of their difficulties and expressed considerable guilt and inadequacy over their performance. Alternatively, if the mother was not overly concerned, helpless and guilty, she could be directly hostile. The final cause for concern lies in the scale of the problem, with estimates of the prevalence of depressive disorders in the puerperium consistently around 10–15% (Cox *et al.*, 1982; Kumar & Robson, 1984; Pitt, 1968).

Several studies have been made on emotional abuse. Research shows that if little is known about the impact on children of parental depression in general, even less is known about the possible effects on infant development that derive from maternal disorders occurring in the puerperium. This omission is striking for several reasons.

First, and most obviously, in the postnatal period and the ensuing months, more than at any other time, the infant's primary environment will, in all probability be the mother herself. Second, it has been suggested that many depressed mothers provide distorted environments for their infants.

A greater understanding of the social and emotional effects of childbirth might avoid many of the problems experienced. It may be argued that society colludes to hide from women the fact that giving birth is not always a joyous experience. On the contrary, for many it is an experience, which seriously interferes with close relationships. This suggests that there are benefits in discussing the issue of socio-emotional strain in the antenatal period and it seems reasonable to suggest that if an illness has sociogenic origins it may also have sociogenic remedies.

Maureen Lawrence (1969) in her book *The Tunnel* described the thoughts which invaded a mothers' head about her killing her infant who was born without any ears:

She took the feet with her right hand and pulled them gently, so that the upper part of the body and the head slipped further into the water, which covered the face; the body convulsed and flailed. Her left hand came down onto the stomach and held it firmly she looked into the red glow of the fire until the splutter and simmer of the water ceased and the child was still. Then she lay the warm dead body on the towel, and flushed the water down the sink.

(pp. 59–60)

Later she wrote:

She bent over the sleeping child. The knife had a shapely wooden handle and a blade curved and pointed. With her brown stained hands she loosened the bonnet and the neck of the child's gown; she tried to lift the chin to find the neck but there was much fat and the chin would not be still[e] .... then she brought the knife to point the place her fingers had sought out. The wide solemn eyes of the child fluttered and the arms waved quietly, but her finger was secure on the place where the knife pointed. She squeezed the handle and pressed down.

(p. 63)

She rested against the gate. It might have been possible to leave the child by the gate, but the cemetery faced the street and there was also the mason. Only in the innermost depths of the place would it be safe to leave it to die, by the grave of her landlady and her two husbands. But there was no way in.

(p. 65)

Effects on society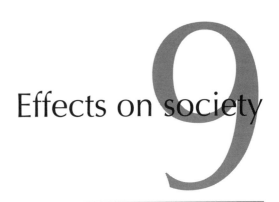

Employment

Traditionally, depression is not well managed in the workplace and is often only addressed in the context of performance. Effective action in recognising and treating depression in the workplace may only occur once it has been accepted that depressive illness is common in the general population. Every year nearly one-third of the workforce will have a mental health problem and some of them are likely to be mothers suffering from postnatal depression. It is not just distressing for the mother but makes them less productive at work. Depression as a general illness is responsible for high rates of sick leave, accidents and staff turnover.

There is no law against refusing to employ someone because they have had depression in the past, but a history of depression is likely to overshadow the mother's recruitment process. It is difficult to determine whether past experience should be explained, with the knowledge that it is easy to misinterpret depression and employers may have misconceptions about mental distress in general. This uncertainty of whether to reveal a history of any mental illness can, in itself, lead to increased stress. The equal opportunities mandate requires applicants to sign a declaration stating that they are not currently suffering from or have not suffered in the past from any 'medical or nervous condition' which could interfere with their ability to carry out their duties satisfactorily. A general practitioner can be removed from practice by other partners if they have been compulsorily detained by the Mental Health Act. Many doctors do not have a general practitioner and therefore cannot access psychiatric help. Psychiatric illness cannot be managed with the self-diagnosis, self-prescribing and casual consultations with which many doctors manage physical illnesses. Doctors who are mentally ill are in a vulnerable position and their rights as patients are easily ignored (Armstrong, 1997).

It is important that each organisation has an interest in the mental health of the workforce and a sound mental health policy. This should ensure a sensitive working environment which enhances all the employees' well-being. There should be an awareness of mental health disorders and a rapid response to the signs and symptoms of mental health issues. This should be coupled with a network of good mental health support and referral. The managers, in particular, should be made aware of the features and causes of depression, including childbirth, and the effects this may have on the employee's ability to work effectively.

All employees, including executives, managers, personnel departments, trade unions and individual employees are encouraged to adopt a positive approach to the overall mental health of the workforce and to understand how that may benefit not only individual employees but the organisation too. There is a plethora of information from non-government organisations and any mental health charity may be contacted for posters, leaflets or information packages.

There would be significant advantage in health education and informing employees of ways in which they may take responsibility for their own stress factors and finding ways in which to reduce stress. The initiation of time out days, time management, assertive training and team building exercises are positive strategies for encouraging good mental health.

The occupational health services in larger organisations are a positive step to enhancing mental health. Educational programmes may be devised for the workforce. They should be responsible for diagnosing and supporting employees with depression. They will understand the importance of confidentiality and job security, coupled with the workplace legislation which would inform the mother of the way in which she would be likely to be treated.

With mental health there may, initially, be minimal days of absence, but these may gradually increase, so the mother's work routine becomes unreliable. Some days they may fail to turn up to work, with no explanation, or take ad hoc days off without prior permission. When they do turn up for work there may be a tendency to be later than normal.

The first warning signs are that the mother does not appear to be her usual self. Her outward appearance may not reflect how she used to dress prior to her pregnancy. Her make-up may be minimal or absent; her hair may be untidy or even unkempt. She may have gained or lost more weight than would have been expected following her pregnancy. Her attitude to work may either be too relaxed or she may have a tendency to be easily upset and a propensity to get into a dispute or argument with colleagues.

The pace at which she works may be noticeably slower and there may be a tendency to make more mistakes than usual. Concentration may be difficult, with an inability to complete tasks to her usual high standard. This is compounded by the lack of confidence in her usual ability to work effectively. She may find it difficult to delegate tasks to other members of staff, coupled with a degree of anxiety about the attitudes of other staff. Important meetings and dates may be forgotten or simple tasks neglected. Although the decline in her work output may be patently obvious to work colleagues it may not necessarily be obvious to the mother. There may be issues around the time she leaves work, if she is working flexible hours in particular, as it may sometimes be less distressing to remain in the workplace than face the turmoil that will greet her at home. It is likely she may feel and behave in the same manner at home.

The mother may lack the insight to understand her depressive symptoms and not understand the situation she is in or is creating. In extreme cases the depressive state may deteriorate to such a degree that she may contemplate suicide. Likewise, she may be acutely aware but would prefer to fight against the adversity as she sees it, anxious that her colleagues may judge her inability to manage as she previously did and like her colleagues manage a home, infant and work. There is the inevitable stigma, which even in today's enlightened society can prevent mothers from admitting they are depressed.

Attitudes of work colleagues

The attitude of her colleagues to postnatal depression is important. If there is already an awareness of the condition there is a possibility it might heighten their awareness of the signs and symptoms. They are in a good position to notice if she is becoming depressed. It can be a difficult subject to broach but sometimes just the acknowledgement of something 'not being right' is sufficient to enable the mother to talk about how she feels, not necessarily in any great depth but perhaps sufficient to understand her own feelings. Should the mother be informed that colleagues are very worried about her and not necessarily her performance at work this may prompt her to seek professional help. It is well known that intervention earlier rather than later can have a more satisfying outcome. This, in turn, may have a positive outcome for the colleagues, who may have the added benefit of preventing their colleague going off on long-term sick leave.

Attitude of managers/employers

Even in minor cases of postnatal depression the mother should be allowed official time for respite. Should the depression be more severe, then an unspecified time should be granted to allow the mother time to recover sufficiently to return to work. This may take several months to occur, particularly if the mother commences antidepressive medication, which, with the new SSRIs, is known to take from four to six weeks to be effective. It would be pertinent during this time to ensure that someone from the department ensured there was regular contact with the mother, as both social and psychological support may be of enormous help and may go some way to reassure the mother that she is not a social or work outcast.

It would also be unreasonable to expect the mother to return any earlier as she may be referred for cognitive behavioural therapy, which may take several weeks to deliver, though there is no reason why if she felt sufficiently well the mother could not return to work whilst receiving both medication and therapy. However, it is also a fact that the mother has an infant to care for and this may justify a review of her working practices. Part-time or flexible working hours may be more suitable and less punitive.

Working mothers

The present inclement financial climate demands that more women work to supplement the family income (Phillips, 1997). Ever since women supported the war effort, they have become accustomed to work outside the home. The modern mother is assumed to be capable of returning to work after a minimum of six weeks following childbirth. Although the time span of maternity leave is not universal, with some companies allowing more generous maternity leave than others, it is possible that women return to work well before either they or their bodies are ready to do so. It has been suggested that over five billion pounds sterling and 80 million working days are lost annually because of clinical depression. This figure is approximately 30 times greater than the number of days lost due to industrial disputes. According to the clinical data regarding the occurrence of postnatal depression, it is quite likely that women will become depressed in the workplace, or at least exhibit the signs and symptoms of the illness. There is also a risk that the women may not be aware of postnatal depression and struggle through the condition because they believe it is all a part of the way they are supposed to feel after childbirth and the extra pressures of work. In addition, there may be reluctance on the part of the women to disclose their feelings as they may feel that this may jeopardise their position in their job and have unfortunate repercussions on their future employment possibilities (Litchfield, 1993).

Fifty years ago the idea of a working mother was condemned and indeed a rarity. Women worked, but when they were childless; now in the twenty-first century it appears to have become a necessity whatever her status. Recent Government statistics have forecast that the NHS spending on each infant is set to fall to £2,416 by the year 2011, which is estimated to be the lowest level for a decade. This will have serious implications for the future of working mothers and suggests that working will continue to be the norm:

> *I thought I could keep on going, managing to get myself ready for work, then my baby, then my husband. Once everything and everyone was sorted I would then begin my day in work. I was exhausted in the evenings and just want to go to bed at 9 o'clock.*

For the depressed mother sometimes the pressures and responsibilities borne by her outweigh the advantages of working. Even when women might prefer to work, as one woman commented, 'Although *childcare facilities are available and there is no excuse to stay at home, the cost of such childcare is prohibitive and in many cases the mother pays almost as much in childcare fees as she earns.*' The benefits of working are cancelled out.

The demise of the extended family and the economic pressures that require a second income have contributed to the present manifestation of the problem. The older female members of the family no longer have a role in raising the infant, nor are they expected to perform the role in which the third generation is cared for by the first. Women can no longer rely on their family for childcare. In fact, for most mothers it is 'Hobson's choice', either they must work and pay for childcare or they stay at home and have to care for their child themselves.

Going to work, in addition to providing a second income also produces a network of relationships that are in themselves a source of personal satisfaction and identity. The birth of a child and the consequent demands upon the mother sometimes appear to be overwhelming. The loss of all, or even part of a second income, will have obvious economic consequences, but the loss of a social network nowadays means a period of isolation.

Often the partner continues to work, which means that there is no one to talk to or to give relief from the demands of a small child. The parents of the mother affected may themselves be working. One does not have to be a psychiatrist to recognise that isolation, loneliness and helplessness can induce depression:

I had to work and I enjoyed it some of the time, but if they had paid me to stay at home I would have[e] ... I think society expects too much of women.

The ideal is fine[e] ... the 'new' man shares the housework and helps with the baby. When you both come home, you roll up your sleeves and get on with it. But it isn't like that. The mother is left to do it all[e] ... cleaning, ironing, dusting, the man may occasionally make food, but that is seen as a favour. I think that 'new' men are very few and far between.

Despite this, often mothers may resent some of the aspects of giving up work because they forfeit their financial independence and loss of status, but equally recognise that some things need to be sacrificed for better mental health. These attitudes may shed some light on the reason why women readily accept the label of postnatal depression. This acceptance provides a legitimate means of exit from the workplace without the penalty of losing all means of financial support.

Working mothers are not exempt from the plethora of problems that can occur with depressive symptoms. One of the main difficulties is suffering from a sleep disorder; when the condition is at its most fierce the mood becomes flat and as a result impairs cognitive behaviour. Everyday tasks become a chore, and the mother should be taken away from the situation that causes the despair. Attempting to function in a workplace which has a strict time regime will cause added distress; then it is practical to allow time off to recover from the condition, allowing both time and space between the mother and the workplace.

So many studies show that changes in lifestyle are inevitable when a child is born. To cope adequately, a mother requires the opportunity or 'space' to adjust. It may be argued that current lifestyles in the Western world are putting too much pressure on some women, causing a form of stress which may have unremitting consequences for her child, her marriage and her economic status. Although lifestyles may change, the emphasis on the needs and demands of young children do not. The current focus on the requirement for some of the mothers to return to work appears to place an intolerable burden of care upon them (Hanley & Long, 2006). They valued the freedom and financial rewards that work brought, but, without appropriate support during the postnatal period, that freedom may also cause intolerable complications and the diagnosis of a perinatal mental health disorder. If a mother is allowed or given the 'permission' to reduce or give up her employment with this diagnosis she then has the freedom to concentrate on the care of her child and deal with the other factors which may have contributed or compounded her condition. The loss of all, or even part of a second income, has obvious economic consequences, but the loss of a social network means a period of isolation.

There is evidence to suggest that working mothers experience significant stress from the tensions arising from straddling the separate spheres of home and work. This may explain, in part, why most women with schoolage children prefer to work part time, if they have to work at all (Phillips, 1997). Attempts to dilute and devolve this responsibility for the home sphere, as in the case of childcare facilities, have sometimes proved to be expensive and difficult. However, it is not always the case that affordable childcare encourages mothers back to work. Research by Dex & Rowthorn (1997) indicates that very few mothers express the desire to work. Perhaps it is time that women challenged the perpetual theories of the Government regarding the working woman and questioned the validity of their usefulness, not just to the State but for their children. There is frequent debate in Government about taxable allowances for childcare and politicians seem aware of the impact working women make on society. Politicians advocate that 90% of women want to work; however, this statistic may belie the truth. Morgan *et al.* (1991) points out that this figure relates to women who wish to work *'at some point in their lives'*. From the study it is plain to see mothers work, grandmothers work, aunties work, sisters work, indeed most women in today's society work (Morgan, 1997).

The Conservative Party has suggested that both the father and mother should be able to take six months paid leave together, which could increase to a year, following the birth of their baby. The ambitious proposals also suggest that paternity leave should be increased. The proposals are based on the experience of cabinet ministers who recognise the strife of sleepless nights which occurs in the first three months. There is also the suggestion that the mother should have at least 14 weeks to recover from childbirth and form a strong bond with the infant. The remaining weeks could be negotiated with both parents. There is also the suggestion that if the mother was the higher wage earner she could return to work while the father has the responsibility of looking after the infant. The plans have been viewed as unrealistic and not cost effective, as the present economic climate demands that at least one parent works. Once again, the evidence suggests that it is not men but grandmothers who need to stay at home. Mothers need mothers, aunties, sisters, grandmothers and girlfriends and if they are all working who is there to help with the feeds and the general childcare?

There have been changes to the legislation in the 'Maternity and Parental Leave and the Paternity and Adoption Leave Regulations 2006', which seek to help both the employer and the employee. The regulations mean that all pregnant employees, regardless of their length of service will be entitled to take up to a year's maternity leave. The current rule, which states that employees have to have 26 weeks service before they are eligible for extended maternity leave, of up to a year, will be abolished. The amendment also allows an entitlement of ten days for 'keeping in touch' with their place of work. These days are designed to help the mothers stay up-to-date with recent developments and changes. It also means she can be phoned at home at any time during this period on work-related matters, with employers safe in the knowledge that they are not harassing the mother. Ideally, the level of contact between the employer and mother should be negotiated to ensure there is 'reasonable contact'. For the more senior members of staff, this certainly means they will be consulted while on maternity leave. The advantage for the mother is that she need not feel isolated or discriminated from her place of work and any contact with the workplace is no longer construed as breaking her maternity leave contract.

The new rules increase the potential for mothers to be absent for longer periods, but the mother is required to give more notice of her intention to return to work. Whereas previously a mother might have given one month's notice, this would double to eight weeks. This may cause a dilemma as it has the advantage of allowing the mother more

time to consider her return to work but may also cause her anxiety as she has to prep
herself for her return too far in advance.

Driving a motor vehicle

There are implications for insurance purposes. Insurance companies will take advice
from the Driving and Vehicle Licensing Authority (DVLA) about a mother's capability
of driving. Under current legislation if a mother is psychotic then the driving licence is
revoked for a period of at least three months. The mother will be allowed a return to
Group 1 driving, subject to specific conditions and following a medical enquiry. This
will include consultation with her psychiatrist to ensure that the medication she may be
prescribed does not affect her ability to drive. In cases of bipolar disorder, particularly
during the hypomanic or manic phase, and where there are repeated changes of mood
state (at least four times during twelve months) driving should not occur until the
mother has been well and symptom free for at least six months. Once again, the return
of the licence is subject to specific medical enquiry (DVLA, 2008).

Life insurance

The application for the necessary life insurance to cover a mortgage also appears to be
problematic for mothers experiencing postnatal depression. There have been reports
of mortgage companies refusing to give out insurance to mothers with a history of
depression, though it is unclear whether this was because of the depression alone.
Some companies will offer a mortgage on the proviso of a medical certificate from the
GP, which states that the mother is taking regular medication or having therapy to
treat her condition, but often the premiums are increased.

For mothers who are diagnosed with either a psychosis or bipolar disorder, the
premiums for their life insurance monthly charges have often been increased as a result
of their illness. Often a clause may be added to exclude any event related to the illness
itself. This means that should the mother die because of suicide 12 to 24 months
after the start date of the cover, because of her depression, the policy will not be paid
out. This clear discrimination means that in effect the mother has to pay double the
premium for not having cover for the bipolar disorder.

Pregnant women in prison

The treatment for mothers in prison is no different from that of mothers in the community. Obstetric care is provided by the local NHS maternity service and the woman may
give birth in a hospital maternity unit. Each pregnancy is monitored and the woman is
cared for in an area of the prison especially dedicated for this purpose and in some instances this is may be a mother and baby unit. Each mother has access to an appointed
mother and baby liaison officer who is able to offer support and advice (Prison service

‧ly, there are seven dedicated units. Two accommodate babies and of nine months, and the others up until the infant is 18 months. ‿on with a mother and baby facility until the infant has reached ‿uths.

‿s the social implications, mental illness has a human cost, in terms of the ‿al situation of the country. A healthy workforce determines the health of the ‿conomy. MIND has estimated that 2% of the gross domestic product (GDP) is lost through mental illness. Other statistics show that mental illness at 34% is the second largest cause of work-related illness, with muscular-skeletal problems accounting for 59%. The Government is making efforts to enhance the work-life balance. Unlike previous generations, there is no guarantee of a job for life, which generates intense competition for the highly skilled and highly knowledgeable jobs. In a developing world these need to be tailored to occupational health protocols, which should be imbedded in the work protocol, aside from any government policies.

Examples of models of good practice are the retailers Marks and Spencer, and Boots, who both have better working practices where the challenges of mental health issues are being addressed. It has been recognised that mental health problems can be broken into four components, with stress the most prevalent at 35%, anxiety second at 28%, 25% with depression and 12% with anxiety and depression. It found that 80% of the section managers' work-related illnesses were either associated with or related to stress and a significant number of those who had stress problems were work related (Macdonald-Milner, 2002). To combat this they have implemented a 'WorkWell programme' the guiding principles of which are to teach cognitive behavioural skills, encourage peer support and help those at risk by counselling or referring for treatment. It was hoped the outcomes would change the number of incidences related to psychosocial ill health and reduce the absence and attrition rates within the workforce. The figures so far are encouraging, as these have been reduced to 1.3% compared to the national average of 8.5%. They also found that 2% reported low job satisfaction compared with the 6% reported in similar groups.

The number of people suffering from mental health problems has escalated alarmingly over the past few years, with an estimated 2.7 million seeking help. In 2002, suicide was the most common cause of death. The World Health Organisation states that mental health is fundamental to the quality of life and produces creative active citizens. It is essential for a vibrant economy.

Social exclusion

The myriad of symptoms experienced by the mother generates irrational feelings of isolation. Many mothers complain they are unable to freely discuss how they actually feel because they are not always encouraged to do so. It is incongruous that at this exciting and precious time those mothers should feel anything but joy. The long awaited infant has arrived safely, in good health with no abnormalities, the home is warm and welcoming there are no financial worries so why would there be any problems? When the mother's feelings are discussed, words like 'guilt', 'hopelessness' and 'despair', may be bandied around but they have little meaning if it is not realised they are tied up with emotions that spell out 'I am and feel like a bad mother'. That may be what the mother truly believes. There may be some response to words of assurance, but often the situation remains so negative that it is difficult for even for a professional to permeate her belief system. In the case of suicidal mothers they may convince professionals that they are reacting to each positive word, but secretly they are harbouring thoughts of falsehoods, or believe that they are being patronised, all of which are without foundation.

The current general assumption is that perinatal mental disorders present with all the characteristics defined by the medical model, and it is convenient to treat them as such. Mothers often have insufficient time for themselves or to allow themselves to time to 'heal'. It is recognised that the fabric of society is continually fragmenting and changing (Phillips, 1997). The emphasis on caring that was once placed on female members of the family and the community now appears to be primarily the remit of social services or the health services. Yet, the majority of mothers will admit to reluctance to accept help from outside services and social services, in particular. Some studies have suggested that mothers welcome the benefits from the support and the interest they receive from health professionals and some of the voluntary support networks. There was little perception that health professionals attempted to take control of the situation and as a result encourage dependency on the services. On the contrary, listening visits and interpersonal therapies helped to empower the mothers. The question is raised of who should ultimately take the responsibility for these mothers, other than the health professionals. It has long been observed that health professionals now manage relationships that were in the past managed by priests and the family.

There is no doubt that a greater understanding of the social and emotional effects of childbirth may avoid many of the problems experienced. Once the mother, her partner and society understand that the mother's behaviour is a recognised condition then the whole process is legitimised and the recovery can commence. It is often argued that society colludes to hide from women the fact that giving birth is not always a joyous experience. For many mothers childbirth is an experience which seriously interferes with close relationships.

Little work has been done to characterise postnatal depression as a social construction, though references have been made to the social causes (Hanley & Long, 2006; Hickey *et al.*, 1997; Jebali, 1993; Morgan, 1997; Sheppard, 1997). The biological symptoms of sleep deprivation, anorexia, isolation, fatigue, despair and poor concentration are the set of characteristics that make up the pathological syndrome of depression, as described in the medical literature. It is possible that some of these symptoms may be construed differently. Brown & Harris (1978) suggest that '*Pregnancy and birth were associated with a greater risk of depression, but that was only in the context of an ongoing difficulty, particularly in cases of bad housing or poor marriage, risk was increased*' (p. 276). Whether these symptoms of postnatal depression occurred because of, or in spite of, the birth of the child has been the subject of much debate. However, as the literature suggests, the biomedical diagnosis appears to have more impact and, as a result, the medical profession is able to exert a very potent influence regarding the knowledge of the condition.

Stigma

The issue of stigma is particularly pertinent because of the unpredictability of perinatal mental health, which in the wake of social science is seen as a means whereby mentally ill mothers become ineffective members of society and are disqualified from social acceptance. Her deviance occurs when the mother fails to conform to the given set of norms which are accepted by the majority of the population (Giddens, 2006). Mothers suffering from the manic phase of bipolar disorder may sometimes be described as 'dangerous' and a threat to society, adding to the concept of their deviant nature.

It is not known for how long mental illnesses have been subject to the suspicion and rejection that occurs when 'normality' in mental health confronts those people who are considered to be 'not right in the head'. Throughout known history, it appears that both the mentally ill and those with learning difficulties have been viewed by others as 'different'.

With the continual growth in knowledge over the years, it has become increasingly important that the public at large should be made more aware of the problems faced by those who suffer in one way or another from disturbed mental functions. Evidence has shown that many of the problems incurred by the mother are exaggerated by the way in which she is treated within her social circumstances. It is only by the process of health education and understanding the deleterious effects of stigma and how mental illness and incapacity is interpreted that this prejudice can be overcome.

In previous years, the mentally ill were housed in large buildings, usually well outside the confines of the cities. Women, who suffered the various symptoms of 'madness', even those who were breast-feeding their babies, were separated from their families without any thought of the disruption that would be wrought. Relatives, in particular, were loath to admit that their loved one was resident in these 'asylums' because of the shame of having a mad person in the family. It was even believed that 'madness' could be contagious. The distances involved in travelling were a deterrent too, as many of the poorer members of the population could barely afford to feed themselves, let alone the cost of a journey perhaps covering many miles, in order to visit a relative or friend. This seeming lack of care on the part of family members must have been detrimental to the recovery of many mentally ill patients in the past.

Over the years the name 'asylum' had come to mean a place where the insane were housed, though the origin of that word, and the original intention of the place had been to serve as a retreat or refuge for those who could no longer function in the outside world because of their retreat into insanity. These asylums were a vast improvement in the care of the mentally ill, who had been accommodated in atrocious surroundings until William Tuke, a Quaker, founded the Retreat in York in 1796. Tuke, and others, had realised that these people were human beings and not animals, as most of their contemporaries saw them.

Asylums, however, became not only refuges, but also a source of damaged and sometimes dangerous people, to be feared by those on the outside. It was thought that 'mad' people were capable of the most dastardly of crimes and, given their freedom, they would perpetrate these crimes on any and all unfortunate people whom they came across. This applied also to those mothers that we now recognise as suffering from puerperal psychosis. One elderly retired mental health nurse recalls the case of an illiterate young woman from a farm deep in West Wales who suffered from this debilitating condition after giving birth, who was admitted to a mental hospital having put her newborn baby on the open fire.

Stories such as this only served to exacerbate the fears of the general public that mad people were unpredictable and liable to harm others if they were allowed their freedom. Most failed to realise that mental ill health is a sickness, and is now probably treatable by drugs and/or therapy. Referring to these people as 'nutters', 'schizo' and other similar appellations is less than helpful, but unfortunately they are still being used. It is apparent that these ideas also preclude many who suffer from varying forms of illness from seeking help. '*I wouldn't tell anyone that I heard voices, or that I saw things*,' said one young mother. '*I was so afraid that I would be locked up forever.*'

The idea still prevails in some circles that the regime of the old mental hospital persists, and that once taken in, one will never be released. Although these ideas may be now mainly moderated, there remains certain and steadfast prejudice against the people who do not fit into society's accepted regime, and there is still very much a 'them and us' situation. Not until society can be educated will this situation ever be resolved.

The advent of television and the making of programmes illustrating aspects of nervous and psychotic conditions appeared to have aroused some interest and made some impact. If reasonable decisions are to be made about issues related to mental illness, there needs to be an understanding of the nature of the images the media mean to portray and how that can shape ideas. In his book *Media Madness*, Otto Wahl takes a critical look at the negative way the mass media exposes mental illness and takes the argument further (Wahl, 1997).

The Government has recently announced their attempt to combat stigma, and one can only hope that this campaign might be the start of a successful fight against stigma relating to mental health. This is being supported by the 'Stigma Project', which has been associated with mental health for many years but recognises that there is still much to be done to educate the public to prevent mentally ill people being denied employment, access to health care, housing, insurance and mortgages. This type of discrimination denies them full citizenship and equal rights. The 'Stigma Project' recognises that the subject is still under researched and poorly understood. In an effort to address this, a Pan-European study, with twenty European countries participating, will look at the impact of stigma on people with a mental illness and their families. It will also measure the interaction between self-stigma, empowerment, perceived discrimination and devaluation. A report was expected in 2009.

Until then all those who are actively involved with mental health issues continue to help to normalise any form of mental illness, which, has been shown, is largely as a result of the society in which we live.

From the findings so far, it may be pertinent to suggest that, to some extent, some forms of perinatal mental disorders may be a consequence of social deterioration, as is postulated by the theorists of functional analysis, rather than a purely physical reaction to the situation of motherhood. It appears that for many women societal factors (which may be an attempt on the part of society to rein in, and therefore control, women if they refuse or cannot conform to the standards set by that society) may exacerbate their experience of mental health (Parsons, 1951). For example, women may on the one hand be constrained by common beliefs and facts that belong to a bygone age;

that is from a functional perspective they may believe that they should stay at home to care for the child. On the other hand they may feel obliged to agree with modern day feminist thinking regarding their 'rights' to freedom and the need to accept this triple role of wife, mother and worker. Whichever way they turn it may appear that women find themselves disadvantaged.

Postnatal depression was, interestingly, uncommon in past years, only coming to the fore during the past 30 years. Those same 30 years have seen significant and in some cases detrimental changes to family structure and values. It is postulated that women of a previous era would have felt the same pressures and stresses had they shared the same lifestyles of today's women. However, women have redefined their role in society in past years and as a result there may be gains and losses which may inevitably affect childcare responsibilities and partnerships between mothers and fathers. It would appear from this study that some women cannot cope with the undue stresses and expectations of today's society.

Presently, it appears to be acceptable to suffer from postnatal 'blues', which is thought to be a self-limiting and acceptable behaviour for a new mother. However, society has limits on the amount of non-coping it can accept, and will castigate the woman who is unable to cope with her position as a mother. Those who fail to cope are given labels. As a result, such mothers may be regarded as deviant and have to assume the sick role to enable them to seek out the support, medical and social help that is required to help them find their place back in society. In adverse social circumstances women are sometimes forced to negotiate their condition by adopting the labels in order that society will accept that something is amiss and respond with appropriate resources.

This lack of support for women does not appear to be intentional; the adoption of a critical theoretical perspective (Gerherdt, 1989) has concluded that there may be a number of factors conspiring to disadvantage new mothers. These have been identified as a medicalisation of normal life events and the current patterns of health care organisation (e.g. early hospital discharge). There are also the professional ideologies that regard the importance of accepting childbirth as a natural event. The societal change in which families have been fragmented and less supportive have brought about new forms of social organisation. Women are expected to work to maintain standards of living and ideologies of equality in which they have sought to build a meaningful life for themselves outside the home.

In the past mothers often had little choice about working because their financial situation dictated that their income was of prime importance to the family. Working outside the family home usually isolated mothers from the home environment. In many cases women were unfamiliar with their female counterparts in the community and were placed in the unenviable position of being forced to rely on support outside their normal social circles if they had need of it. Previous support systems appear to have deteriorated, as statistics show that 4.7 million of the workforce have dependent children and the majority of the workforce in the older age bracket are women. As a result, some women appear to have more commitment to the workplace than the home.

Perinatal mental illness has made some of the women in the study re-evaluate their lifestyle and in a few cases significant changes were made, which included ceasing full-time employment or re-examining their family construction. This raises the question of why women should be forced to such extremes before they are able to instigate radical changes in their lives. Perhaps there is a need to re-examine the existing social supportive structures and find out why their function has been radically diminished. Certainly it would appear that further research could be encouraged to reveal why so many factors prevent women from recognising the poverty of their daily lives.

Management of postnatal depression

Once thought to be a time of emotional well-being for mothers, it is now known that pregnancy may not 'protect' women from the persistence or emergence of psychiatric disorders. Several studies have suggested that rates of mood disorder during pregnancy are equal to those in matched non-pregnant women. Further data suggest that pregnant women with recurrent mood and anxiety disorders have a high risk of relapse following discontinuation of antidepressants (Appleby, 1991).

Marcus *et al.* (2005) found that over 5% of mothers will reduce or stop their antidepressants once they realise they are pregnant and yet research suggests that the requirements for antidepressants will increase as the pregnancy progresses (Hostetter *et al.*, 2006).

When a mother presents with the symptoms of postnatal depression it is pertinent to conduct a routine medical examination to rule out any possible physical causes. In the light of recent research it would also be applicable to test for levels of thyroxin in the blood and hormonal levels. The reality is that in most clinical practices mothers are routinely prescribed an antidepressant drug. If the mother is breast-feeding this is usually a tricyclic or one of the newer selective serotonin reuptake inhibitors (SSRIs).

Tricyclic and related antidepressant drugs (TCAs) and SSRIs are the two main groups of antidepressant drugs in common use in general practice. Tricyclic antidepressants were first introduced in 1959 and until recently were the most commonly used. Newer tricyclic and related drugs have subsequently been developed which are generally less toxic and have modified side effects.

The prevalence of clinical depression in pregnancy is estimated to be around 7–12% (Bennet *et al.*, 2004). The decision about whether to treat pregnant mothers with medication for their mental disorder is complex and requires careful consideration of the many possible adverse effects of untreated depression. There are concerns that mothers, whose symptoms are neglected and where medication is discontinued, may lack any motivation to attend antenatal clinics. As their symptoms develop there are fears that they will neglect their general health and in particular their diet. In an effort to seek solace they may resort to the calming affects of alcohol, tobacco or illicit drugs, all of which may have a far more harmful effect. In extreme cases they may be liable to self-harm or contemplate suicide (Appleby, 1991; Zuckerman *et al.*, 1989). It is recommended that each case is considered individually and the positive effects of the medication weighed against the adverse effects of more serious maternal depression.

The increased prescribing of selective serotonin reuptake inhibitors (SSRIs) has attracted some criticism and in recent reports the pharmaceutical companies have urged consideration when prescribing SSRIs in the third trimester of pregnancy as they have been found to carry the risk of neonatal withdrawal/serotonergic syndrome (an overdose of serotonin). However, despite this there is no compelling evidence to suggest that medication should be withdrawn or weaned off.

Research has shown the foetus is exposed to significant concentrations of the medication, and although there is a very slight risk, this has been linked with persistent pulmonary hypertension in the neonate. The most common symptoms reported in the infant following delivery are persistent crying, screaming, irritability, changes in body temperature, difficulty in settling, feeding and sucking problems, and jaundice. Those side affects, which have been reported, have been found to be both non-specific and self-limiting (Bonarie *et al.*, 2004). Studies do not suggest that there is an increase in any congenital abnormalities following medication (Bonarie *et al.*, 2004).

Despite some alarming facts, the SSRIs are less toxic than the tricyclic and related antidepressants and they are relatively less expensive. Despite their poor press there have been reports of a significant rate of success with this treatment, which has encouraged their popularity and demand.

Trials conducted in primary care show that a range of tricyclic antidepressants can be effective in the treatment of major depression when it is used in stipulated therapeutic doses. Amitriptyline has been extensively evaluated and produces a 50–100% improvement, compared with a placebo. However, studies have found that low dose regimes are less effective and may not always be superior to the placebo (Hollyman *et al.*, 1988). Treatment with tricyclic and related antidepressants produces a parallel reduction in anxiety and improves sleep (Thompson & Thompson, 1989).

Mothers with mild forms of depression do not appear to respond well to tricyclic medication (Elkin *et al.*, 1989; NICE, 2004). The more severe the depression, the better the response is to the treatment (Llorente *et al.*, 2003). In the majority of cases, major depression resolves with treatment, but around 12–15% of women continue to be depressed for up to two years (Scott, 1988). It has been suggested that relapse after one year is also a serious possibility. This may occur even if the original depression was resolved. This necessitates continuing the medication, even after the symptoms have resolved.

Wisner et al (1997) reviewed the literature on the use of antidepressants and breast-feeding; there were adverse effects in infants whose mothers had been prescribed the drugs doxepin or fluoxetine during breast-feeding. There were no adverse effects shown by any of the other prescribed antidepressants. The collective serum level data suggested that infants older than ten weeks were at low risk of adverse effects of tricyclics and there is no evidence of accumulation.

Haberg & Matheson (1997) found that fluoxetine has a long half life and a higher transfer and that sertraline and paroxetine are better alternatives. However, the latter has not been studied in repeated doses. It was recommended that breast-fed infants should be monitored for side effects of any antidepressant drug.

Appleby *et al.* (1997) conducted trials to study the effectiveness of fluoxetine and cognitive behavioural counselling in postnatal depression and to compare fluoxetine with a placebo. The study entailed comparing six sessions of counselling with only one session, and compared it with a study which combined both drugs and counselling. A highly significant improvement was seen in all of the treatment groups. The improvement in the mothers receiving fluoxetine was significantly greater than in those receiving a placebo. The improvement in the mothers' mood after six sessions of counselling was significantly greater than after a single session. Interaction between counselling and fluoxetine was not statistically significant. Differences were evident after one week and improvement in all groups was complete after four weeks. It was concluded that both fluoxetine and cognitive behavioural counselling, given as a course of therapy, are effective treatments for non-psychotic depression in postnatal women. After an initial session of counselling, additional benefit results from either fluoxetine or further counselling, but there seems to be no advantage in receiving both. It was therefore postulated that the women made the choice of treatment themselves.

Antidepressants are generally effective in the treatment of major postnatal depression. It is not unusual for some women to discontinue the treatment, primarily because they are unable to cope with the feelings of being out of control, or they may acquiesce to family pressure to stop their reliance on drug therapy. Once treatment has been discontinued without medical advice, there is evidence of relapse. Over two-thirds of women with a history of current depression will relapse after pregnancy if their antidepressant medication is discontinued prior to or early on in the pregnancy (Cohen *et al.*, 2006).

Breast-feeding and medication

Mothers need to understand the potential risks of drug toxicity to their infant and the importance of monitoring their baby's behaviour. All drugs given to mothers will enter the breast milk but the levels will vary greatly. There is little evidence about the amounts absorbed and specific effects of these on the neonate. Several studies have concentrated on the use of antipsychotic and antidepressant drugs during pregnancy and followed the progress into the puerperium. Evidence is now emerging about the transmission of these drugs into the breast milk and there is continuing research into the implications for the lactating mother.

It is understood that because antidepressants are lipid soluble they are excreted in breast milk. Once ingested by the infant they are metabolised by an immature liver and excreted by the kidneys, which are also immature, though the function of these organs rapidly develops in the first few days following delivery. It is probable that the immaturity of these major organs leads to an accumulation of the drugs.

The values for the daily dose per kilogram ingested by the breast-fed infant is less than 1% of the maternal dose and minute amounts of antidepressant drugs have been detected in infants' plasma and urine. The brain tissue, however, is lipophilic and it is possible that the drugs will concentrate here. Studies have highlighted few problems and the risks appear minimal. The findings to date suggest that provided infants are healthy at the outset then it is likely that the benefits of breast-feeding will outweigh any potential problems, if the mothers are taking antidepressants at recommended doses. There is less evidence, however, about the risks of treatment with SSRIs.

In bipolar disorder it is generally felt that the drug lithium is contraindicated for breast-feeding mothers. However, whatever the drug regime or recommendations it is important that the risks of taking the medication are balanced against the benefits of breast-feeding.

The usefulness of transdermal oestrogen (Gregoire *et al.*, 1996) for mothers with major postnatal depression was evaluated but it was found that the effect of oestrogen was modest. The side effects of the treatment included the possibility of embolism but because it diminishes the supply of breast milk it would not be the drug of choice.

The treatments that have been developed to combat depression have been mostly pharmaceutical. There may be a philosophical argument about the administration of antidepressants, which is the continued administration of a set of old laws that seek to control the distribution of dangerous products. Perhaps it is worth noting that opiates were used to combat depression – *vide* Thomas de Quincy. Originally the concern was with the use of opiates but since that time the majority of pharmaceutical products have been classified as being 'only available upon prescription'. The doctor is thus part of the legal system of restriction, a set of laws, like so many others, that have been passed in order to protect society.

The question may be raised about who actually benefits most from the manufacture of pharmaceutical products. One of the problems that besets major manufacturers is the fact that of every thousand products that start life in their research laboratory, only two or three will eventually reach the pharmacist's shelf. Of those three, only one will be a major moneymaker.

Drugs to relieve depressive disorders, as an area of pharmaceutical research interest, are relatively recent and, for a few major producers, they have proven to be massively profitable. The money earned is not siphoned off into profits; indeed, the current returns to shareholders in this sector, whilst steady, are not spectacular. The research component of their work is fearfully expensive which is why any manufacturer of a new product has at least seven years of protection against thousands of small companies who do no research but merely copy. It is how they do the research that begs the question.

Depressive disorders, for these companies, have to be seen as some sort of chemical imbalance, abnormality or dysfunction, which may then be remedied by another chemical. That is perhaps an oversimplification of their approach but it does describe their intervention in this field. Serotonin diminution and Prozac are a typical example. This means that their research has to treat the depression as a reaction to something else, for example diminished serotonin, and that something else has got to be treatable by one of their products.

In terms of the classical research method this implies that the depression is a dependent variable that can be explained by the occurrence of the abnormality. For treatment, the sequence is reversed. The depression is now the independent variable that can be influenced by a dependent variable – the pharmaceutical preparation. This is not a conspiracy but rather the way in which ethical pharmaceutical products are developed. If the rules of scientific research are not followed then dangerous drugs with unknown side effects will come onto the market and years of litigation may ensue.

There is the possibility that the depression and the pharmaceutical product might both be variables of the same kind. If the depression itself has occurred as a result of events outside the sufferer, fear of the future, loneliness, isolation, rejection, then a pill is not going to remedy the problem. You cannot take a pill to change the behaviour of an uncaring partner, but no pharmaceutical company is ever going to investigate such a cause of depression. If it were possible to prove conclusively that serotonin diminution occurs after something else, and if it were possible to prove that a pharmaceutical company knew this, then the conspiracy theory is proven. If a depressed mother presents herself in the surgery then the doctor must attempt to deal with the depression. If the doctor knows that an antidepressant drug will ease the condition, then his/her own humanity may lead him/her to prescribe it.

Electroconvulsive therapy

This treatment continues to raise much controversy amongst the general public and medical professionals alike. Some feel it is barbaric, its application is archaic and clumsy. The short-term side effects are loss of memory and confusion, but even though it has been in use for over sixty years there is little research data on the long-term effects. It is unusual for ECT to be used against a mother's will, even where it is used extensively (Wheeldon *et al.*, 1999).

ECT was developed in 1938 and was an effective treatment for multiple psychiatric conditions, particularly severe depression. As psychiatric medications and antidepressants became more sophisticated, the popularity of ECT waned and its use diminished significantly. However, during the 1970s the management of the equipment was revised and improved. Particular attention was paid to the use of a more effective anaesthesia and the emphasis was on increased safety and comfort.

ECT is most commonly used to treat patients with severe depression who fail to respond to medications or who are unable to tolerate the side effects associated with the medications. ECT may also be the treatment of choice for patients who need a more rapid response than medications can provide. This would include mothers who are severely agitated, have hallucinations and delusions, have stopped or declined eating or drinking, or have serious suicidal thoughts. It is also very effective with mothers who exhibit the features of catatonia. Its use is not limited to the treatment of depression and may be used to stabilise bipolar illness during extreme episodes of mania or depression. Additionally, ECT can be used to diminish psychotic episodes associated with schizophrenia. Appleby (1991) found that major puerperal depression and psychosis is particularly sensitive to treatment with ECT, but it is not recommended for mothers with less severe forms of depressive illness.

Prior to any treatment, the mother is given pre-medication which will help to alleviate any anxieties about the treatment. Even though her condition may cause both apathy and lethargy it is still possible to have impending doubts about the methods of this treatment. It is the responsibility of the nursing staff to ensure that the mother is comfortable and that all pre-operative procedures have been acknowledged. Any sharp objects, jewellery, false teeth and nail varnish should be removed. The mother lies on a couch and is wheeled into the clinic where a Venflon is inserted into a vein and an intravenous infusion of anaesthesia is administered. Brain waves, heart rhythm and blood pressure are recorded.

There are two types of electrode placements used in the delivery of ECT. One or each side of the brain is stimulated, the timing of the response in unilateral delivery is longer and the potential side effects are said to be less. In the case of bilateral treatments, electrodes are placed on both temples and a brief electrical pulse is applied via the electrode box. This pulse excites the brain cells, which causes them to fire in unison and produce a seizure or fit. This fit lasts approximately three to five seconds, but it is usually ten to twenty minutes before the mother is fully awake.

The course of treatment normally ranges from six to twelve treatments over six to eight weeks. The average number of treatments is nine. The severity of the symptoms and the rapidity of the response usually determine the number of treatments. It usually takes six treatments before major improvements in symptoms are noted. These may include an increase in the level of activity, improved and more satisfying sleeping patterns, and a mild increase in appetite.

Common side effects following the treatment may include nausea and headache. Often there is acute confusion, possibly resulting from a combination of the anaesthesia and the ECT treatment. This typically lasts for an hour or less. The loss of short-term memory is more distressing, but usually resolves after a few weeks. There have been cases of memory impairment were memory recall is patchy and in some extreme cases there has been severe memory loss. Dulling of the intellect and subtle changes in personality were further features which have been noted.

There are multiple theories to explain why ECT is effective. One theory suggests that the seizure activity itself causes an alteration of the neurotransmitters. Another theory proposes that ECT treatments adjust the stress hormone regulation in the brain, which may affect energy, sleep, appetite and mood. In recent years there have been developments in neurosurgery with the advances in the stereotactic techniques and the development of reversible and adjustable neuromodulatory technologies; these include deep brain stimulation and vagal nerve stimulation.

Any surgical intervention raises the spectre of Jack Nicholson's experiences in *One Flew Over the Cuckoo's Nest*, despite the success rates of frontal lobotomies for patients with unretractable and severe depression in the past. Bilateral deep brain stimulation electrodes conjure up similar repulsion. However, when they were implanted into severely depressed patients' brains the results were encouraging as the patients' moods improved and there were no significant side effects. The less invasive vagal nerve stimulation also proved to be successful. It has been noted that at the present time the evidence for the use of both techniques is still underdeveloped (Henderson, 2007).

Non-invasive therapies

There is evidence that indicates that the management of the doctor/patient consultation coupled with certain prescribed medications has a positive effect before the medication is claimed to 'kick-in'. It also suggests that the human intervention,by voluntary or statutory agencies does have a beneficial effect, as demonstrated by Gruen (1990), Eliott (1990) and Pitts (1995) in their advocacy of support groups.

Cognitive behavioural therapy (CBT)

Prenatal and postnatal women frequently present with symptoms of anxiety and panic, such as global diffuse anxiety; intrusive, obsessive thoughts and panic attacks. The result is a perception of lack of control in their lives, low self-esteem and low maternal confidence, and accompanying depression.

The intervention therapy CBT was introduced by Aaron Beck during the 1950s. Research into other populations has indicated that cognitive behavioural therapy and guided relaxation may be as effective for the treatment of these types of symptoms as are psychotropic medications. These interventions also provide an attractive alternative for pregnant and breast-feeding mothers who are reluctant to take medication. Using these techniques can both enhance treatment, when combined with medication, and provide short-term relief of symptoms as well as developing long-term life skills.

Mothers, as part of the depression, may feel locked into their problem situations. Ellis & Dryden (1987) in their 'rational-emotive' therapy and Meichenbaum & Genest (1987) in their 'cognitive-behaviour modification', understand the need to challenge the inner or covert experiences and behaviour that sustain self-defeating patterns of overt behaviour. Both have developed methods for helping clients to overcome what can be called 'self-limiting' or 'self-defeating' internal dialogue or self-talk.

Challenging women's self-limiting ways of thinking can be one of the most powerful methodologies for behavioural change. Cypert (1987) and Fordyce (1983) believe that negative thoughts stand in the way of problem solving; therefore, positive thoughts can greatly contribute to managing problems and developing opportunities.

Some of the more common beliefs that Ellis (1987) believes get in the way of effective living are feeling powerless and not in control of situations, almost assuming a passive stance. The philosophy of being a 'bad' mother is a typical example. Because the mother feels that she is a poor mother she must be incompetent. This will make her disliked and as a result, unloved. The least traumatic way to deal with these feelings is to avoid any responsibilities and almost become a victim to the terrible feelings of hopelessness and helplessness. Ellis (1987) suggests that if any beliefs are violated in a person's life, then the experience may be seen as terrible, awful or even catastrophic.

The research into postnatal depression and other perinatal mental health conditions has indicated that most depressed women will experience many, if not all of these feelings. This renders everything in their life 'out of control', as indeed most depressed mothers will admit. Distinctions may be made between blatant and obvious irrational beliefs, and those that are subtle and tricky.

An example of a blatantly irrational belief is: '*Since I strongly want to be approved of by people I find significant, I must have their approval otherwise, I am a worthless and unlovable person.*' The more subtle or 'tricky' belief is:

Because I strongly desire to be approved by people I find significant, and because the lack of their approval makes me behave so badly, my dysfunctional behaviour proves that I absolutely must have their approval.

Irrational beliefs appear to correlate with a variety of psychological problems which include depression and lack of assertion.

Pointing out to depressed women that there is some logic to their behaviour, even though this appears to be ultimately self-defeating, challenges their view of themselves as being irrational. Women with postnatal depression are challenged to find whatever they feel is the logic embedded in their distorted thinking, and to use this logic to manage problem situations, instead of perpetuating them.

The most common process is to create five stages to enable the problem to be more manageable. A 'situation' is identified, which could be a single event or something that is foremost in the mother's mind, and 'thoughts' and 'emotions', which surround it, are discussed. An attempt is made to identify the 'physical feelings' which accompany it – stomach cramps, nausea etc., and then be able to 'evaluate' why these feelings occurred, what impact they have had and what actions can be done to reduce or even alleviate the problem to make it more manageable.

It is easy for the mother to be overwhelmed by negative thoughts and translate the actions of others as disapproving or judgemental. CBT helps her to re-evaluate and re-interpret those feelings.

It is usual to have five to twenty therapy sessions each lasting between 30 to 60 minutes, depending on the mother and the therapist relationship. The evaluation of a treatment programme with educational, social support and cognitive behavioural components by Meager & Milgrom (1996) showed that following treatment, there was a significant improvement in the mother's mood state. It was suggested that a cognitive behavioural group programme might be effective as a treatment in the post-partum period. A diagram of the CBT cycle is shown in Figure 10.1.

There are arguments, however, about the wisdom of introducing cognitive be-havioural therapies into a mother's life when there are so many life events and changes, but the evidence of the effectiveness appears to outweigh the doubts. An added dif-ficulty is the availability of appropriate therapeutic services. In the majority of areas around the UK there is a dearth of qualified CBT therapists, and waiting times for mother's appointments are prohibitive. However, with the NICE recommendations this shortfall should be addressed.

Non-directive counselling (listening visits)

This is derived from the clinical theories of Carl Rogers (1957) based on years of therapeutic practice. His theories were logical, pragmatic and with the basis for broad application. Rogers viewed everyone as basically good. Good mental health was viewed as the normal progression of life and mental illness, criminality and deviance as the distortion of natural life.

He postulated that there is a motivation in everyone to develop and reach his or her full potential. Rogers acknowledged that people thrive on 'positive regard', which is nurtured by the feelings and actions of the attention, affection and love that is offered and/or given by other people. This is further translated into the phrase 'positive self-regard' which demonstrates the positive self-worth or self-esteem of a mother which is created and developed by encouragement and belief in her by someone else.

Occasionally there are conditions that govern the encouragement given by people, but Rogers argued that conditions are very powerful and have the ability to fracture beliefs, which may ultimately lead onto a dysfunctional relationship. It was with this

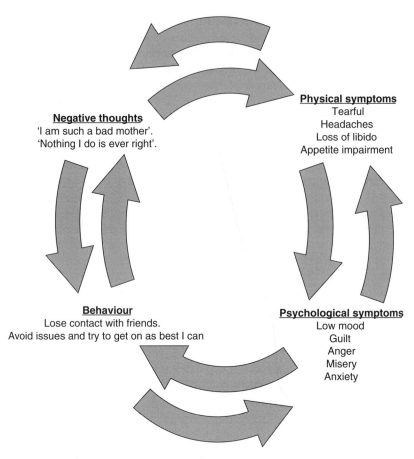

Figure 10.1   CBT cycle

in mind that he developed 'unconditional positive regard'. This concept encourages the counsellor to accept the mother for what she is, not to judge her but to treat her as a worthy and capable being, even though her self-esteem may be low and she may feel unworthy. By showing this unconditional positive regard and acceptance by both actions and words, the counsellor is providing positive conditions for her personal growth. To allow a therapeutic relationship to develop the counsellor provides feedback, checking how the mother feels and if there has been correct interpretation of her feelings.

The several differences between directive and non-directive counselling are that 'directive' implies giving advice and information to the mother and demonstrating what to do, whereas non-directive is more concerned with helping the mother to understand her situation and explore possible options and explanations for her situation. Holden *et al.* (1989) developed the concept of 'listening visits'. This approach is offered by briefly trained healthcare professionals and often takes place in the mother's home.

In the primary care setting, non-directive counselling and cognitive behaviour therapy have both been shown to be significantly more effective clinically than usual GP care in the short term. King *et al.* (2000) discovered there were no differences between these three treatments in either clinical outcomes or costs at twelve-month follow-up. Compared with usual GP care, no differences in overall costs were observed.

There are relatively few such studies comparing cognitive therapy with less specialised psychological interventions, but Milgrom *et al.* (2005) demonstrated that all of the interventions were superior to conventional routine care. Harvey *et al.* (1998) in their study of counselling in primary care found no difference in either functional or mental health outcome for the patients that were offered access to counselling and those given usual care by their GP.

However, a study by Pearlstein *et al.* (2006) found that mothers preferred to have interpersonal psychotherapy rather than antidepressants or a combination of therapy and medication.

Interpersonal psychotherapy (IPT)

This was developed by Klerman *et al.* (1984) for the treatment of depression, but has since been extended to include other mental disorders. It has been described as a '*discrete, time limited, structured psychological intervention derived from an interpersonal model of affective disorders which focuses on interpersonal issues*'. It involves collaboration between the therapist and the mother where they are able to recognise any conflict she is experiencing during the transition to motherhood. This may include grieving the loss of her previous status and ascertaining which social skills have gone and what, in turn. has heightened her anxiety. Facilitated by the therapist, the mother learns to understand recent events in interpersonal terms and explore alternative ways of coping with these situations.

Gestalt therapy

Gestalt therapy can be used on women suffering from postnatal depression at any stage in the illness as it poses little threat to the psyche. It is about the 'here and now', and although there is great emphasis on this it also includes how the mother describes her story as well as what she describes. A therapist listens to the mother's story, which is described in Gestalt therapy as the 'field'. As the therapist listens, he/she may comment on the phenomenology of what he/she hears, observes, experiences and senses. The therapist is also willing to enter into a dialogue with the client called 'the I and thou' of the relationship, which demands the therapist to be congruent. Postnatally depressed mothers will frequently find it hard to make contact with the therapist. The Gestalt 'contact cycle' will pinpoint where the interruption in this contact process occurs, to make the most appropriate interventions.

Support groups

Current literature suggests that support groups are one of the most important and effective treatments for women suffering from postnatal depression. The most common approach appears to be to offer ongoing and 'open-ended' groups. A social group has several definitions and indeed several functions.

A group has been defined as a situation in which the members share common motivation or goals. The members join the group with the hope, or belief, that in doing so they will fulfil some need. Some feel that a group has organisational properties, with group members having certain roles and status. As a result, the relationships tend to be more structured than is the case with individuals drawn together on a random basis. The group can also generate interdependence of group members where individuals believe that if something affects one person, then it also affects others. The significance of so-cial interaction between group members enables them to communicate with each other on a frequent regular basis and this interaction tends to be face-to-face rather, than indirect. Sustained face-to-face interaction requires both common motivations and a degree of organisation of relationships between group members. Furthermore, a degree of interdependence between group members seems to be a more likely consequence of sustained face-to-face interaction. Groups help to satisfy the individual's basic need to affiliate with others.

Mothers' support groups

There appears to be overwhelming support for group intervention to help the de-pressed mother. As the research has indicated, groups have made a significant impact by decreasing the severity of the depression. One purpose of the group situation is to homogenise feelings and thoughts about the highs and lows of motherhood, and not to concentrate on the depths.

If the group is organised by health visitors, and has a structure, they can be both cost effective and efficient (Gordon *et al.*, 1995). Although the actual philosophy behind group work in the prevention of postnatal depression has not been measured, factors indicate that the self-esteem and mood state of women have been greatly enhanced. As each mother is an individual, so each mother's emotional response will be different and group membership will not suit everyone's needs. A skilled worker should be able to introduce certain elements of psychotherapy or use a therapeutic system to enhance the group function as a whole. This would complement the group and perhaps appeal to more mothers. If the main component of the group is to share experiences and benefit from each other's examples, this will be therapeutic in itself. As in most life situations, the threat of exposing innermost feelings to strangers is not always welcomed.

Pitts (1999) described the success with her health visitor-led group. Her evaluation suggested that the majority of mothers found discussion and having the opportunity to empathise with their peers a positive factor, coupled with the advantage of an alternative to their domestic isolation. The overall running of the group was both effective and cost-efficient in helping women through postnatal depression. A few mothers complained that the group situation made their symptoms worse but the positives outweighed the negatives. These findings are further supported by Gutteridge (2001) and an American study by Ugarriza (2004) that consider that as little as three sessions may be sufficient for mothers.

There is sound evidence to support the role of group exercise to help reduce levels of depression May (1995) used the technique of exercise and relaxation to examine mothers' perceived benefits. The aim of the group was to teach depressed mothers how to tone up muscles, using exercise and lively music to enhance their well-being and reduce stress levels. The programme was specific, coordinated and involved the help of a physiotherapist and a dietician to discuss healthy eating habits. Evaluation of this programme showed that although some mothers felt apprehensive about meeting strangers, most reported an improved feeling of well-being as a result of the exercise and half of the mothers said they exercised at home as well as in the group. However, the opportunity for discussion as an activity was rated higher than both the exercise and relaxation, as it is this that improved the feeling of well-being. The majority of mothers reported that their partners had noted a positive difference in them, since joining the group. The study concluded the importance of peer-group social contact is that it provides the opportunity for women to have baby-free time for themselves.

Field *et al.* (1996) described a group of postnatal adolescent women who received ten thirty-minute sessions of massage therapy or relaxation, over a five-week period. Although both groups reported lower anxiety levels, following their first and last therapy sessions, only the massage groups showed behavioural and stress hormone changes, including a decrease in anxious behaviour, pulse and salivary cortisol levels. A decrease in urine cortisol levels suggested lower stress following the five-week period for the massage therapy group.

Support groups are usually successful in engaging first-time mothers and in reducing their prevalence of depression. However, meetings for second-time mothers are sometimes poorly attended as some women may feel the group situation is more damaging than helpful and may avoid it in the initial stages of their condition. It must also be remembered that the emotional state of the woman may cause her mood state to be lowered. In this situation, her cognitive reasoning will be impaired and therefore her suitability for group participation is questionable. Nevertheless, it is important to recognise that a fairly simple programme has a significant impact on the prevalence of depression in the first three months after childbirth.

Men's support groups

The prevalence of men's support groups tends to be sparse and this is particularly sobering when the lack of them has been reported in studies (Huang & Warner, 2005). Morgan (1997) described a group programme for depressed mothers and their partners in Australia. Here the issues surrounding anxieties and feelings about their partners, mothers and infants were addressed. The men expressed the opinion that the added responsibilities towards their new situation only resulted in an increase in tension and family strife. The object of the programme was to help men understand the reason for this behaviour as well as looking at strategies for dealing with it. A psychotherapeutic and cognitive behavioural approach was used. The results showed an increase in men's self-esteem and a decrease in their levels of distress.

Alternative treatments

Hypericum perforatum (St John's Wort)

There are few specific studies which examine the effects of *Hypericum perforatum* (St John's Wort) on postnatal depression but studies of the general population have shown it improves the mood state, sleep patterns and appetite in cases of mild or moderate depression. One study failed to support the efficacy of *H. perforatum* in moderately severe major depression. It was acknowledged that this may be due to low assay sensitivity of the trial, but the complete absence of trends suggestive of efficacy for *H. perforatum* is noteworthy (HDTS Group, 2002).

St John's Wort contains concentrated plant extract; however, there is neither regulation nor standardisation on the quantity of extract in each tablet. As it is sold as a food supplement it is not subject to the rigorous safety checks of other forms of medication and treatment and its use is unregulated (Linde & Mulrow, 2004).

Although most of the chemical constituents have been identified there is still uncertainty about the rest. There is a possibility it may enhance the neurotransmitters, of which serotonin is one, and that St Johns Wort may reduce the supply of the protein interleukin 6 which has the propensity to reduce levels of certain hormones (NCCAM, 2007). Common side effects include nausea, diarrhoea, confusion, dry mouth or tiredness. In some instances headaches and a loss of libido has been noted (Shelton *et al.*, 2001).

The lack of rigorous research means St John's Wort as a treatment is not recommended by any medical or national guidelines. As there is a dearth of information on the effects on the foetus or infants, it is also not recommended for pregnant women. As there is little known about the interaction with other drugs and data on its safety during breast-feeding is limited, it cannot be recommend for breast-feeding mothers (Hendrick, 2003). Ideally, mothers should be advised to inform their general practitioners should they choose to take St John's Wort.

Dioscorea villosa (Wild yam)

It has been claimed that the addition of plant sterols and sterolins to the diet is a proven treatment of postnatal depression. Scientific research and clinical trials suggest that yam is capable of improving health and well-being. The whole dried root helps to maintain a balance of hormones. Yam contains plant hormone precursors, which help in the production and balancing of progesterone and oestrogen. The application of wild yam cream, which it is claimed mimics the structure of progesterone, is suggested to alleviate the symptoms of postnatal depression. Further evidence suggests that yam consumption can normalise the production of the adrenal cortex hormones. The essence of the action of yam appears to be in facilitating the production of dehydroepiandrosterone. There were, however, no scientific studies to support the claims.

Geranium

Geranium was once planted around homes to keep evil spirits at bay and was considered an excellent healing plant. It is reputed to balance the emotions, and also have the ability to act as an antidepressant as it can uplift the body, mind and emotions. It may be used either as a bath or massage oil, or as a vaporiser. Its properties make it useful for the menopause and PMT, as well as having a tonic effect on the liver and kidneys.

Light therapy

Treatment using 'bright light' was advocated in one study. There is no evidence of adverse effects in pregnancy, making it a suitable alternative to medication in the antenatal period (Oren *et al.*, 2002). In the open trial, 16 pregnant mothers with major depression were treated with three to five weeks of light therapy. They were exposed to daily bright light therapy (10,000 lux) for 60 minutes, starting during the first ten minutes of awakening. The light therapy was well tolerated, with only two patients developing nausea, but this diminished when there was a reduction in duration of light exposure. The study demonstrated that morning bright light therapy had the propensity be an effective treatment for antenatal depression. When compared with people who suffered from seasonal affective disorder (SAD) the mothers appeared to have a more gradual improvement in depressive symptoms. The study found, however, that after three weeks of treatment remission rates were similar. This posed the problem of an ideal length of time of the treatment and further study has been recommended.

To develop the theory further, light bulbs which do not transmit blue light rays have been manufactured for use in the nursery, with the intention of helping to help prevent post-partum depression. It is postulated that melatonin, produced by the pineal gland, starts to flow at night, during which time the eyes are closed. The flow increases to reach a maximum peak approximately halfway through the night. Should the mother have to wake during the night to attend the infant, then a light is switched on and the production of melatonin is suppressed. The continuous disruption of the sleep pattern alters the flow of melatonin and may totally disrupt the circadian flow, which has been known to lead to depressive symptoms. However, it is only the blue rays in the light which cause this and once they are obscured the pineal gland can continue to work. Researchers have worked to develop not only light bulbs but glasses for mothers to wear which block out the blue rays (Mackenzie & Levitan, 2005).

Exercise therapy

Exercise therapy has its critics as to whether it is a realistic option for pregnant mothers. The literature is sparse, but it has been argued that it may be more effective when used with other conventional treatments (Manber *et al.*, 2002). It is becoming more popular to prescribe exercise for mothers who suffer mild to moderate depression. Some primary care teams have established contracts with local leisure centres in a bid to encourage mothers to become more active within the community by joining a gym or taking part in group exercises. There have been few side effects reported and the benefits appear to outweigh any negative ones.

It is well documented that physical exercise which results in weight loss can help to reduce the risk of developing heart disease, stroke and diabetes by 50% and the risk of premature death by up to 30%. Maintaining an exercise routine is recommended as part of the management of a healthy lifestyle. Exercise is becoming increasingly popular as a treatment for depression. The Department of Health has recognised that people who lead an active lifestyle have a reduced risk of suffering from depression, though there is evidence to suggest it can also improve other forms of mental disorders. It is believed it can improve mood state and anxiety as the act of physical exertion can improve sleep patterns and improve mental as well as physical agility. People who go to the gym on a regular basis report that it is one of the most effective ways of improving mood states. Those who are physically active are said to be more satisfied and happier with their lifestyle.

The effect of exercise has been the subject of research for several decades and there have been several reasons proposed about why it should benefit depression. In 1992, Veale *et al.* looked at the efficacy of two aerobic exercise programmes which were combined with the traditional treatment for depression. It was found that there was no specific improvement in the patients in either group nor was there any correlation between the extent of their physical fitness because of the exercise or an improvement in their condition. A later meta-analysis by Craft & Landers (1998) found that exercise was indeed beneficial. Whatever the findings, exercise appears to be growing in popularity with both men and women as leisure centres become more sophisticated. It is not only the exercise machines which are attractive but the other leisure activities and treatments which are available, all designed to enhance the body and soul.

It is a paradox that although it may not have been the main purpose for the institutions and mental asylums, they did offer the solitude and comfort that could not have been gained in the towns or villages. Today many of the old buildings are occupied by health clubs and complexes which are designed to entice healthy men and women to the promise of a more relaxed and regenerated body, offering the wealth of alternative treatments to repair and restore, something that was denied to the chronic patients whose 'home' it was for many years.

'Exercise on prescription' not only encompasses a treatment for physical ailments but is now included for mental health disorders, in particular anxiety and depression (Hawkins, 2001). It may act as a distraction from negative thoughts or the social interaction with other participants may enhance well-being. There may also be physiological effects of the changes in the endorphin and monoamine concentrations. Fox *et al.* (1997) found that in the UK the rates of compliance with exercise on prescription vary greatly between 20% and 50%.

Lawlor & Hopker (2001) presented the findings of their study that also confirmed similar findings to the previous meta-analyses. They found no association between the exercise and the variation in the results between the studies, which indicated that aerobic and non-aerobic exercise has a similar effect. Work by Annesi & Westcott (2001) demonstrated that the immediate short-term improvement in mood following an episode of supervised exercise can predict the likely improvement in mood state after a ten-week training programme. It is difficult to replicate this type of study accurately because of the conflicting variables. Their study confirmed that it was not possible to determine the effectiveness of exercise in the management of depression from the evidence which was available. However, exercise as a form of therapy should not be discounted as the social and emotional, as well as physical well-being should be considered. Physical benefits may include an increase in the endorphins and serotonin, which will enhance sleep patterns, improve the mother's memory and help the level of depression. The cerebral blood flow and core temperature is increased and there is a reduction in any muscular tension and neurotransmitter efficiency. The benefit to her emotional well-being will include an improvement in her perception of confidence or a confidence about her body and its capability. The advantages are an improvement in the mother's body image which can facilitate a desire to continue with the programme and finally a sense of achievement. This might be one of the only areas in her lifestyle that the mother is able to control.

Intensive training programmes are recommended but the actual type of programme has to be tailored to meet the needs of the mother. However, it is worth remembering that the symptoms of the depressive condition experienced by the mother may make physical exertion difficult and any failure to comply with or fail to complete any prescribed training programmes may make the mother feel even more guilty and further damage her self-esteem. However, despite the minority of side effects, exercise appears beneficial and there is no doubt that exercise is relevant and probably effective in some form in most depressive disorders.

Green therapy

Following on from the importance of exercise it appears that 'ecotherapy' is increasingly becoming one of the more popular suggestions for improving mental well-being and the treatment of depressive symptoms. It is based on the concept of taking gentle exercise in an area which is surrounded by greenery (Pretty *et al.*, 2007). It could be a walk in the park or a trip to the countryside, where trees and green fields dominate. It is postulated that one of the main reasons for seasonal affective disorder (SAD) is the lack of green during the autumn and winter months.

The colour green occupies more space in the colour spectrum visible to the human eye. It is pervasive and is used as a background for many other colours. Colour therapists suggest green translates as peace and tranquility and it is recommended as a background for living rooms to help alleviate nervousness and anxiety.

A visit to a 'care farm' has already been prescribed throughout some parts of Europe, where a holiday at a farm is believed to have a therapeutic effect. 'Green care' is defined as the utilisation of farms as a base for promoting mental and physical health. It is intended that the constituents of a farm, the animals, fields, woodlands and gardens are used for recreational and work activities. Currently, the main clients are people with learning difficulties, mental health problems, or those suffering from social exclusion. The idea is gaining popularity across Europe and the number of care farms is increasing. In the Netherlands it is estimated that the number of farms have increased by 500% in the past five years. Care farming is still in its infancy in the UK and there are approximately 43 existing farms. The National Care Farming Initiative is an organisation which has been developed to support new and existing farms.

In the absence of care farms, alternative means are recommended. There is growing evidence which indicates that exposure to nature can make a positive contribution to health and help people to recover from existing stressors. In the study by Pretty *et al.* (2007) the majority of people felt less tense, had decreased levels of depression, and felt their self-esteem and mood state had improved following a 'green' walk. This contrasted with people who felt their mental state deteriorated when they spent time in an urban area. There are ways of benefiting from ecotherapy without being outdoors. Looking through the window at a garden, viewing a picture depicting a country theme, or looking at a photograph with plant images are all reputed to help to improve mood states. The most powerful therapy, however, is actually participating in an activity which includes gardening, horse riding or taking a bike ride in the country.

Although it may not always be practical for a mother and her infant to visit green space, they might be encouraged to visit a park or garden to help boost self-esteem and well-being if only for a limited amount of time. If this could be supported on a regular basis, it is suggested that there might be long-term benefits. All of this is emerging research and there is little definitive proof that it works, but mental asylums were rarely built in urban areas and the majority were distributed within the surrounding countryside. Each was self-contained and managed with its own farm on which the patients, particularly the long-term patients suffering from chronic conditions, were expected to work. Patients often had the liberty to roam freely in the extensive, usually well maintained grounds.

Mental health organisations are recommending ecotherapy as a valid treatment for mental disorders and that general practitioners should consider prescribing it as a treatment option, as they currently do for exercise programmes. It is also advocated that there should be reflection about how the future of mental health is managed and consideration given to the part that care farms will take in this concept. The notion that mothers will benefit from a care farm is probably impractical, but perhaps a more sophisticated escape to green spaces may be considered in the future, particularly as it is forecast that within the next decade the number of homes in urban areas will exceed those in rural areas.

Pram walking

Probably the most effective and most natural form of exercise a mother can take is to push her infant in a pram. Pram walking with a supervised group of peers may provide an alternative or complementary therapy. It is postulated that pram walking intervention programmes have the potential to enhance personal and emotional well-being. However, there is limited published research on the effectiveness of an organised pram walk for postnatal depression. In an attempt to address this, Armstrong & Edwards (2004) assessed the benefits of a pram walking as an intervention programme for those mothers who had experienced postnatal depression compared to similar women with no symptoms of depression. The findings showed that the mothers in the intervention group improved their fitness levels and also reduced their symptoms of depression significantly more than those in the other group. It was suggested that the exercise had a direct impact on the mothers' well-being.

The popularity of pram walking is increasing and most mothers view it as a social event as well as a therapeutic session. Many groups are springing up around the country. In some areas it has gained the reputation of being a 'power push' or a 'run for fun'.

Lullabies

One tradition that appears to have faded into the annals of time is soothing or singing an infant to sleep. Research is emerging which suggests that this has a therapeutic effect on both the mother and the infant. There is a plethora of information about the importance of music as a mood enhancer and stabiliser. Music therapy appears to be gaining in popularity throughout residential homes and long-stay wards in hospitals. It is part of a regimen of treatment in psychogeriatric and geriatric wards, in particular, but also where there are people with head injuries, severe mental illness and special needs. It is intended to help those who find it difficult to communicate verbally to express themselves in a variety of different ways.

Feelings and emotions can be expressed through the music, without the use of words. In a safe environment it is then possible for the patient or client to express any repressed or complex emotions in a contained and therapeutic way, allowing them to face their fear or anger and then to manage it more effectively. The interaction and relationship between the therapist and the patient helps to promote communication and as a result enhances self-esteem, self-awareness and ultimately improves well-being.

The therapy involves the use of percussion instruments, a bongo drum, triangle, cymbal, maracas or any instrument that will be easy to play, hold and move. It does not involve learning to play the instrument, just to understand how music and rhythms can be produced and helping to understand how this makes the patient or client feel. Often sessions do not require the use of a musical instrument and the therapist and client are able to sing and listen to each other. The music is often chosen to suit the individual's needs.

A study, which used music therapy with people suffering from a severe mental illness, found that music increased the quality of their life (Grocke *et al.*, 2006). They were able to enjoy leisure opportunities and had a more social environment. One major improvement was a significant improvement in the ability to make eye contact. The group composed a song, which they recorded and while they found this relaxing and enjoyed the experience, they also expressed a real sense of achievement.

Everyone has an innate ability to appreciate and respond to music and if the theory of music therapy is correct then a mother singing to an infant listening to a lullaby must have positive effects in a number of ways. The mother who sings her infant to sleep, the mother who perhaps sings for herself and the infant who is soothed by the singing both partake in the engaging ritual where the mother can gaze into her infant's eyes as he/she falls asleep.

The word lullaby originates from the French word *berceuse*, meaning 'cradle song'. The traditional lyrics often portray tranquil moments, *'when the wind blows, the cradle will rock,'* or *'rocked so gently by thy mother's arms'*. The words also help the movement of rocking back and forwards, a proven way of helping infants to sleep, if not by research, then by mothers' experiences. *'Slumber slumber, sweetest dearest treasure,'* *'Golden slumbers kiss your eyes,'* *'Bye Baby Bunting,'* are words that are meant to soothe and placate a troubled infant whereas *'hush a by baby'* or *'hush little baby'* have the rhythmic sounds of a heart beating, which infants find comforting. The actual wording of the lullaby is often a complex pattern of phrases.

For the music purists, the lullaby is typically written in a triple or compound meter. Tonally, they are simple and alternate tonic, the first note of a musical scale and dominant, the fifth degree of the scale and harmonies, with the intention of initiating sleep.

Mothers have the ability to attune their singing in response to their infant's needs. It is important to acknowledge that the infant is in distress and equally important to ensure that the infant is aware of his/her mother's empathy. This may be achieved by singing with a strong volume and vocal pitch. *'Hush little baby don't say a word mamma's gonna buy you a mocking bird[e] ...'* deliver a strong message of *'I am right here with you, I understand how you must be feeling[e] ...'*

One mother described it as: *'When my son used to cry loudly, I used to sing even louder. I think he was shocked that I could make more noise than he did[e] ... then he calmed down and I was able to lull him to sleep.'*

This connection with the infant's emotional state meant the distress was recognised, understood, acknowledged and accepted. Baker & Mackinlay (2006) in their study found that the mothers chose the same selection of lullabies to sing to their infants to familiarise them with the tunes, but more importantly to associate them with a safe and secure environment, which was conducive to helping the infant to sleep. There were also personal reasons for choosing the lullabies as well as their efficacy for their infant's needs.

The natural, naïve voice of mother and the simplicity of the words all provide a safe and secure environment for the infant. Lullabies heard by the younger children will also be remembered as a form of familiarity, warmth, time and probably love. Most people will associate and remember past emotional events with the words and tune of a favourite song rather than the words of a conversation. Dissnayake (2000) wrote of the importance of musical interaction between the mother and infant because the synchronisation produced between the couple enhances the feeling of harmony and contentment. While Field (1998) has suggested that interventions such as music and massage therapy have the ability to alter the mood of the mother and soothe the infant.

There are also therapeutic benefits for the mother, as she is able to relax and relieve her own anxieties. One mother described her embarrassment at singing to her infant:

> You don't hear people throwing out a song these days unless it is in front of the karaoke machine in the pub or they want to get onto a reality show. I could not sing in public, but when it is just my baby and me I can sing for as long as I like.

Custodero *et al.* (2003) suggested that musical interactions with children appear to be linked with the mother's mental state. They found that the more emotionally distressed parents were the less likely they were to engage musically with their children. Non-depressed mothers were nearly one and a half times more likely have a rapport with their children musically, than depressed mothers. It was also found that parents who sang or played music with their children were less likely to report depressive symptoms, be less frustrated and more responsive to their infants' crying. It may be postulated that the more musical interaction there is between mother and child, the more improved their emotional well-being.

The decline of the singing mother has seen the upsurge of commercial recordings, all proclaiming to enhance the infant's intellect, by improving sleep patterns and stimulating cerebral functions. A CD containing an arrangement of symphonies, especially for babies, is being marketed with the intention of playing them in the nursery or car. Papousak (1996) has argued that infants do not have the prerequisite cognitive skills to translate these complex harmonies and rhythms. However, the infant's perceptual capabilities when listening to music are said to be similar in terms of consonance, dissonance and recognising changes in the tempo (Custordero *et al.*, 2003).

Many of the classic lullabies have been recorded in the style of more populist music. The Beatles' *Good Night* and Billy Joel's *Lullaby (Good Night My Angel)* are a couple of the current ones.

Lullabies are common throughout cultures and each has its familiar, traditional version. In Southern India and Sri Lanka a lullaby is known as a *thaalattu* and in the Philippines it is called a *huluna*.

The results of a study by Custodero *et al.* (2003) found that over 60% of parents daily engage with a musical activity of some sort, but that this figure was disappointingly low and parents should be encouraged to participate in some form of musical input. It might be suggested that parents require education on the benefits of singing lullabies or sharing songs and music with their infants. Singing lullabies and communicating through the medium of song may be a positive way to empathise with their infant's emotional well-being and might enable mothers to cope with the pressures and stress of parenthood.

There is the danger that the art of singing and remembering the lullaby will be lost if mothers are not encouraged to use them, and pass on the art to their children. Often mothers do not even think about their use as, along with the reciting of nursery rhymes, they appear to have fallen into disuse. There is evidence to show that children who learn nursery rhymes learn to read more quickly but the efficacy of lullabies is lacking in sound research. However, if, as is now being discovered, there is a positive therapeutic effect of music then there is probably some great merit in singing infants to sleep, coupled with all the non-verbal rituals of holding, caressing, eye contact, tone and volume of song, pace and, most importantly, warmth. For the depressed mother this may be a difficult job to contemplate, but once achieved may have a very positive effect and is possibly more satisfying than putting on the vacuum cleaner or washing machine to create the background noise that is apparently so effective.

Swaddling

The practice of swaddling an infant to make it feel safe and keep it secure has been used for centuries. There is a succinct history of its use and there have been many versions and types of swaddling used. Examples can be seen in paintings of the Madonna and Child. One of the earliest references to swaddling was in the New Testament where the birth of Jesus is described thus: '*And she brought forth her firstborn son, and wrapped him in swaddling clothes and laid him in a manger; because there was no room for them in the inn*' (Luke: 2: 7).

In Ancient Greek and Roman civilisations the excavated tombs of mothers with their infants have revealed the infants wrapped in swaddling. Although the custom appears to have fallen out of favour in the Western world, many Eastern cultures and traditional societies still use it. It is thought it was originally intended to keep the infant's limbs wrapped in a cocoon to restrict movement to prevent them from flailing around with purposeless movement and hurting themselves (Ferber & Makhoul, 2004). There was also the presumption that the tightness of the wrapping would ensure the limbs would remain straight which would ensure that they grew correctly.

The infant is swathed in a cloth which is pulled tightly. It creates a slight pressure around the body which is designed to give infants a sense of security. It is supposed to mimic the pressure of the amniotic fluid, and recreate the familiar environment of the womb.

The benefits of swaddling must rely on the experiences of mothers who have testified to their infants sleeping and feeling more relaxed. However, a few studies have confirmed there are greater benefits. The most comfortable position for a swaddled baby in the crib is to be placed on the child's back. This conforms to the current advice to nurse infants on their backs to prevent cot death. It also sustains the infant's sleep and reduces the frequency of spontaneous waking and when they are awake the infants are generally more alert (Franco *et al.*, 2005; Gerrard *et al.*, 2001).

The traditional way of swaddling is simple and with a cooperative infant is easy to apply. A small (preferably) cotton or lightweight sheet is placed on a hard surface with one corner folded over. The infant is placed on its back with the neck resting against the fold. The left hand corner of the sheet is wrapped around the body and tucked underneath. The bottom corner is placed over the feet and the right hand corner is wrapped around the body, leaving the neck and head exposed. This was only meant to be used when the infant was placed in the crib for the night.

There have been arguments against its use as the cloth prevents the skin to skin contact so necessary for cortisol production. A further study found that when rats were swathed in cloth they had depletions in their serotonin and dopamine levels which caused them to become aggressive.

Today, the receptacles used to carry infants employ a length of cloth, dynamic tension and metal or plastic rings through which the cloth is secured. The cloth, usually strong, lightweight cotton, calico or silk, is wrapped around the mother's body from one shoulder to the opposite hip around the back and over her other shoulder. The end is threaded through the rings to make a buckle effect. The infant is placed in the pocket that is formed and the physics of the tension caused by the infant's weight allow the rings to lock the sling into position to accommodate and support the infant in a comfortable position. The position may be altered by pulling the fabric through the rings. The adjustability of the sling allows easy access to both the infant and the mother's breasts to assist the process of breast-feeding. A correctly fitting sling ensures the infant does not sag away from the mother's body, is no lower than the hip line and does not feel claustrophobic by being held uncomfortably tight.

The use of the sling on one shoulder is limited, as when the infant grows there is an asymmetrical distribution of weight and this can create an uncomfortable strain on the back of the mother. The better the fit, the ability and the quality of the fabric to carry the weight, the more evenly the weight is distributed around the back and shoulders, the greater the length of time the sling may be used. The wrap and Welsh shawl (Fig. 10.2) appear to meets those requirements. The length of fabric is longer (approximately two metres by one metre wide) than the sling but the type of fabric used is of the same quality and performs the same functions. The shawl is draped over the left shoulder of the mother, and while she is holding the infant the shawl is wrapped around the infant and pulled into the right hip and held in the mother's left hand. The other piece of the shawl is pulled around the mother's waist and tucked under the infant's body. The weight of the infant will stretch the fabric downwards but at the same time forming a comfortable pocket. This method of carrying babies enables both hands to be free and mothers are able to do domestic chores and carry their infant at the same time.

This tradition, found in Wales and some parts of the north of England is now unfashionable, yet many of the older generation will testify to the fact that it is still one of the most effective ways of soothing and nursing a fractious infant. This is evidenced by some grand and great-grandmothers who are seen walking the streets at night in an effort to calm their grandchildren. One mother admitted she often gave her daughter, now eight months old to her grandmother to help get her infant to sleep and allow her some respite. Many of the young mothers are reluctant to use this method as they view it as a cumbersome practice yet it appears the benefits outweigh any fashion statements.

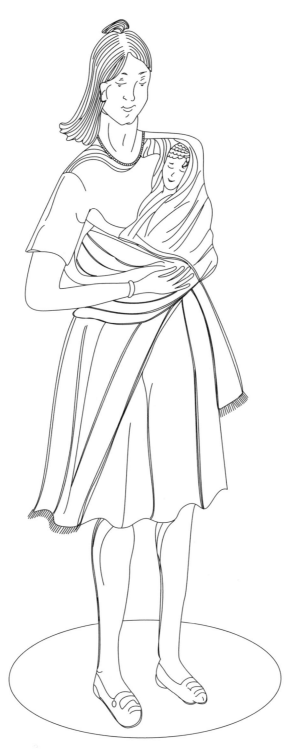

Figure 10.2 Welsh shawl

IVERPOOL JOHN MOORES UNIVERSITY
LEARNING SERVICES

This method of carrying an infant remains popular throughout other cultures and is seen in countries as diverse as Sweden and Africa It is not unusual to see an infant swathed in a cloth carrier being carried on a mother's (or father's) back, in the front, pressed against the breast or suspended just above the hip. In Africa they are called kangas, in the West Tiny Tush, Robojox, LittlePods (trade names) to name but a few.

Naturally, there are adverse factors for carrying an infant with a sling and other means of wrapping and there is a danger that if the carrier is incorrectly, insecurely, unsafely or inappropriately used the infant may fall out, collide with other objects, and risk being scalded with hot beverages held by the mother. Concern is often expressed that excessive nursing will make the infant overly dependent on the mother, or 'spoil' them.

The benefits of a correctly fitting wrap, however, are numerous, not least because it allows a closer, physical interaction between the mother and her infant. She is free to use her hands, or is able to breast-feed without encumbrance, which in turn leads to successful breast-feeding. It also allows the mother to tend to the needs of other children. The sling has the ability to support the back and shoulders and eases any discomfort in the mother's arms if this is the sole means of carrying the infant. Logistically it is easier for travelling and access as the mother and infant are one; therefore, hauling prams and other forms of baby carriers from cars or onto buses becomes unnecessary.

The infant can feel and capture the security of the mother's warmth and if held near to her heart may feel comforted by the rhythmic beat of it. The infant is also able to have a view of what is around them; this state of quiet alertness allows the infant visual exploration which is also vital for enabling social contact. It has been suggested that the more upright position of the infant improves the oxygenation of the infant. There has been concern about the risk to the infant's spine or hips but there is no definitive research around this and there is some evidence to suggest that if the older infant's legs are splayed around the mother's hips, this will assist in helping to prevent hip dysplasia.

When used shortly after birth swaddling helps to contribute to the infant's efforts to regulate themselves in terms of motor systems, balance and sleep organisation during the transition from womb to the their outside environment (Ferber *et al.*, 2002). It also improves infant growth and development through vestibular stimulation.

Research is emerging which supports the use of such methods of carrying an infant as an aid for reducing postnatal depression as it allows an increase in mother-infant interaction and assists in a positive bonding process. It has the added attraction of calming the infant, which must lead to the mother feeling more competent and satisfied with her parenting skills.

Feldman *et al.* (2002) looked at the impact of 'kangaroo care' on a newborn. This describes the process of skin to skin contact with their mothers – mimicking the way in which a kangaroo carries its infant in a pouch. They found that this had a very positive impact on the infant's perceptual-cognitive and motor development and on the parenting process. As the mother's mood and her interaction with the infant were improved it was postulated that this contributed to the infant's neurophysiological organisation and in turn improved infant development. It was suggested that this method had a direct impact on infant development. Other studies which examined the effects of holding infants found that the longer infants were held, the less they cried and as a result they were more alert.

Swaddling may also be a simple, non-pharmacological remedy for colic. There have been suggestions for the cause of colic, ranging from pathological to a healthy way of relieving stress. Recent research has found a correlation between colic and mild gastric reflux. This engenders the argument of whether the colic is exacerbated by the excess crying or the gastric reflux itself. Many health professionals will be familiar with the history of the occurrence of colic in the evening time, usually around the time of the television soaps *Coronation Street* or *Eastenders*, and it has been dubbed 'Coronation Street colic' It has been found that these are some of the programmes most enjoyed by mothers at the end of a stressful day. There has also been a study outlining the correlation between colic and postnatal depression (Akman *et al.*, 2006). It was found that mothers with insecure attachment style had a higher risk of having a baby with infantile colic. The mother may be less attentive to her infant's needs and provide poorer quality interventions. This may be misinterpreted by her infant who may become increasingly distressed, until he/she becomes almost impossible to console. Here swaddling may help to comfort and soothe the infant.

The act of crying itself is an adaptive behaviour designed to promote the mother-infant proximity. If an infant cries the mother will respond by coming over to the infant. This in itself provides the opportunity for social interaction. When the infant is being carried the proximity of the mother renders crying less of a necessity, therefore the infant will spend less time crying and more time being comforted. It is well known that excessive crying in infants can cause negative reactions in the mother and can erode any positive emotions and coping skills. If it is ceaseless it has been found that mothers tend to be less responsive and when they do respond their responses are more abrupt and of poorer quality.

Baby massage

Several studies have outlined the problems of mothers and their inability to interact with their infants from an early age. These children are penalised in later life as there is evidence to suggest that both their behaviour and intelligence are often affected. It may be argued that one of the factors missing from the early interactions with their mother was her inability to relate to and connect appropriately with her infant. Being helped and supported to take part in the process of baby massage might be one of the more positive ways for a mother to learn to understand, stimulate and as a result be able to feel, or display her fondness and ultimately affection, for her infant. At the same time it will enable her to see this as a pleasurable, even enjoyable experience.

One study which investigated the benefits of baby massage for mothers with postnatal depression and their infants found the results were unremarkable; however, there appeared to be better interactions with their infants (Higgins *et al.*, 2007). Conversely, Fujita *et al.* (2006) found that infant massage had a positive effect on the mother's mood state.

Small trials have found that just by attending infant massage classes the mothers felt there was a significant effect on the way in which they reacted with their infant and a considerable reduction in the level of depression they experienced (Higgins *et al.*, 2007). It is the opportunity to interact with their infants that appears to attract mothers to learn how to massage their infant and although there is little evidence on the long-term effects, anecdotally in the short term it appears to be enjoyed by mothers and infants alike.

It has been found that baby massage can be beneficial in other ways. Rice (1997) has claimed that massage can improve the infant's neuropsychological development. Scaffidi *et al.* (1990) found that touch therapy or massage simulated and improved the growth and motor maturity of preterm infants. It also helped the circadian rhythm to mature and increased the melanin secretion. This has been supported by work by Field *et al.* (1996) and Agarwal *et al.* (2000). Although there is little supporting evidence, it has been suggested that massage of the abdomen can relieve colic and constipation. Massaging the jaw can help the infant to feel more secure about swallowing or taking solids, whilst massaging the gums may alleviate teething pains. Gentle massage around the nasal passages can unblock tear ducts.

The method of massaging is not innate and many mothers have to learn the experience of massage. It is recommended that massage instructors follow the philosophy of the International Association of Infant Massage (IAIM), founded by Vimala Mc-Clure in 1986. Two instructors usually work together, one supervising the mothers and the other educating them. The instructors demonstrate massaging techniques on dolls which allows the mother to understand the skills and procedures before massaging their own infants. They acquire the skills of controlling the way they respond to the non-verbal signals from their infants to understand what is pleasurable and relaxing.

Massage has several therapeutic factors for infants as it appears to help colic and teething. It is also proven to help premature infants by improving muscle tone and stimulating the growth hormone.

Baby massage classes may be held in health centres or complementary therapy clinics. Often the courses last for five weeks, whilst others may offer a drop-in clinic where techniques may be learnt. Some simple guidelines may be accessed on websites (Netmums, 2007).

The method for massage is uncomplicated and can be easily carried out in the home environment. It is important to choose a time when there are no outside pressures, mealtimes or visitors. A dedicated time for each session can help to ensure that there are no stressors, usually shortly after the baby has been fed and both the mother and infant are relaxed. The room should be conducive to relaxation: warm, dimly lit and with calming music.

Grape seed or almond are the preferred oils. The infant should be placed on a changing mat, which has been covered with a towel, and stripped down to the nappy. All the mother's jewellery should be removed from her hands and the oil should be poured into her palms and her hands gently rubbed together to warm the oil.

The mother's hands are placed on the infant's shoulders and then gently stroked to the feet. This should be repeated about six times. Then the palms of the hands are placed on top of the infant's chest and stroked upwards towards the collarbone, shoulders and along the arms. This process is also repeated six times. The tummy is massaged in a clockwise direction with the fingertips and then the sides of the tummy are stroked from the umbilicus outwards. The legs are massaged in a similar way, moving from the top of the thigh to the foot, again repeating several times. The infant can then be turned over and massaged again. The shoulder to feet massage is repeated six times, after each section of the massage routine. Once the massage is complete, the infant should be wrapped in a warm towel.

In a Cochrane review on massage for promoting mental and physical health in infants under six months, it was suggested that there was some evidence on the benefits of the interaction between the mother and the infant and there was sufficient evidence to support the use of the procedure, particularly where the stimulation of infants may be poor. The review showed no evidence of any effects on cognitive or behavioural outcomes, infant attachment or temperament.

Despite the findings of the study there tend to be numerous benefits of infant massage, but most importantly it is the interaction between mother and infant to develop skills at determining the non-verbal cues given by the infant. The intimacy and relaxed manner of the procedure encourages both dependency and a mutual understanding between mother and infant, which appears to help the depressed mother to feel more positive about herself and her capabilities.

The role of laughter

In 1906, Israel Waynbaum, a French physiologist, published a radical theory explaining the function of facial expressions. This was a theory that defied conventional thought about emotions, including Darwin's dominant idea discussed in the *Expression of the Emotion in Man and Animals* (1872). Darwin argued that emotional expressions are innate and evolved from lower life forms. He gathered evidence which demonstrated that individuals express the same state of mind by the same movements. Waynbaum's research indicated that the facial muscles used for expressing emotions, for example smiling, anger or disgust, trigger changes in the brain blood temperature. He believed that the act of smiling had a positive effect on hormones, whereas the other expressions, like anger or disgust, had a negative one. Anything that an individual can do to change the hypothalamic temperature has subjective effects. Laughter is reputed to lower the levels of the stress hormones, cortisol, adrenaline and noradrenalin, which in turn boosts the mood and relieves stress. It also produces the chemical dopamine which has a role in motivation, desire and pleasure.

Researchers in the USA have recognised that laughter can help as a distraction for children who may have to undergo stressful or painful events in the hospital ward. The pilot study recognised the importance of humour for healing (Stuber *et al.*, 2007) and a programme is being piloted around the country.

Laughter usually occurs around four months of age. Stimuli which promote laughter may be auditory, social, tactile or visual. As the child becomes older the potency of the stimulation may become less effective, while other types become increasingly successful. The visual game 'peek-a-boo' and the auditory game 'boo' have limited appeal, and are often only enjoyed by infants. The stimulus makes greater cognitive demands on the infant and the changes in the forms and type of laughter often denote a meaningful interaction between the infant and the environment (Sroufe & Piccard Wunsch, 1972).

Young children generally enjoy surprises, pranks and the absurd. It makes them laugh with delight. They also revel in being tickled or swung around by the arms. Funny stories, rhymes and songs make them laugh and giggle as they learn to understand the importance of not being afraid. The cognitive factors seem to play an important role in the suggestion of whether they should emit fear or laughter. Children learn that the surprise that initially caused them to be fearful will dissipate when they feel safe and know that no harm will come to them. It allows the discharge of tension and is a learned way of coping with anxiety. This is why children enjoy the repetition of the experience. A similar experience is found in adults when they encounter the rollercoaster or see a horror film.

The added assurance of the parents helps to restore their faith and reduce anxiety. When an infant cries he pulls away and turns from the stimulus, yet when laughter occurs or there is a joyful social interaction the infant turns towards the stimulus. This occurs in adult life too. The importance of laughter and having the ability to laugh are fundamental and mothers should be encouraged to seek stimuli which would make them laugh. A video, film or television programme that invites comedy can only be therapeutic and have a positive effect on emotions.

The multidisciplinary team

The role of the nurse

In an ideal world every mother and her family would be aware of the potential dangers of suffering from postnatal depression or any other perinatal mental health disorder. They would also be aware of the management and treatment programmes available that make postnatal depression one of the most researched and studied conditions in the early maternal mental health period. However, the stigma of mental illness persists and despite the attempts of the more informed professionals the detection of the condition remains elusive. There is limited evidence for the reticence of mothers and the perceived barriers that prevent them seeking help.

A survey by Netmums (2007) and studies by Shakespeare *et al.* (2003) and Robinson (2003) found that when completing the EPDS (Appendix 2) mothers admitted to providing inaccurate information. They tended to avoid the negative answers, which were more likely to obscure their actual feelings. Poole *et al.* (2006) has suggested that the evidence that women find screening acceptable is ambiguous. The study by Netmums (2007) emphasised the fact that the EPDS questionnaire facilitated discussion around feelings they would otherwise have hidden, whereas previous research by Shakespeare *et al.* (2003) found that mothers preferred to discuss how they felt rather than completing a questionnaire.

All this ensures that for a multitude of reasons the mother may not have the opportunity to be rescued from her inner turmoil. It is in these situations that the perceptiveness of the nurse in primary care is invaluable. It is possible that the signs and symptoms of depression may not be particularly obvious until a full history is given from the mother. She may, however, present for a clinic appointment complaining of constant or chronic symptoms which have no obvious physical cause. These may be persistent headaches, which necessitate medication, or there may be vague stomach pains, usually consistent with the presentation of general psychosomatic conditions.

More probably, there may be excessive concern and a preoccupation with her infant's general well-being. She may complain about her infant's failure to thrive, the incessant crying or difficulties in feeding her infant. These may include difficulties taking bottle feeds by failing to suck properly, gulping or showing little interest in feeding. In some instances, discussion around the type of colic the baby suffers may be the precursor to discussing the mother's general well-being. This occurs in an otherwise healthy infant and the symptoms include intense, angry crying, where the infant becomes red and flushed in the face. The fists may be clenched, the back arched and the knees drawn up. They are often inconsolable and crying may persist for several hours.

There is little research into this phenomenon, yet anecdotal evidence from health visitors and other professionals indicates that the incidence of colic may be one of the first indicators that a mother is not coping. It often occurs during the evening and has been dubbed 'Coronation Street colic' as mothers often complain they are unable to watch their favourite television programme because their child is upset.

It is estimated that between 10 and 20% of all infants will suffer from colic. It usually occurs during the first few weeks and most cases will only continue until weaning occurs. The cause of colic is unclear and although there are several theories, scientists are unable to agree on one single cause. There is no specific treatment plan.

The most popular theory is that the infant suffers from stomach cramp, precipitated by an overactive gut which is too immature to fully digest food. Another theory is that the infant is rushed with their food, teat holes may be too large and milk pours out of the infant's mouth or the infant is forced to suck particularly hard, as the teat holes may be too small. This may not only tire the infant but cause unnecessary air to enter the bottle. The mother may forget, can't be bothered or does not recognise the importance of winding the infant to remove any excess or build up of air in the gut.

There is a possibility that the infant is sensitive to the lactose, found in cow's milk or in the case of breast-feeding mothers, any of the substances she may have eaten. However, there is little evidence to support these theories (Kalliomaki *et al.*, 2001; Lucas & St James-Roberts, 1998).

The important factor to be aware of is that the treatment and management of colic in all instances suggest that once all obvious causes have been eliminated the infant should be soothed and comforted. This is important not only for the infant but the distressed parents. Often the infant will react to the over anxious responses of the mother, and may in some instances become even more distressed, which in turn perpetuates the pain of the colic. The vicious circle continues.

The most effective suggestions have been to take the infant for a walk in a pram, as they appear to react to the slow steady movement. If this is not practical then often a drive in the car has a similar effect. There is no research into the effectiveness of the non-specific background noise, but often it has been found, and is recommended by several baby websites, that a running vacuum cleaner or washing machine left next to the infant's cot can have a calming result.

For the mothers and fathers it is suggested that they are diligent about their own well-being as an infant suffering with colic can be both exhausting and distressing, but also it is possible to be depressed and helpless. When the situation is acute, it is suggested that the mother lies the infant safely in the cot and leaves the room, where she is unable to hear the crying. This 'time out' enables the mother to relax and gather her thoughts. It is also advisable to enlist the help of family and friends, particularly when there have been chronic periods of crying. This may include leaving the infant with a grandparent overnight or having a friend to stay to take over the night feeds.

However, if no help is available or sought it is possible the intensity of the problem may escalate, if not add to, the myriad signs and symptoms of depression. Complaints of chronic colic or an inability to cope with the condition may be an indicator of the mother's mood state.

Another worrying sign may be that the mother may confide and complain that other health professionals, in particular the general practitioner and or the health visitor, are critical of her parenting skills. There may not have been any actual indication that she has been diagnosed as depressed, but she may feel that if she admits to any depressive symptoms there is a strong possibility her infant will be taken into care. The findings of one study by Kawamura *et al.* (1999) indicated that there is the potential for parents who are experiencing stressful situations and who have elevated scores on the EPDS (Appendix 2) in the post-partum period, to physically abuse their infant.

The nurse has several options to help the mother. The most effective is engaging in conversation in a non-threatening, yet non-colluding manner. It is important that the nurse does not give the mother the impression that the opinions of the other health professionals are misguided. The instigation of social as well as emotional support may also be relevant.

Until women's mental health is taken into the mainstream of care the management of the condition will depend on the commitment and enthusiasm of the primary care team. The current organisation of perinatal mental health services is inconsistent across England and Wales, and recommendations are often fragmented. However, it is hoped that the implementation of the NICE guidelines in 2007 will rectify this and allow for a more national coordinated approach.

The role of the general practitioner

Within their generic role of caring for mothers and their children, the general practitioner (GP) has an overall view of any previous or existing problems of mental health that may be present and may be in a position to detect and diagnose postnatal depression. There is simply no answer to the complex problem of diagnosis. The one luxury the GP does not have is time. In a surgery, which is dictated by a specified time per patient, it is difficult to extrapolate information within a seven-minute timeframe. Mental illness is insuperable. A prescription for a pill, which takes less time to swallow than for a therapeutic intervention to take place, is the more obvious solution. There are certainly chemical answers for most situations and it would appear that the treatment is the same as for psychotic episodes, but in smaller doses and in less time.

If a mother is mildly to moderately depressed then an antidepressant is not normally prescribed and other therapeutic interventions are considered. However, if a mother presents with a major or life-threatening depression then antidepressants have a very valuable role and are generally well tolerated. There is little evidence about efficacy or the overall effectiveness of antidepressant drugs for postnatal depression and little systematic data upon which to base decisions about the safety of breast-feeding while taking these medications. It is for these reasons that most manufacturers' data sheets carry warnings that antidepressants should not be given to nursing mothers.

This lack of research and the contradictory nature of the available data, often leads general practitioners to advise mothers not to stop breast-feeding. This raises the paradox of the added distress this may cause the mother. An alternative suggestion is to delay or reduce any pharmacotherapy. Any reduction in dosage has the potential to be ineffective. There are many confounding factors, for example the sampling methods used for drug levels, milk fat variations and timing of assessments, making the establishment of definitive treatment guidelines tenuous. There have been very few attempts at controlled, longitudinal investigations (Yoshida *et al.*, 1999).

Women with postnatal depression can be treated with fluoxetine which, when used with CBT, is equally effective in the short term. However, the long-term effects of antidepressants are not known, which is particularly important in breast-feeding women and their infants.

It appears that there is no clinical indication for a breast-feeding woman not to receive a tricyclic antidepressant (TCA), with the exception of doxepin, provided the infant is healthy and their progress is monitored. However, the ideal TCA for breast-feeding mothers is non-sedating with a shorter half-life, reduced anticholinergic effects, no active metabolites, highly protein bound and one that has been studied clinically in pregnancy and women who breast-feed. The TCA most closely meeting these criteria is imipramine. The use of SSRIs paroxetine, fluoxetine, and sertraline has been reported in breast-feeding mothers. Paroxetine is associated with low or undetectable serum concentrations in infants and may be preferable to other SSRIs in breast-feeding mothers.

Pathways of care and protocols are being established in the more enlightened surgeries and there is a clear idea of what to do next for the mother. The liaison between the GP, the health visitor and other members of the primary care team appears to be of the utmost importance. A study by Aitken & Jacobson (1997) highlighted the remarkably low level of knowledge, skills and familiarity with the Edinburgh Postnatal Depression Scale and suggested that there was significant evidence that GPs required training and development in this area. Over the past few years GPs have achieved a greater understanding of motherhood and the potential problems of childbearing. Many recognise the need for multidisciplinary working and are mindful of potential problems.

Most mothers are prepared to consult a GP and discuss the intimacy of their problems. Often when they felt their condition had been sanctioned and given a label by the GP they felt they could safely be 'depressed' (Hanley & Long, 2006). Their genuine need seemed to be to get well as swiftly as possible by whatever 'respectable' means were available and mothers will accept the medicalising of their condition.

It is ultimately the GP's responsibility for the mother and her infant. To that end it is important to secure a good outcome whether it is by pharmaceutical or psychotherapeutic methods. It may be argued, however, from a social perspective that the problem does not lie in the doctor's surgery because it may already be too late for all but a small minority of sufferers.

Some of the most commonly asked questions are:

(1) Can I take antidepressant medication when I am pregnant?
    This is usually not prescribed during the first trimester, except in exceptional circumstances where the mother may be suffering from bipolar disorder or a psychotic episode.
(2) How long should I talk the tablets for?
    Usually they should be taken for a minimum of twelve weeks and sometimes it is possible to be on antidepressants for a year.
(3) Can I breast-feed while I am taking them?
    Yes, in the majority of cases, though in some cases mothers feel so poorly it is better to discontinue breast-feeding and continue with the medication.
(4) What is the most common drug prescribed for postnatal depression?
    There have been good results with fluoxetine (Prozac), which comes from the SSRI group or the older form of antidepressants, which are the tricyclics TCAD group, e.g. Prothiaden.
(5) Can I stop taking the tablets as soon as I feel better?
    It is better not to stop them as soon as you feel better as sometimes the symptoms may return. It is advisable to complete the course of tablets and see the GP when they have finished. The GP will be able to discuss how you feel and either reduce the dose or the number of times you take the pills. If there is no improvement, the GP may increase the dosage of medication, suggest you see the health visitor for more help, or refer you for counseling or CBT.
(6) Are they addictive?
    No.
(7) What are the side effects?
    These depend on the type of drug prescribed and usually only occur within the first few days. You may feel tired, groggy, or your mouth may be dry but after a while any unwanted symptoms die down.
(8) Will it affect my ability to look after the baby?
    No, if you had no problems before. You may require some help for the first couple of days, though, to help you to get used to the medication.
(9) Am I more likely to get postnatal depression again?
    It is likely but at least you will be aware of the symptoms and will be able to get help. There is a 30% risk of this.
(10) My friend is on 20 mgs and I am on 100 mgs.
    They might be different types of drugs and so the doses may vary. Medication affects different people in different ways, so the doses may have to be higher for some.

The role of the health visitor

A health visitor is a trained registered nurse, with an extra year's training for the Diploma in Health Visiting. Some have the additional qualification as a midwife, paediatric nurse, school nurse, district nurse or psychiatric nurse. Since nurses have undertaken training within universities and now hold degrees, the health visitor may hold either a BSc (Hons) graduate diploma or MSc in Public Health and Specialist Public Health Nursing (SPHN) in order to be admitted to the third part of the Nursing and Midwifery Council register. The current training prepares practitioners to work in diverse ways. They need to apply knowledge, understanding and skill to prepare them for multi-agency collaboration and to enable them to respond to rapidly changing environments. They are also required to adapt to, initiate and lead practice development for implementing new systems of service delivery. These include a public health approach to promote health and well-being throughout the population. They undertake diagnostic investigations, health screening, health surveillance and evaluate specialist health care interventions to promote population health. It would therefore appear that they are well qualified to respond to the needs of mothers who have perinatal mental health disorders.

It is suggested by the *National Service Framework for Mental Health* that health visitors can contribute significantly to the management of postnatal depression by the early detection and treatment, which in turn could prevent serious mental illness. This of course only refers to the symptoms of a postnatally depressive condition and not the myriad of other mental health disorders that a health visitor may encounter, but it is understanding what is a 'normally healthy' situation for the mother that helps the health visitor identify and detect what and how a new mother is feeling.

It has been argued it is the innate ability, 'intuition', or even experience that helps the health visitor be vigilant and perceptive about the mother's general health. It is to this end that there has been argument about the introduction of the Edinburgh Postnatal Depression Scale (EPDS) as a means of detecting depression, as some may feel that it does not enable them to use their intuition. Often intuition itself is insufficient and studies have revealed that sometimes the judgement and detection of depression in mothers is unreliable. Briscoe (1986) found anomalies in some of the diagnoses offered by health visitors. In a similar study by Hearne *et al.* (1998) over ten years later the results were just as worrying, with 13 mothers regarded as depressed by the primary care health professional, whereas in the same cohort over 30 were found to be have signs of a depressive condition after completing the EPDS.

Often health visitors will claim they instinctively know when a mother is depressed. In the majority of cases this is probably true, but also it has to be remembered that there are still mothers with what they feel are chronic episodes of depression, levying criticism at health professionals for not recognising their plight in the early stages. This quote is probably a typical example of what mothers feel if they have been disappointed by their health visitor's lack of concern: '*My last health visitor was useless, I never saw her.*'

This probably reflects the fact that those who need a health visitor don't want one and those who want a health visitor don't need one. It is an unenviable conundrum. However, the main consensus of opinion is that the EPDS itself is enabling as it facilitates open, and if used correctly, free discussion with the mother about how she is really feeling. The tenth question in particular, if asked in a sympathetic and non-judgmental way, allows the mother the freedom to explore her feelings of self-harm.

It must also be remembered that health visitors have varying degrees of expertise in the management of postnatal depression. The EPDS has been translated into 28 languages, making it available to most mothers. This means the mother should be able to complete it independently, without the aid of the health visitor. However, if one of the questions is answered ambiguously the health visitor can check the answer with the mother. This is particularly important with question 10, which asks about self-harm. This can open up an honest discussion which might not have occurred if the health visitor had to ask the question. One mother found this very useful:

> *I'm glad it was spotted[postnatal depression]before I went completely mad. I didn't know who to turn to. When I started to fill in that form [EPDS]I knew I couldn't lie about how I felt anymore. The Health Visitor and I had a short chat. She asked to see me in a few days when she could spend more time with me. I saw her every week for 8 weeks, Thank God we did. I sorted out a lot of my life, thanks to her.*

Most mothers find the use of the EPDS acceptable and if a health visitor is distracted will often seek her out to verify or confirm the results of the 'test'.

If a mother should refuse to complete the form then this leaves an ethical dilemma of who actually owns the form and the primary purpose of completing it. Is it to determine the mother's emotional distress or establish her suitability as a mother? For a minority of mothers it is the latter and because of that they choose to falsify the results. Brown & Bacigalupo (2006) found that although health visitors believe they have identified mothers with postnatal depression that is not always the case, as sometimes they have contacted other services for help as they fear the health visitors may be more concerned with child protection issues and work in collaboration with social services to this end. Indeed, health visitors feel that this question has child protection connotations and, as has previously been discussed, it does raise some important questions. What if the mother is threatening to harm herself or the child? The most obvious answer is that this must be handled sensitively and put into perspective, otherwise how can mothers ever trust health visitors with their innermost feelings and know that they will be dealt with appropriately. Discovering the reasons for their distress and understanding what can be done to alleviate the situation will often be sufficient to prevent any escalation of the mother's feelings and any act she would otherwise perpetrate. In an effort to tackle any misconceptions about their intentions the majority of health visitors in the Brown & Bacigalupo (2006) sample reiterated their role as being concerned with family working not solely child protection.

> *I needed someone to talk to but I didn't know who. My husband said I had to see someone, but I knew if I went to the doctor, he would send me away to the hospital. When I went to the clinic, it was something the health visitor said about how I was feeling that upset me I burst into tears, I can't explain why, I just did. We got talking and then she explained to me what I was going through. I didn't feel afraid anymore.*

A leaflet has been produced from the evidence from a survey carried out by Netmums.com, which found that mothers were reluctant to admit to 'failing as a mother' because of the perceived consequences. The survey also recognised the importance of establishing a close relationship with the mother. The leaflet suggests that health visitors ask simple questions about the mother's lifestyle to establish if she feels isolated or anxious and to offer simple preventative measures like joining a support group, exercising or just being encouraged to talk while the health visitor listens.

How the EPDS is administered is as important as why. The form should be given to the mother and ideally she should complete it in the presence of the health visitor. It should not be given to the mother to take home as there is little guarantee that the mother will complete it, rather than someone else doing it for her. Neither should it be completed in the clinic situation where there is the risk that the mother may become emotional in a public area. The mother deserves to have the findings analysed in a sensitive and empathetic way, directly after she has completed the form.

The whole process should be calm and unhurried, allowing the mother space and time to complete the form. It usually takes a few minutes to fill in but at least ten minutes should be allowed for the feedback and a clinical interview to elicit what exactly the mother meant when she said 'I worry unnecessarily' or 'without good reason'. This often requires further analysis of what the mother really meant by those statements. Seeley (2001) recommends that using the EPDS '*going through the nine symptoms from the DSM1V to tease out more of a mother's experience and the effect on her life, in particular the persistency and pervasiveness of the depressive symptoms,*' will allow a more accurate assessment of the mother's mood state. It is equally important that it is not filed away in a drawer, in the hope that a more experienced health visitor will feel more confident and competent at interpreting the results.

Mothers who score just under 12 are offered listening visits and negotiate whatever help and support they feel is necessary. Cox *et al.* (1987) has proved that health visitors can deliver the intervention effectively and some health visitors are trained in the art, but not all. Some health visitors may offer open discussions, which have no set agenda, others may adhere strictly to a protocol devised by the trust or primary health care team, others may be somewhere in between.

Currently, in some practices the liaison between the general practitioner and the health visitor appears to be of profound importance when managing mothers' mental health. When the mother's care is undertaken successfully the general practitioner appears to have a greater understanding of the mother and some of the problems surrounding her depression. The majority of women when interviewed in studies do not express any anger or irritation when advised to consult the general practitioner and there was little resistance when complying with any antidepressant or other prescribed medication. In one study by May (1995) 90% of the mothers said it was beneficial to have a health visitor because they appreciated the support gained from this group of professionals. Gordon *et al.* (1995) also suggest that mothers trust the judgement of health visitors and are willing to be guided by their expertise. When all three worked in partnership, that is the mother, health visitor and general practitioner, the mothers reported that they felt the illness had been 'sanctioned' and given a label so that they could safely be 'depressed'. She was given permission to be ill. The purpose of this is to highlight how intervention of one informed person can, in some way, assist in managing the mother's depression. The fact that some professionals are not as competent as others may raise the possibility that the person might be more important than the professional role.

Of course there is the need for a holistic approach to the condition and it is the health visitor who, with the mother, is able to assess what her greatest needs are and how best she and her family can be supported. The help of a voluntary agency, such as Home-Start may be initiated or if that service is unavailable, a referral made to Sure Start. Social services may be contacted to provide family support. For the depressed mother with a toddler the opportunity for her child to attend a crèche for a few mornings a week might be the solution if she needs to have extra rest or respite. She may be eligible for financial support or home help services. In some areas the mother may be referred to a postnatal group, which is facilitated by the health visitor, and in some areas groups specialising in postnatal depression may be available. Other therapeutic approaches may also be considered. Encouraging pram walking, green spaces, aromatherapy sessions, herbal remedies, exercise and dieting can all be a part of the effort to help and support the mother while she is recovering from her postnatal illness.

Although there are pockets of excellent practice which offer mothers a first class service, on the whole it would appear that nationwide there are no clear organisational care pathways. There is a lack of awareness and coordinated approaches. Since the welcome introduction of the NICE guidelines on antenatal and postnatal mental health there appears to have been an overall effort to develop the existing mental health services in the delivery of care. Its aim is to establish collaboration within the professionals in primary and secondary specialist services to provide accessible and appropriate services for mothers and their families.

A report, *Towards Better Births: a Review of Maternity Services in England*, surveyed 5000 maternity staff and 26,000 mothers in England. It found that 42% of the trusts do have not access to a specialist perinatal health service for mothers with postnatal depression. The report also noted that there was inadequate staffing and there was little evidence of teamworking within this area. There is the added impact of the reduction in the numbers of health visitors (Adams, 2008) in the UK. This lack of mental health support for a mother suffering from postnatal depression and other perinatal mental health disorders is compounded by this shortfall in services. It appears that emotional well-being remains an area which requires greater investment, not only in time but in commitment. With an ageing workforce in health visiting and a deinvestment in services, the overwhelming evidence suggests that it is an area that requires immediate attention.

The role of the midwife

The midwife is either a registered nurse with a degree or diploma in midwifery or has a degree in midwifery.

Midwives have been identified as having a role to play in screening for and educating about perinatal mental health disorders. Yet there are still few studies into their experiences and preparation for supporting mothers. Research by Stewart & Henshaw (2002) identified that although midwives had some knowledge of the prevalence of perinatal mental health disorders and most felt they had a role in its management, they felt that their practice needed to alter and they would require more training to take on the role more fully.

Midwives may come into contact with a woman who has a pre-existing mental health disorder who would like pre-conceptual information or is already pregnant. A clear understanding of the woman's motives and her perception of the pregnancy are important, particularly if she has a history of bipolar disorder or a psychosis. The woman may have a history of self-harm or an eating disorder and each type of condition requires careful consideration on the management and treatment outcomes. It is a difficult task for the midwife to undertake, particularly when there is the burden of physical care. Nevertheless, the role is probably one of the most important in the primary care team as it is the midwife who is the first to establish a rapport with the mother. It is the wisdom of the midwife, which will often determine the best outcome for the woman and her foetus. Risk: the risk of relapse, the risk of medication, the risk of the physiological changes in the woman's body and the risk to her mental state are all considerations for the midwife. There is the added pressure of doing this in a culturally sensitive way which de-stigmatises the condition but also helps the mother to understand that if she should get pregnant or continue with the pregnancy, she and her family will receive all the possible help and support that current services will provide.

The family and partner may be aware of the mental health status of the woman but as has been previously discussed, the mother may not have disclosed the extent of her illness and this is something they may need to be made aware of in order to continue to support the woman during and after the pregnancy.

Whether the midwife is aware of any existing mental health condition or not, it is important that in communication with the mother the midwife asks if there is history of a mental disorder and if there is what type of disorder and whether a diagnosis was given. This is particularly important at the booking visit as any referral can allow sufficient time to alert all of the relevant specialist services and agencies. The woman may be able to give specific information about her treatment and past management which would make the referral process easier, but in the first instance the woman should be referred to the general practitioner for referral onto other services.

It is also important to enquire about the relationship between the woman and her current partner, the father of the baby or any other relationships within the nuclear family. In the light of research into mothers' coping mechanisms following the birth, it is also relevant to explore the relationship with the female members of the family, or anyone who is likely to be supportive during this time. Although this information does not need to be shared with the perinatal services, arrangements could be made with other agencies, such as social care and housing departments to alleviate dire social circumstances.

It is recommended by the NICE guidelines that in order to detect any form of mental disorder the two following questions are asked by the midwife at the booking clinic:

1) During the past month have you been bothered by feeling down, depressed or hopeless?
2) During the past month have you been bothered by having little interest or pleasure in doing things?

If the mother answers yes to both of the questions then a third question is asked:

3) Is this something you feel need or want help with?

If there is any doubt about the mental health of the mother then one of the self-report measures such as the Hospital, Anxiety and Depression Scale (HAD), or Patient Health Questionnaire 9 (PHQ9) could be administered.

If there are any concerns about the overall state of the woman's mental health then the midwife can discuss this with colleagues who may be more familiar with the mother's history or have greater experience in the field of mental health issues. If the concern continues then this could be raised with the general practitioner who will refer on to the secondary services. Any interventions or referrals should be recorded in the woman's notes. Once the woman is referred, the midwife continues her responsibilities and is able to offer a caring and supportive role. She is able to normalise the process for the woman and the non-stigmatising way in which she works will help not only the woman but the family to cope and come to terms with any future outcomes.

It is the responsibility of managers and senior staff to ensure that there is a clearly specified care pathway ensuring that all primary and secondary health care professionals know how to access assessment and treatment. All midwives should be acquainted with the types of mental health disorder and it is important that managers ensure that the midwives have the appropriate training, supervision and support. The implementation of the NICE guidelines in the future should ensure the ease of transition of the referral system and the care of pregnant women in general.

It is estimated that there is a 5000 shortfall in the number of midwives needed for the future care of mothers. With the increase in the number of migrants over recent years there appears to be an underestimation in the numbers of babies who will be born. In 2007, the Government underestimated the number of deliveries by 40,000 and already it has been reported that midwifery units have been forced to turn away mothers because of the rising demand. In 2002, 584,000 babies were born, but in 2011 the number is expected to rise to 660,700. Already the average amount of money spent per child is £2570, but there is disparity in the amounts around the country. In East Anglia it is £2061, whereas in the East Midlands it is £3,177. In 2006/2007 the Government invested £1.6 billion on maternity services and in 2008 extra funding totalling £330 million was promised over the next three years. As in all Government manifestos they believe the money will ensure that mothers have access to the best possible care and are guaranteed a full range of the choices available.

The role of the community psychiatric nurse

A community psychiatric nurse (CPN) is a registered mental nurse who holds an approved degree, advanced diploma, or diploma of higher education in nursing (mental health branch). A CPN is a fully trained staff or charge nurse who has had several years of experience working on psychiatric wards in hospitals and receives further training within an educational institution. The CPN may be trained in counselling techniques, relaxation therapy, art therapy, music therapy, relaxation techniques and how to develop coping skills and stress management skills.

During the 1950s the community psychiatric nurse (CPN) was a ward based nurse who was sent out into the community to follow up patients who had been discharged from psychiatric hospitals. Their remit was to administer medication and monitor the patient's progress. Since that time there has been a revolution in the way CPNs work in the community. Originally they worked with a consultant psychiatrist based in hospitals, but now work more autonomously, taking referrals from the primary care team as well as the psychiatrist. They now work in case management as a method of service delivery.

Understandably, CPNs primarily considered mothers with postnatal depression as part of the worried well and not within their remit. However, with the working of collaborative services it is now possible to have a much more joined up approach, with CPNs working in partnership with midwives and health visitors to deliver therapeutic care to mothers. Many CPNs will now see mothers with postnatal depression as part of their generic work. Health visitors who need advice, information or support when caring for a depressed mother can refer to the community psychiatric nursing service. Their wide exposure to mental health problems will enable the CPN to understand and make a sound judgement on the prognosis of the mother's condition, the interventions that may be necessary and advise on referral to the appropriate agencies.

It is envisaged that the CPN will be involved with the midwife in obtaining a psychosocial history in early pregnancy. Detailed information should be obtained on the circumstances surrounding the present pregnancy and the implications for the rest of the family. Examples could be overcrowding or financial hardships. In this way women who are at risk may be identified early on and their mental health can be monitored closely.

In the case of more severe depressive symptoms or if the mother develops a psychosis, the health visitor may feel threatened or limited by her capabilities to help the mother. Ideally, the psychiatric team will be aware of any mother who has a history of bipolar disorder or schizophrenia and systems for therapeutic support and medication will already be in place. The psychiatric team may have been alerted by the midwife of any history of a psychiatric disorder or potential disorder the mother may have had. Once again, they may have made arrangements to monitor the mother's progress to ensure that the mother has access to continuing support. Occasionally, the system breaks down and the health visitor may inadvertently be exposed to a severe situation that she feels she is unable to manage.

In severe depression or acute disorders the CPN can be the key worker. A CPN usually visits mothers in their home but they also have clinics based in health centres or GP surgeries. They monitor the mother's progress and ensure she takes her medication and observe for any side effects or deterioration in mental state.

The CPN has the key skills of being able to establish and sustain a therapeutic relationship with the mother by using interpersonal skills and counselling techniques. They can monitor anxiety and stress levels. They are also able to refer the mother on to an appropriate system of help. This may require admission to a mother and baby unit, whose staff include psychiatric nurses, or arranging for a domiciliary visit by a psychiatrist. Often a joint visit is arranged with both the CPN and the health visitor. They are able to see the mother in her home and take a team approach to discuss, with the full involvement of the mother, her needs and how she and her family may be supported. CPNs are also a valuable support when there are postnatal support groups arranged specifically for depressed mothers. Here the CPN can offer suitable, useful suggestions about how the group should be run and what to consider, ensuring it provides a safe, therapeutic haven. The CPN's support is not limited to the midwife or health visitor and can include all members of the primary care team.

Where the mother fears issues of child protection, she may feel that disclosing her feelings to the CPN is a safer option, although the rules of child protection procedures also apply to CPNs.

There is sometimes the danger that once the mother is referred to the psychiatric services other agencies will absolve themselves of their responsibilities. This is when there may be a failure of communication and responsibilities can fragment and confusion prevails.

If the mother is unable to function properly the CPN can help her to attend a day centre, day hospital or community mental health centre, where she will be able to meet with others in a safe, secure and non-threatening environment. Some centres offer exercise classes, or creative pursuits such as painting or pottery, which offer a form of relaxation coupled with a sense of achievement. For mothers who have been acutely ill and who need to return to work there are work projects which can provide retraining or help to develop existing skills. For the more seriously ill there are specialist rehabilitation services.

Mothers with schizophrenia may benefit from a care programme approach (CPA) which is specifically designed for them. A care cocoordinator is responsible for the whole organisation of the care and treatment plans.

CPNs will also be able to engage with other family members and provide current information about the course of the illness and what the prognosis is likely to be. They will be in a position to help with the more practical daily chores and be an advocate for the family when they have to deal with other agencies. Often the CPN becomes the mainstay of the family and when working in multidisciplinary teams are very valuable resources, providing information about mental health issues, not only to the family but also assisting and advising other members of the team.

Sometimes there is blurring of roles between the general practitioner, health visitor and CPN, but this has it advantages and disadvantages. The mother may benefit from the wider perspectives of care and support which may help to address the uncertain causes of postnatal depression whilst, at the same time, focusing on the complexity of the problems which present for the mother and her family (Hardy & Parke, 1996).

The role of the occupational therapist

Occupational therapists (OTs) have a BSc degree or postgraduate qualification in occupational therapy. This will take either three or four years to achieve on a full-time basis. They may work either privately or in the NHS. Occupational therapists are often a part of the community mental health team and mothers who are severely or chronically ill may be referred to them as part of the care plan. This care has strategies designed to help if the mother's condition deteriorates or there are logistical difficulties.

One of the main aims of the occupational therapists is to actively engage mothers in purposeful activities which will help to promote, regain, maintain and maximise her mental health and well-being.

A thorough and valid assessment is the basis for all interventions by the occupational therapist, to determine the needs of the mother and her goals and expectations. A mother suffering with the more severe forms of postnatal depression may find it difficult to manage daily activities. The occupational therapist works with her to help her accomplish everyday tasks. Occupational therapists can help develop existing skills and assist with socialising the mother back into the community, particularly if they have been depressed for a significant amount of time. Planning achievable activities is one of the main goals. Agreed goals that have measurable outcomes are established and these are linked to the objectives of the care plan.

Usually the community mental health team has meetings, approximately every three to six months to review the care plan. These often involve the mother, carers or members of her family, as appropriate, the psychiatrist, care coordinator and other agencies concerned with her care.

The role of the perinatal psychiatrist

The psychiatrist is a trained doctor with an additional six years in speciality training. A perinatal psychiatrist has an interest in the management of antenatal and postnatal mental health disorders. This is a relatively new speciality and perinatal psychiatry is a developing area, with services being established around the country.

Perinatal psychiatrists work in outpatient clinics with assessment and follow-up of patients referred to in the service. There are regular reviews of inpatients in the mother and baby unit, and the general wards or the day hospital. They provide information to GPs on the use of psychotropic drugs during pregnancy and whilst the mother is breast-feeding. Urgent assessments are performed on pregnant women or mothers who have recently delivered a baby if the obstetric team or the GP have concerns about the mother's mental health. The perinatal psychiatrist has an important role in education, both in the professional and public arena. Perinatal psychiatry was a special interest group within the Royal College of Psychiatrists until recently, when it became a section of the college.

Specialist perinatal mental health services

In the UK over half of the primary care trusts have identified a clinical lead or manager responsible for overseeing care in perinatal mental health. There are a similar number of trusts who have a protocol for the care of women with an existing mental disorder, and nearly three-quarters of them have a policy to enquire about the mental health status of the women during both the antenatal and postnatal period. Only one quarter of primary care trusts have a fully developed and implemented policy for ante and postnatal mental health (NICE, 2007).

Inpatient treatment is also variable. A significant majority of trusts have access to either a mother and baby unit or a specialised service within their catchment area. Many, however, have to use psychiatric beds outside the trust which, in many instances, are general beds with a facility for admitting infants.

For a mother with a mental health disorder either during her pregnancy and/or the postnatal period, the current specialist service provision around the country is very patchy. The sizes of specialist perinatal teams also vary. Some may have over five or more members whilst others may have less. The composition of multidisciplinary agencies varies considerably as some teams may not have access to a psychologist or psychiatrist on a regular basis. Some teams have specific protocols for the types of disorders which are managed, and in some instances that does not include alcohol or drug related problems. Some teams have a limited capacity on the number and duration of home visits that they are able to offer, whilst others may visit the mother for up to a year postnatally.

The majority of mothers who have a mental health problem initially present to the GP or at the health centre, where they may be seen, assessed and usually managed by a health professional. The role of the professional has been discussed previously but the key message is that if the mother is seriously unwell or unable to be managed in the community without disruption to her home life, a referral should be made to the specialist perinatal team. Additionally, if the health professional feels the management of the mother's condition is beyond their or any members of the primary health care team's capabilities, then it is important that an appropriate referral is made to the team. This might be for advice, for example, on psychotropic medication, or for her continuing care to be managed by the specialist team. Mothers may be managed by the general mental health services, mental liaison services, perinatal specialist mental health services or any combination of these services (NICE, 2007).

The specialist mental health services are able to provide a service which is relevant to the needs of the mother either following the birth of her infant, during the pregnancy, or prior to conception. This is particularly important if the mother has a history of bipolar disorder, has a psychosis or has had a psychotic episode, has a history of depression, or self-harm, or drug, alcohol or substance abuse, or an eating disorder. The mother may not have been hospitalised in the past, but usually her mental state merits sufficient concern to ensure that her progress is frequently monitored and assessed by the team.

For mothers who wish to become pregnant for a second or subsequent time there is the provision of specialist consultation and advice to provide her with the best possible options for her and her infant. The mother will be made aware of the risks she may encounter. A reduction or increase in medication may be necessary to stabilise her mood state and this may have negative effects on her infant. The care and support the mother can expect during this period may also be outlined. This may include the provision of intensive interventions following the birth of the infant, whereby the perinatal psychiatrist, obstetrician, community psychiatric nurse, midwife and maternity services, and primary care services, which include the health visitor and GP, collaborate as a team to formulate a pathway of care which supports the mother, her infant and her family during the initial days. Depending on the needs of the mother, a longer term strategy is employed, whereby there is regular liaison with members of the team and the mother to discuss and monitor her progress and plan for future care.

Mothers who have no history of mental disorder but present with a mild to moderate disorder following the birth of their infant are also considered by the team, particularly if she has been on medication but is not responding to the regime she has been prescribed. Should she require hospitalisation her care may be managed either in a specialist perinatal unit or a general ward with specialist perinatal support.

For mothers with moderate to severe mental health problems who need to be hospitalised, the team can liaise with the maternity and primary care services to ensure the continued well-being of both the mother and her infant. Discharge planning is of equal importance to ensure the mother has access to any social or voluntary organisations she should require when she leaves hospital.

The NICE guidelines (2007) recommend the following principles when considering the service for the future.

The detection of any perinatal mental health disorder should be effective, assessed and referred to the appropriate services with the minimum of delay. Ideally, there should be collaboration between the primary care, mental health and social care services, allowing the mother free access to all services, which are located in fairly close proximity to the community in which she lives. There should also be an element of choice, which allows the mother to select the service which is the most appropriate to meet her needs and that of her family.

Treatment plans should be evidence based, with the mother given accurate information about her medication and how it may affect her, her infant, her family and her wider social circle. She should also have sound advice on her disorder so that she may understand the wider implications and mentally prepare for them, if necessary.

Professionals should have the opportunity for further education and development to understand the social and psychosocial implications of a perinatal mental health disorder. Further training in the use of screening tools to detect disorders and to increase the provision of psychological therapies is also recommended.

In order for this to be achieved it is recommended that there is a specialist perinatal service in each locality. It is important to engage with local commissioning partners to commission and develop a managed clinical network for perinatal mental health provision. It is suggested there is a coordinating board to monitor referral and management protocols. Each professional should have a clearly defined role and be competent in their area of expertise. There should be an unambiguous pathway of care for service users with no service barriers.

It is recommended that there should be provision of units specifically designed for mothers and infants. It has been estimated that there should be approximately six to twelve beds in the mother and baby unit, available to a population which has between 25,000 and 50,000 live births. Each unit should have the full range of therapeutic services which are closely integrated and coordinated with the community mental health, maternity and primary care services.

Social services

A registered social worker (RSW) is required to register with the General Social Care Council (GSCC) and then regularly update their training. They can have post-qualifying awards in specialist, higher specialist and advanced social work. They work with people who have been socially excluded or who are experiencing a crisis. Their generic role is to support and enable autonomy for service users.

The health visitor, along with other agencies, works closely with social services. If the health visitor or the mother feels that extra help with social support is necessary, this can be arranged by a social worker. A referral is made, either by telephone or letter and the social worker arranges to visit the mother and her family at home. The number of services which may be applicable to the mother's needs can be negotiated.

Family aides are paid workers, employed by some social services. A family aide will work with families who are socially excluded or have specific needs. In the case of a mother with a perinatal mental health problem they will be able to help with domestic chores or help with child care issues by encouraging and enlarging on the appropriate parenting skills shown by the mother.

Should the mother require some respite care from either her infant or other younger children to allow her a period of rest or opportunities to complete any unfinished household chores, this can be provided by a registered childminder who can take care of the child on specific days. Social services may sponsor a place at a local crèche for a few mornings a week, or for older children they might arrange for them to go to a local nursery or playgroup placement. If transportation is a problem, this can also be arranged and paid for by social services or a charitable organisation.

In times of crisis the older children can attend summer play schemes and often holidays are arranged for children in need and the children may be eligible to go away for a week to a seaside resort or into the country.

Together with the health visitor, the social worker can arrange regular visits to monitor the progress of the interventions and to decide whether a reduction is required or whether the services should be increased. If the mother's concentration is impaired or she has difficulty in focusing on official paperwork, the social worker can offer her practical help to complete forms or help her to write official letters.

Stigma remains a problem and there is little that distresses a mother more than knowing she may be referred to social services, but once the mother understands that this is non-threatening she can benefit substantially from the services which are available. The social worker can often be an advocate for the mother by understanding her needs and liaising with other agencies. One of the main focuses of the social services department is the the Children's Act 1989 and the Children's Act 2004, *Every Child Matters*.

The Children's Act 1989 stipulates that the welfare of the child is paramount, whether they are within their family, whether families are not living together, or whenever the local authority is providing support for a family. Parents have a responsibility to care for and bring up the child. The welfare of the child must be protected. This responsibility diminishes as the child develops sufficient understanding to be capable of making up his or her mind on matters requiring a decision.

There are specific principles for the provision of services, which indicate that there should be a partnership between the parents and the child, each of the child's identified needs should be met and all of these should be appropriate to the child's ethnicity, religion, language and culture. Finally, social services should be able to draw upon effective collaboration between different agencies, including those in the voluntary sector.

The role of the cognitive behavioural therapist

Cognitive behavioural therapy (CBT) has been shown to be effective in the treatment of anxiety and depressive disorders. It is also more effective at preventing relapse, as the mother learns to be aware of the triggers which could initiate a return of her original condition. The success of the therapy has resulted in a reduction in the number of visits to the general practitioner, and unnecessary referrals to secondary or specialist care. It has become the preferred treatment of choice for many practitioners and mothers alike.

The NICE guidelines recommend that anyone who suffers from anxiety or a depressive disorder which causes distress should be offered a form of non-invasive therapy, such as cognitive behavioural therapy (CBT). As the effectiveness of CBT increases, so does the popularity for the treatment and the need to be seen by a qualified therapist. If the statistics are to be believed this means that there are over six million people in the UK who require help and support. It has been estimated that currently there is

…ained therapists per 250,000 population. Logistically, the demand is …ghing the supply and at the present time there is a serious shortfall in …ained therapists.

…pro-active way of delivering a service it has been recommended that therapists work more effectively in teams that are lead by a senior therapist. The formation of teams will ensure there is continuity in the care pathways, that facilities are in place for supervision, in-service training is current and updated, and there is scope for a career structure.

Ideally, most therapies should be delivered within easy commuting distance and it is not unrealistic to expect that clinics could be held within health centres or GP clinics, though there is little reason why the therapy cannot be held in any community centre, hall or charitable establishment such as a Home-Start centre. This will not only be less of an inconvenience but also make the therapy sessions more of a social event and take away the stigma of medicalising the condition.

There are fairly strict controls on the way in which treatments are implemented. The therapist is required to record the sessions with the mother through a client care pathway. The aim of this is to assist in the decision making, clinical review and discharge planning. It will also help the therapist to monitor the mother's progress and help her to recognise where she has been, what she is feeling and what she is likely to feel in the future.

There are two forms of CBT and CSIP (2008) and NICE recommend a tiered approach to both types of treatment. For mothers with mild to moderate depression it is proposed they begin at step two, which consists of a relatively brief, low intensity intervention. This would mean no more than six sessions of psychological interventions and involve a form of guided self-help. This could also include the use of computerised cognitive behavioural therapy.

For those mothers who are more severely depressed and cannot respond to the milder form of therapy, step three is advised. Here there are more intensive sessions, with face-to-face intervention and the treatment time is prolonged and may last for up to twenty sessions.

The training of cognitive behavioural therapists is important too, as it is dependent on the quality of the training as much as the types of people who apply. It is has been recommended that therapists who deliver low intensity treatment can be recruited from those people who are interested in pursuing a therapeutic career and who have an innate interest in people and an ability to communicate effectively. This may involve those who already have had some experience in the area of counselling or who are university graduates. It is envisaged the course would be one day a week for a year, in a recognised establishment and include time dedicated to working with clients, under professional mentorship.

For the more intense therapy it is suggested that psychologists, psychotherapists, those with a mental health background and established counsellors, and those who are employed in the service, are encouraged to have two days a week training in an established institution for a year. Working with clients, under clinical supervision, will also be a requirement (CSIP, 2008).

In 2008/2009 the Government has allocated £33 million to support the first phase of the implementation process. This will include training costs, salaries and additional costs.

Once all of the training measures and quality standards are in place it is hoped there will be a substantially improved service in the provision of cognitive behavioural therapies. It is anticipated that the services will be more accessible, waiting times will be shortened, the treatment plan will be appropriate to the client and most importantly there will be an improvement in the well-being of the client, which will help develop a healthier society.

In the meantime there are severely depressed mothers who are reluctant to take any prescribed medication and as a consequence remain without any form of satisfactory treatment. This only perpetuates their suffering and that of their families.

Voluntary organisations

Home-Start

Home-Start was founded in 1973 in Leicester by Margaret Harrison. It is a nationwide voluntary organisation and the schemes are rooted in the communities in which they serve. Home-Start is also working with families in the British Forces in Germany and Cyprus. The Home-Start network consists of Home-Start UK and has over 340 affiliated schemes. They are managed at local level by a Home-Start supervisor but the support is offered by the national organisation that offers training, information and guidance. This ensures there is consistent and quality support, friendship and practical support for parents and children. Each local scheme is an independently registered charity and has responsibility for raising the funds to support it; this is supported by a board of volunteer trustees. In areas of high economic deprivation and where Home-Start has agreed to set up a base, the funds are often supplemented with a social services agreement. The constitution of the local schemes is based on the nationally agreed model which is adapted to suit local circumstances. This structure is commonplace in the voluntary sector where independent schemes adhere to a national framework for core functions, standards, policies and good practice, but stand alone financially and in terms of local accountability.

The Home-Start mission statement states that the organisation: '*believes that children need a happy and secure childhood and that parents play the key role in giving their children a good start in life and helping them to achieve their full potential*'.

Home-Start relies on volunteers who are recruited either by word of mouth or in response to a local advertising campaign. The prerequisites are that the volunteers are parents themselves and will therefore will have some understanding of the trials and tribulations of bringing up children and experience of the difficulties that may be encountered by all social groups. Any family who has a child less than five years of age is eligible for the services of the organisation. Primarily, the schemes are situated in areas of high socio-economic deprivation, but that does not mean that mothers who are in higher income brackets are not eligible for a volunteer.

The referral of mothers to the scheme comes from a variety of sources. The mother may refer herself, but the majority of referrals come from health visitors, social services, midwives or other non-government or voluntary organisations. One reason for the referral from a professional might be because the professional is aware that the mother has a previous history of suffering from postnatal depression or that the mother is exposed to some of the risk factors which make it more likely she will be prone to it.

Often the needs of mothers and their families are very diverse but all will require a particular type of support. The main reason for a referral to Home-Start is the specific way in which the organisation engages with mothers and offers constructive help that is user-friendly and often does not have the connotations of the 'fascist' approach often linked with statutory agencies or organisations. This is particularly important in mothers who have emotional or depressive difficulties and whose needs are more sensitive than others.

A volunteer is able to help the mother with the practical domestic and childcare issues in a caring and, most importantly, non-judgemental way. The aim is to alleviate the mother's distress by encouragement and support, and enhance the overall functioning of the family. The key to achieving this is the quality of the relationship which develops between the volunteer and the mother. If the relationship is successful the volunteer will become a confidante and someone the mother can rely on to give an honest and focused opinion. This can only be achieved with the skills of the volunteer who develops a process of listening to the mother with an empathetic ear. He/she may be able to identify with how it feels to be in a similar situation and offer solutions, based on experiences, about how to resolve any difficulties, which are practical for both the mother and her infant. The volunteer might have the ability to put things into a clearer perspective. The volunteer often emulates the role of a female relation or family friend and, as has previously been discussed, with the fragmentation of family life this role is probably more important now than ever.

It is essential for a successful relationship that both parties establish boundaries. Times and interventions are negotiated to ensure that the mother has an opportunity to choose the type of help she requires and when she would like it. Often, however, quite the reverse is true, as financial constraints mean that the service is restricted to only a few hours per week and if they are utilised in taking the mother and her infant shopping or helping with the laundry, the quality of time spent talking and listening is severely limited.

There may be situations where confidentiality is compromised and the mother may confess to behaviour which has threatened or harmed the infant and asks the volunteer to maintain the confidence. The volunteer has the support of her manager and the organisation and has a code of conduct in child protection matters, which means she has to report any untoward circumstances to the appropriate authorities.

There are recorded case scenarios where the mother had a history of mental illness and was supported by Home-Start. The following is one example:

The mother was anxious about the possibility of postnatal depression and feared harming her infant. She was socially isolated with poor family support and was reviewed by a psychiatrist every three months. Home-Start ensured there was contact with the mother prior to the birth to help to ease her anxieties. She was visited once a fortnight and telephoned in the intervening week. The volunteer was able to listen to her and makes comment on how the mother appears to 'adore' her baby. This affirmation of the mother's ability to convey emotion helps to raise the mother's self-esteem. The partner is relieved to know she is being cared for, he is able to help more and discussions with the volunteer help him to recognise premature signs of depression. The mother saw the benefits of the service as she could felt she was able to ring and say she was 'losing it' without feeling guilty or judged. Her mood state improved and psychiatric visits have been reduced.

(Everingham, 2006)

This mirrors a similar study which also looked at mothers with postnatal depression and recorded their views on the services they received from Home-Start (Hanley, 2001). The majority of mothers in the study were appreciative of the friendship and support they received from the volunteers:

I recognise she can only come to the house once a week and then only for two hours but they are the two most important hours in my week[e] ... She and I usually go shopping with the kids[e] ... It is lovely to have the company. My mother is working and can only come over on the weekend, my husband is around then so I feel I have to divide my time between them all[e] ... My volunteers are more like friends than people in a 'working relationship'[e] ... Sometimes she comes to visit me during the week, on her way to another job[e] ... She will also baby sit for me if I am stuck. The kids love her, she is so patient with them.

Another volunteer provided childcare for the children of a depressed mother to enable her to attend a therapy session:

I couldn't see how I was going to get to counselling otherwise[e] ... It was pointless taking my daughter with me as she would wake or something during the session, so then I would have to spend time with her and lose the track of what I was saying about myself[e] ... It is such a luxury to be able to have the time to self-indulge, just talk about me – not babies, children, nothing, just to talk about me.

The impact of Home-Start on a mother who is depressed is encouraging. The non-stigmatising nature of the service and its ability to provide a confidante at a time when the mother is at her most vulnerable is a relief for anyone who has engaged with the skills of a volunteer. Some communities facilitate postnatal support groups and in some areas these have been the only keystone for depressed or mentally unwell mothers who require more intensive, specialised help. It provides a paradigm for the way in which society should show more compassion for new mothers and mothers with mental health issues in particular.

Sure Start

This differs from Home-Start as it is a major Government initative which was set up to eradicate child poverty and enable children to achieve their full potential by creating opportunities for a better start in life. It attempts to bring together early education, childcare, health and family support.

Sure Start originated in 1999 as the result of the *1998 Comprehensive Spending Review*. Nowadays centres and programmes are found nationwide. It covers a wide range of programmes, both universal and those targeted on particular local areas or disadvantaged groups. Sure Start local programmes are an area-based initiative. The aim is to improve the health and well-being of families and children. Initiatives can take place in the antenatal period and continue until the child is four years of age. Anyone with a child under four is eligible for help. Sure Start usually concentrates on areas where there are high levels of socio-economic deprivation. Catchment areas cover the 20% most deprived wards (Index of Multiple Deprivation). Although specifically designed for particular areas, there are often drop-in centres which enable anyone who has a need to join in the groups which are held there. It is envisaged that all Sure Start local programmes will eventually become children's centres, with a variety of services exclusive to that area. There is usually an agreement with local authorities to implement local Sure Start programmes. Part of the remit of Sure Start is to support and help mothers who have been diagnosed with postnatal depression in a culturally sensitive way, and examine a way they may be cared for which is of benefit to the mother and her infant. One of the main strengths of the Sure Start programme is the mentoring project which focuses on the support of families in the community by promoting and providing a 'Positive Parenting' service. The principles of the service are guided by the recommendations made by Government health policies, with the aim of improving access to healthcare, improving health and reducing those inequalities which cause ill health.

Trained volunteer parents, usually trained to level 2, work in unison with the mother's health visitors. The interventions take place in the formative years of children from 0–3 years of age. The aims of the mentoring project are to specifically provide an easily accessible, equitable and non-stigmatising service. The main strength is the community befriending scheme.

Volunteers provide support to promote the early bonding between parents and their children, which has been proved to improve their social and emotional development. This area is particularly important, as has been previously discussed, as the process of the mother-child interaction in mothers suffering from postnatal depression is severely compromised. If the mentor is made aware of the implications of this shortfall, then they have the opportunity to negotiate with the mother ways in which they can engage with the infant and encourage the mother to partake also. They can also support parents to make informed decisions, allowing them free choice but also supporting them if they make an incorrect decision. This, in turn, will help to increase the motivation of the mother and ultimately her self-esteem.

If the mother is allowed to learn by example she will gain increased confidence handling her infant and children, not only physically but also psychologically and emotionally. Once the mother feels more secure in her positive parenting skills she can then, with the help of the mentor, learn to develop them. Once empowered, the mother has the opportunity to take control of and manage her own welfare, which in turn will help to reduce family stress.

Referrals are accepted from midwives, health visitors or through self-referrals. Following this the Sure Start health visitor completes a home assessment and a pre-service questionnaire, which includes a behaviour management questionnaire and the EPDS. Trained volunteers, recruited and supported by the Sure Start health visitors, work closely with the parents in the family home. The volunteers are fully supported and supervised by the health visiting service, with supervisory sessions every four to six weeks.

The Sure Start health visitors provide training on postnatal depression, communication and interpersonal skills, positive parenting, behavioural management, play, basic parenting skills, confidentiality and child protection.

The care is holistic and the mother is given the opportunity to decide which type of service would be most beneficial for both her and her family. Each volunteer is closely matched to the family's needs by the Sure Start health visitor. Volunteers have a code of conduct and confidentiality is acknowledged where necessary. The proposed outcomes when working with a family are to help to relieve family stress through befriending, support and listening. This is of course of particular importance if the mother feels isolated or is suffering from postnatal depression. The skills of listening appropriately, being patient, being sensitive and having empathy are necessary to develop a relation-ship of trust and confidence. Mutual respect and integrity between the mother and volunteer is fundamental.

The role of the volunteer is also practical and it is often this that mothers find the most acceptable. They can accompany parents and encourage the use of local facilities. These may include the family centre, playgroups, or to keep clinic appointments. In some areas Sure Start facilitate support groups, primarily using a multidisciplinary approach.

The Marcé Society

The principal aim of the Marcé Society is to promote, facilitate and communicate about research into all aspects of the perinatal mental health of women, their in-fants and partners. This involves a broad range of research activities ranging from basic science through to health services research. The Society is multidisciplinary and encourages involvement from all disciplines including: psychiatrists, psycholo-gists, paediatricians, obstetricians, midwives, early childhood nurses, physiotherapists, occupational therapists, community psychiatric nurses, community nurses and health visitors.

The society also encourages the involvement of consumer and carer (self-help) groups. The society holds an international meeting every two years hosted by the President of the Society. The meetings with the high quality scientific content bring together researchers, clinicians and consumers from around the world. Much of the research cited in this book has been carried out by scientists, academics, clinicians, practitioners and users who are members of the Society.

Access to information on perinatal mental health via the Web

There are several websites now available for the mother to view, to access information and share stories.

Netmums.com

Netmums states on its website that it *'is a unique local network for mums (or dads), offering a wealth of information on both a national and local level'*. Following registra-tion at a local site it is possible to access a plethora of information. It has a chatroom where it is possible to share any issues about childcare. Netmums is informative about postnatal depression and holds regular surveys to establish how mothers feel about issues that matter. A recent major survey looked at 'happiness and well-being'. Over five thousand mothers responded to the questionnaire and the findings concluded that in the twenty-first century mothers feel '*lonely, isolated and even unwell, because of the pressures they face and the lack of local community support*'. The survey also revealed that over half of the mothers surveyed felt that they had suffered from some sort of perinatal depression.

This website is for all mothers, with nearly half a million members accessing the site, and not exclusively for depressed or ill mothers; nevertheless, its section on postnatal depression appears to be very successful and the information it generates is useful and educational. There is a section which discusses the management and treatment of postnatal depression and the EPDS is featured, which helps to expel the myth of it being a child protection 'test'. An interactive page allows mothers to share how they feel. Over two thousand people visit the site each month.

Netmums is also proactive and founder members are keen to raise awareness of postnatal depression and the implications it has for all mothers, by lecturing to researchers, clinicians and practitioners on a national scale. The organisers are keen that information on the condition is heard, not only by the public but by Government and funding bodies which can make a difference to mothers. There are regular press releases to inform the public about what is happening to the services, the plight of health visitors and the plight of mothers who have suffered or are suffering from postnatal depression.

Fatherhood Institute

A website, this time dedicated to fathers, is the Fatherhood Institute (www. fatherhoodinstitute.org) which describes itself as the UK's fatherhood think-tank.

The website describes the functions of the Institute as:

- Collating and publishing international research on fathers.
- Using different approaches to engaging with fathers by public services and employers.
- Helping to shape national and local policies to ensure a father-inclusive approach to family policy.
- Injecting research evidence on fathers and fatherhood into national debates about parenting and parental roles.
- Lobbying for changes in law, policy and practice to dismantle barriers to fathers' care of infants and children.

It claims to be the UK's leading provider of training, consultancy and publications on father-inclusive practice, for public and third sector agencies and employers. The vision of the Institute as stated on the website is '*for a society that gives all children a strong and positive relationship with their father and any father-figures; supports both mothers and fathers as earners and carers; and prepares boys and girls for a future shared role in caring for children*'.

This website has a section dedicated to fathers and postnatal depression and offers research findings into the father's own depression, the factors that are linked with paternal depression and the impact of fathers' depression on infants and children. It also discusses ameliorating the impact of a mother's depression on infants and what postnatal depression means to fathers. The Institute is keen to broaden this section and raise the awareness of postnatal depression and the impact it can have on men and society.

Scott (2005) postulated that the use of Google as a diagnostic aid is valuable, particularly when it comes to diagnosing difficult cases. This is supported by Tang & Hwee Kwoon Ng (2006) who believe that googling for a diagnosis is a useful aid as it has the advantage of being easy to use and is freely available at any time of the day. Providing the user has the correct search terms it should not be difficult to access a website which will provide a list of symptoms to match the ones the mother is experiencing. The majority of the websites on the Internet have a sound description of the symptoms of postnatal depression and most have a structured section which discusses appropriate interventions. Most will suggest the mother seeks help from her doctor, health visitor, nurse, psychiatrist or counsellor. Some will have practical advice, all designed to help and support the mother, to prevent her from feeling isolated and alone. It will help her to understand that a significant number of mothers can also relate to the feelings. However, for some mothers it may be difficult to differentiate the symptoms she is experiencing and she may be confused if some of the language she encounters is medically based.

A Google search is quick, efficient and accurately finds factual information. It has been suggested by Tang & Hwee Kwoon Ng (2006), however, that Google searches by a medical expert have a better yield as they may enter more accurate search terms. Google allows users access to more than three billion articles on the Web, which exceeds PubMed as the search engine of choice for retrieving medical articles. Twenty five million people in the UK were estimated to have Web access in 2001, and searching for health information was one of the most common uses of the Web (Powell & Clarke, 2002).

Access to media resources and technology

Videos

For every practitioner who has facilitated parentcraft classes or initiated postnatal groups, one part of the overall teaching programme has often required the use of a video to enhance the presentation. This could help to illustrate more clearly the pertinent issues around feelings and emotions which mothers may feel when they are anxious or depressed. A video may also act as a trigger to allow discussion to develop. Despite the newer concept of DVDs, the video recorder still remains one of the more accessible and inexpensive aids. It is not always easy to locate a current, appropriate and technically sound video or DVD on perinatal mental health. There are videos available on postnatal depression but accessing them is not always easy.

The use of videos on perinatal mental health can create a complex network of images that have the capability of portraying cultural constructions and resonance, which are usually understood but are not actually explicitly acknowledged. Videos are an effective way of representing performative aspects of culture, which are in the broadest sense the symbolic aspects of everyday life. They allow some insight into the sense of the emotional impact or allow viewers the opportunity to provide their own interpretations or explanations for the behaviour that a commentator may fail to do (Hanley & Long, 2006).

Images speak louder than words and the facial expressions, intonations and pauses may allow a greater understanding of the nature of the condition. A video may also serve as a supplement for written material, but it is recognised by educationalists that a video should not be used in isolation and should serve to complement a teaching or educational session. Pink (2001) commented that: '*Video is not simply a data collecting tool, but a technology that participates in the negotiation of social relationships and a medium through which ethnographic knowledge is produced.*'

In one study, English speaking videos from the USA, South Africa, Australia and the UK were located. All of the videos centred around postnatal depression, some spoke of bipolar disorder and one concentrated on the death of the five children of Andrea Yates in Texas USA, who is known to have suffered from post-partum psychosis.

It is not known if there have been other such studies on perinatal mental health, but the art of critiquing videos is certainly not new in the field of anthropology. It has been suggested that the timing of a video is crucial and the concentration span for a visual impression is three minutes; therefore it is important for the scene to be altered frequently to capture the viewer's attention (Crawford, 1993). In the better videos there were short engaging interviews, with views of the children, mothers and groups of mothers. Some of the scenes were facilitated by a commentator who usually explained the condition and its onset, and made reassuring gestures of understanding and support. One video from South Africa had short vignettes, which although interesting, became repetitive and as a result tedious. All of the videos were of good quality, and issues were addressed both sensitively and constructively. There was no evidence of patronising or paternalistic dialogue.

Music was a further important component. It was mostly non-diegetic; the viewer was not conscious of its presence but it was a primary vehicle for the narrative. There was a relationship between the images and narrative which the music helped to nurture and construct. Some of the music was emotional and imparted quality to the images, which if they had not been supported by it might have imparted different meanings. However, it may also have the opposite effect and the viewer might link it too tenuously with past associations (Barbash & Taylor, 1997).

All of the videos viewed were evidence-based research. The health messages, the description of the symptoms in minor and major depression, risk factors, types of medication and suggested therapies were all presented by a health professional, usually a psychiatrist or psychologist. Only the American videos mentioned the difficulties associated with bipolar disorder and obsessive compulsive disorder. Suicide and suicidal tendencies were not discussed in any great depth in any of the videos.

One Australian GP described his consultations as: '*You have a glowing happy mother with the perfect new baby that you see in a magazine[e] . . . at the other end you can have quite severe depression that requires a lot of treatment – most women fall somewhere in between.*'

The earlier videos, in particular the American and South African videos, advocated a medical approach and discussed the effect of hormones, sleep deprivation and poor self-care as the prime causes of postnatal depression. Medication, primarily, and/or counselling were suggested. Although the South African videos subscribed to this view too, the use of support groups was very evident, where mothers talked freely about their condition. The later videos were based on the social model of help and though the treatment included medication, the emphasis was on seeking social support to share the burden of motherhood. In videos where the analysis was more specific, the images were sometimes swamped with words.

All of the videos were concerned with raising awareness of postnatal depression and simplified the content to make them more acceptable for public viewing.

The use of the Edinburgh Postnatal Depression Scale (EPDS) (Cox et al., 1987), was absent from the American and South African videos and only mentioned in an old Australian video. Two British videos clearly illustrated the use and management of the EPDS (10).

Mothers were the focus of most of the videos. Loosely structured interviews allowed them to disclose and to share their experiences in their own metaphors and verbal effusion. The lack of scripts, actors or sets captured the essence of the mothers' fears, distress and ultimately, calmness. One noticeable observation in the Australian and South African videos was the implication of discreet sexual innuendoes. This may be construed as an effort to focus attention away from them as depressed mothers and to allow a more empathetic reaction towards them as sensual women.

Mothers spoke about stigma and a society that did not value motherhood and failed to expose the truth about the hardship of childbearing. Suicide was mentioned but not discussed in depth, but there was the belief that if they admitted to suicidal thought the infant would be taken from them. The majority recognised the value of sharing problems in the form of support groups or talking therapies, even art therapy was mentioned in one British video.

All the videos examined the effect of postnatal depression on the nuclear family but only one British and one Australian video explored the attitude of the extended family. One British video looked specifically at the problems of being a teenage mother. There were several videos available for ethnic minorities.

As has been discussed in a previous chapter there is a dearth of literature on the partner's attitude to postnatal depression. During the videos the fathers were interviewed both in the antenatal and postnatal period. Similarly to the mothers, they also freely discussed their anguish and frustration at not understanding the condition and not being allowed to be involved; despite this there were instances of humour and levity peppered throughout the interviews. This might be how they think they should respond in a difficult situation and may be seen as their way of coping with the enormity of the condition and the influence it had on their lives.

What was interesting about the videos was that although they were from several different continents the sentiments about postnatal depression from both the father and the mother were similar. All of the videos conveyed positive messages reinforcing that mothers would recover, they would get better and they would enjoy life again. The most important point was to seek help and treatment. The use of videos may be seen as an empowering visual medium which offers the mothers and their partners a chance to reproduce, understand and interpret postnatal depression, as opposed to any dominant representation that may be depicted in the mass media. Mothers with postnatal depression viewing the videos might be interested to look at 'images' of themselves reflected in the eyes of other mothers (Rony, 1996).

The value of these videos should not be underestimated. There appears to be a need for further exploration into the effectiveness and theoretical rigour of videos on postnatal depression within health education. The application and creation of video libraries focusing on particular groups could include teenage mothers, mothers from ethnic backgrounds, fathers, and grandparents. Particular topics to include are: post-partum psychosis, bipolar disorder, sexual issues and suicide. These may be useful for health professionals and mothers alike, to enable them to be more specific in the way their needs are targeted (Hanley *et al.*, 2007).

YouTube

YouTube was created in 2005 by three former PayPal employees, Chad Hurley, Steve Chen and Jawed Karim, and bought by Google in 2006 (Jefferson, 2005). It is a video sharing website where short original videos, TV film and music videos are shared with anyone who is able to upload them onto their computer. Registered users, over 18 years of age, are permitted to upload an unlimited number of videos. There are strict controls on the types of videos that may be used as their content is monitored. Any which are thought to be offensive are prohibited (Jefferson, 2005). Prior to its formation there was a limited means of accessing free view videos which were made by the general public and were available to the general public.

This is a further form of visual art, which for mothers with a computer is one of the most accessible forms of information. It is accessed by the search engine Google. As the volume of videos is so extensive it is impossible to monitor them all. Many are downloaded without authorisation and as a result some of the content can be offensive. However, it is possible to capture the subject matter of the video within the first few frames, enabling a choice to be made as to whether to watch them or not. The danger is because they are unregulated anyone can say anything about perinatal mental health issues. There is a possibility they may not be evidence based or totally correct. However, there is also the possibility that they express the frank and honest feelings of mothers who have suffered from the condition.

There is an extensive range of clips and typing in the words 'postnatal depression' will show videos made by mothers who have suffered from it. One clip is made by 'Maxine'. It shows pictures of Maxine's infant daughter; overwritten with words, and the background music *The Reason* by Hoobastank. This is an attempt to demonstrate the anguish Maxine now suffers when she recalls her behaviour towards her daughter when she was an infant. This poignant video explains how she was '*too proud to ask for help[e] ... I had been so cold, so numb to her*,' she explains. '*All I needed to do was ask for help.*' Other clips, of five minutes duration or less, were similar to the longer videos available for sale and included health professionals discussing the course and management of the condition. Postnatal depression for men was also included. One video clip on bipolar disorder (My Story) described the stigma of being '*mentally ill*' and portrays the symptoms which made them believe they were invincible '*I felt I had worked out theories[e] ... I wrote to the Pope, Presidents, the Prime Minister[e] ... felt at times I had no control over my body[e] ... Heard music all the time.*' There were a few comic videos which mocked mothers with postnatal depression but the comments which were posted made it quite clear that this form of comedy would not be tolerated in a sensitive area. In one video with two men discussing post-partum depression one of the men concluded that his lack of sexual activity was '*post-partum depression – a fancy way of saying your repulsive!*'

The viewing figures are in the billions and it is estimated that approximately ten hours of video are uploaded every minute. The popularity of this new culture suggests this is one way of targeting people with the facts and management of perinatal mental health disorders and having the opportunity to be creative in the way it is presented. However, this lack of regulation also means that erroneous messages may also be uploaded and the effect this may have on mothers is yet to be calculated.

Global cultural practices

12

United Kingdom

There is little doubt that the concept of motherhood as a carefree, highly pleasurable experience has been accepted by the majority of mothers in the West. Many are able to experience the fulfilment of motherhood and do subscribe to the notion that it is a wonderful occurrence and compares to nothing else in their life. For others, however, this image of contentment is something mothers strive for but fail to attain and because of this failure they often feel excluded from the mainstream of society.

When examining the history of motherhood in the UK it would appear that although it was far from the ideal, and mothers did not have the money and technology that is available today, it was probably a more satisfying existence for the majority of mothers. There was little choice but to rely on the subsistence gained from the land and the communities consisted of those who toiled alongside each other. Children were seen as important assets to assist with the chores and help maintain the land, which provided for their future too. Therefore fertility was a blessing and motherhood was a highly valued position in the community, which ensured that the children were not only produced but were also loved and nurtured in a stable, comfortable home environment. The mother was assured of her position in society and for the most part it was certain.

Throughout the world pregnant women have held a twofold presence. They are considered to be most powerful, in that they are the 'life givers'. Only women are able to reproduce the species, and only they can ensure future generations. They are also considered the seducers of men, the evil ones who distract man from the worship of his god. The pregnant woman is untouchable and unavailable, but she is also to be feared. The myths and legends appended to her state are manifold and attempts are made to contextualise these, bringing them into focus in present day thinking.

The process of bearing a child was fraught from the outset and relied on well-meaning folk to predict the outcome as well as the process of the pregnancy. If the belief was strong the mother could have a troubled pregnancy from the onset, not from a physical prospect, but from the anxiety caused by the predictions. In order to determine the sex of the foetus, a needle threaded with white cotton was suspended over the pregnant mother's abdomen. Depending on which way the pendulum swung the observer would tell what sex the baby was. The decision was made, whether it was what the mother wanted or not, and for the rest of her pregnancy she was forced to worry about the female or male child she was obliged to bear. The English nursery rhyme '*Monday's child is fair of face/Tuesday's child is full of grace*' was predictive of the type of lifestyle the infant could expect and though little could be done about the delivery date it nevertheless must have caused concern to a new mother to have her infant born on a Friday knowing that '*Friday's child is full of woe*'. Another old adage states '*Blue ring around the nose/Never wears his wedding clothes,*' a prognostication which must have been very upsetting for the joyous new mother who had to endure the fact that her child was destined to die at a young age.

It was suggested that to secure a positive fate for her infant the pregnant mother should avoid stepping over graves, tying a cord too tightly around her waist or dipping her fingers into dirty water (Owen, 1987). There were other precautions, albeit based on superstitions that are still practised today. The parents should not procure a perambulator or other expensive requirements, but only the equipment and clothing deemed to be necessary until the child was born. Any contact with strawberries, either touching them or eating them during pregnancy was supposed to be responsible for that type of birthmark on the unborn child (Priya, 1992).

It was also thought that the mother playing with flowers ensured her infant would have a keen sense of smell. It is still believed in some parts of Wales that should a child clutch an offered coin they will never be short of money, and the converse, that should they refuse the coin they will remain poor all their life.

Only a few generations ago the Christian ceremony of 'churching' was still practised. New mothers were encouraged to attend their local church in order to be 'cleansed' and blessed. A thanksgiving service was performed, giving thanks for the survival of the mother. The ceremony has been attributed to the Bible: Leviticus 12: 2–8, where women are said to be unclean after birth. The ceremony draws on imagery and symbolism. The usual date for 'churching' was forty days following the birth of the baby. According to the Old Testament a mother who had born a child was considered unclean for seven days and was to remain for thirty three days '*in the blood of purification*' (Leviticus 12: 2–8). Sometimes it was more convenient for the churching service to be carried out in the home. If the mother chose to go to the church it was important that she wore a veil or some form of headdress to cover her head.

Until the service was performed the mother was unable to have contact with anyone as it was considered unlucky and impure. Her condition did not allow her to prepare food or socialise. This practice presumably ensured the mother rested and recovered from the ordeal of childbirth until she was able to attend church. In some parts of the UK it was believed that new mothers who had not been churched were attractive to fairies and were in danger of being kidnapped by them.

Global issues

In other parts of the world various foods were thought to have deleterious effects on the unborn child. For example, a mother should not eat shrimps because the baby might develop a humped back, or eat chillies as they might burn the baby (Priya, 1992). Privations such as these might well be cause for anxiety, especially if these items happened to be part of the staple diet.

In China, it was believed that should the mother eat light coloured food her child would be fair-skinned. Whether or not this would have a deleterious effect on the mother is not clear. The Chinese pregnant mother had to have a knife or other sharp instrument under her bed in order to discourage evil spirits. During pregnancy she had to guard her thoughts, as these would have an influence on her unborn child. Similarly, she read poetry, listened to soothing music, but she was not to gossip, laugh loudly, look at clashing colours, sit on a crooked mat, or lose her temper. No construction work could take place in the home, and sexual intercourse was prohibited. A glass of water would be placed under the infant's cot to deter evil spirits. No name would be given to the baby for at least three months after birth so that evil spirits would be thwarted. It was felt that all these precautions would help to stabilise the mother's total state of mind and help to prevent any symptoms of anxiety or depression.

At the birth of Sikh children, no visitors would be allowed. If any should arrive they would be required to 'shake off' evil spirits in another room before being allowed to visit.

In recent years in the UK and other Western civilisations the use of henna has become popular, especially among the younger generation. This practice has been known for many years in the Middle East as well as North Africa and India, and many pregnant women and neonates are decorated with this preparation. The feet are generally the subject, and whilst they are adorned in this way, the new mother is encouraged to save the decoration by keeping her feet up off the ground. This of course results in the mother having to rest and recuperate after her labour. As well as deterring the 'evil eye', the henna decoration ensures that the mother is freed from the chores of housework, whilst her extended family and friends help out. In Nepal also, henna is used, together with *kohl* and *swak*, the latter being a lip stain made from walnut root intended to deter evil spirits. It is interesting to note that the incidence of postnatal depression in these countries is notably low (Jones, 2002).

In Rajasthan, as in some other parts of the world, the birth of a girl would be treated with great sorrow and grief, and there would be anxious prayers for another child. The birth of a boy, however, would be the cause of great rejoicing. The woman in late pregnancy would be decorated with henna and *rangoli*, and at the eighth month the *Athawansa* ceremony would be performed. She would be bathed in scented water and scented oils applied to her body. Henna, applied to hands, feet, wrists and ankles in beautiful traditional patterns were meant to provide protection from evil spirits. Seated on a *cauki*, a ceremonial wooden seat, her lap would be filled with sweets, fruit and coconut in the ceremony known as 'the filling of the lap'. The floors surrounding her were ornamented with *rangoli* (called *Athvansa-ko-cowk*), and all these rites and ceremonies were meant to promote the health and well-being of the mother and her child, as well as inviting protection from the evil eye. This eight-month ritual provides a social safety net within the community and purges pollution after childbirth. If this ritual is not performed, it is felt that the mother may not recover, but if she should die, the ceremony would ensure her entry into paradise (Jones, 2002).

African native women were required to observe four to five days seclusion, with only close relatives allowed to visit during that period. In Morocco in North Africa to give birth was considered a blessing. The term *Baraka* means blessedness. The use of henna, together with incense, amulets and ritual actions are also performed in this part of the world. In Jewish Morocco a large sword is waved in a magic circle through the air around the woman in labour to ward off evil spirits (Jones, 2002).

Throughout labour and postnatally the mother is kept covered up, with only her midwife having access, to prevent the evil eye from being able to view the mother's genitals. Henna is applied seven days after birth, the mother remaining secluded and attended by only the midwife who works behind a curtain to keep her safe from the witchcraft that could cause illness, depression and even death. This was continued for ten days to allow the hormones to stabilise after the disturbances of pregnancy and childbirth. Neither the mother nor the child was washed with water during this period, only oil and henna were used for cleansing. On the seventh day, the child was washed and given its name. Henna was applied to the child's head, neck, navel, feet, fingernails, armpits and between its legs. The mother was now dressed wearing slippers on her feet, with her head and body draped, leaving only her eyes, nose and mouth free. Women sang *zgrit* several times when a boy was born, but not so many times when the child was a daughter. The celebration lasted for seven days, during which the mother was dressed in fine clothes after bathing in rosewater and oil, and again henna was applied. All these preparations ensured the mother's rest and the transition phase lasted for forty days, with the saying 'her grave is open'. No sexual intercourse was allowed during this period, although the husband could share his wife's bed after seven days. The child was never left on its own during this time (Jones, 2002).

Romany folk (gypsies) were considered impure during pregnancy and after birth until the child was baptised. If the birth took place within the home that, too, was considered to be impure and any objects had to be discarded. It is assumed that the premises were also disinfected, though the itinerant life led by this nomadic people probably meant that their homes were easily replaced. All knots had to be undone, even hair ribbons, to prevent the umbilical cord from knotting. The new mother could not touch anything for the first month after birth and if this was not possible, she had to wear gloves to detract the evil spirits (*tsinivari*) from herself and her baby. It is interesting that only other women were allowed to attend to the needs of the mother and child, and only they could protect the mother from the evil spirits (Crowe, 1996).

These methods were to ensure that signs were to be of benefit for the mother and baby's welfare, and similar ideas were held in the UK. In Wales, for example:

> *Children born when the moon was new would be eloquent; those born during the last quarter would have excellent reasoning powers[e] ... If a baby held its head up during the ceremony it would live to be very old. If the godparents came from three different parishes the baby would live to an old age.*
>
> (Owen, 1987).

These forecasts were most likely to be of great relief to the expectant and new mother and would be of great help in her recovery from childbirth.

In the beliefs of the peoples of the Eastern countries already described, and those optimistic old adages of the UK, the mother would have more confidence that her baby, and indirectly she, would live healthy lives, thus improving her mental welfare. The necessary precautions, if adhered to, would help to stabilise the mother's anxiety or depressive symptoms and thus reduce the risks of postnatal depression that seem so prevalent in present day Western society.

In today's society motherhood is something that is done as well as something else and many would argue that the title of motherhood has been superseded by something more to do with the workplace. Social life has changed dramatically in the last fifty years, when to return to work less than three months following the birth of the baby was less common. The norm was to remain at home with the infant. Today it is perfectly acceptable to return to work and juggle the work life balance. For the majority of mothers although the financial burden of motherhood is so overwhelming there is no choice but to work outside the home.

This Western ideal appears to be filtering across other cultures and countries, where the woman's unique position is being threatened. However, the cultural practice of valuing motherhood still persists and as a result there is different interpretation of the sadness and anxiety that may follow childbirth.

International studies, however, using the Edinburgh Postnatal Depression Scale have identified mothers with postnatal depression across the globe. Eberhard-Gran *et al.* (2002) in their Norwegian study found that there was a higher risk of depression for women in the post-partum period. The risk factors identified were a history of depression, a current somatic illness and multiple pregnancies. Danaci *et al.* (2002) studied immigrant mothers in the Manisa province of Turkey. They found the factors that caused mothers to suffer from postnatal depression were linked to the problems of living in a shanty and having to share accommodation with the parents-in-law. Although this practice was traditional in that part of the country, it was the quality of the relationship that had more impact on the mother's mental health. Further risk factors included the size of the family the mother had to care for and her anxieties over her sick infants.

Chaaya *et al.* (2002) found in their study in Lebanon that social support, breast-feeding and a stressful life were not confirmed as risk factors in their study as these were all common to the mothers. What their study noted was the place of residence, which influenced the type of delivery they received. The women in the provinces feared having a Caesarean section, whilst those in the city saw it as a preferable option. There was a suggestion that mothers were unprepared for the role of motherhood and had little understanding of their own emotional needs. It was further suggested that women needed more preparation for the type of obstetrical procedure they would receive.

In Heh's (2001) study on Taiwanese mothers it was found that they were less depressed if they stayed in their parent's home and their mother took care of them. The greater the level of care received by the mother the less likely she became depressed. It is common practice for the woman's mother-in-law to accompany her for the first postnatal month. Those mothers classed as suffering from depression attributed this to the unwanted support from the parents-in-law. The findings of Jadresic & Araya (1995) and Risco *et al.* (2002) in Chilean studies showed a correlation between the depressive symptoms exhibited by mothers and an unwanted pregnancy, too many children, living in crowded conditions and having a poor or no relationship with the father of her child.

An overview of women's perinatal mental health

Poor perinatal mental health appears common to all cultures; however, the social construction of the condition varies tremendously despite the fact that the signs and symptoms are similar. At the present time, Western society has constructed perinatal mental health within a medical framework and there is no doubt that the recognition and treatment of the conditions have been very beneficial in some instances. Whilst there is no intention to denigrate the contribution medicine makes to the treatment of this condition, the construction of mothers' mental health within a critical framework is claimed by some to provide an alternative option for intervention. This option illustrates how externalising the effects of the condition may help women to recover more quickly from their experiences.

A more sophisticated interpretation of social structure might be strengthened by the neo-Marxist views of 'critical theory'. It is argued that certain aspects of society are capable of maintaining the status quo of the superficiality of that society by persuading people that they should be satisfied with the more trivial aspects of their lives. They are fed a diet of consumerism and led to believe in the importance of issues incorporating fashion and fad. This ephemeral life diverts attention away from the real, more important changes in society and persuades people not to challenge or be critical of deeper issues in the social system that may significantly direct their lives. Marcuse (1964) felt so strongly about this issue that he suggested that the masses are subjugated by a pre-packaged set of ideas spread by the 'culture' industry. Critical theorists maintain that modern society is irrational, oppressive and takes away the basic features of modern life, particularly the ability to transform the environment and make collective rational choices about life. It seeks to demonstrate that everything is open to criticism and if society accepts this knowledge then every system is capable of social change. It assumes that critical appraisal of good quality and competitive arguments will ensure that fact emerges as well as truth and this will stem from a consensus of opinion. It is postulated that an overall awareness of the barriers that prevent current change will encourage people to aspire to make that change. Therefore if women cease to believe the prevailing concept that 'perfect happy motherhood' is possible without an appropriate network from society, they might begin to recognise that these factors may be a threat to their own and their family's emotional well-being. As a result women may be empowered to challenge the current policies and structures which direct and impoverish their lives.

The problem with this approach is that it assumes that somewhere, somehow there is a conspiracy. First, there has to be a 'victim', which in this case is the newly delivered mother. She is 'depressed'. It is often argued that the medical profession is the perpetrator of this victimisation and it is often accused of having hijacked the condition. The implications are that during the past thirty or forty years, an august body like the BMA or one of the Royal Colleges, deliberately 'medicalised' perinatal mental health along with any other form of depression that is difficult to explain and manage. However, the likelihood of this occurring is extremely remote, if not impossible.

If there is such a thing as a 'conspiracy theory' then there may also be its polar opposite known colloquially as 'cock-up theory'. This appears to have more relevance than does conspiracy theory. The sequence offers a more likely explanation. A woman finds herself in a situation in which her life is going to change almost irrevocably. Pregnancy involves a series of physiological and psychological changes that are truly within the medical domain. Advances in clinical medicine have radically improved the morbidity and mortality that one hundred years ago made childbearing hazardous. In some countries it still is hazardous. It is the processes of psychological adaptation to new personal and social roles that seem to be in question.

Motherhood is supposed to be a joyous fulfilling event which mothers accept gladly. With much the same reasoning the end of childrearing is supposed to be a liberating event that allows mothers to take up new and satisfying roles in order to achieve all that they have foregone whilst being a 'good' mother. Unfortunately for many, this is not the case. Pregnancy is a slow debilitating process. Movement becomes more difficult, there are an increasing number of restrictions on what the woman can and cannot do, ensuring that even simple household chores become tiresome burdens. This is just the consequence of carrying a child and until we achieve the brave new world where children are born in bottles, it will continue to remain so. There is also the distinct possibility that once the child is born everything else will have to change.

If there is a conspiracy it must therefore be somewhere in the Department of Health. In fact it is not a conspiracy at all but rather the continued administration of a set of old laws that seek to control the distribution of dangerous products. Perhaps it is worth noting that opiates were used to combat depression, *vide* Sherlock Holmes. Originally, the concern was with the use of opiates but since that time the majority of pharmaceutical products have been classified as being 'only available upon prescription'. The doctor is thus part of the legal system of restriction – a set of laws, like so many others, that have been passed in order to protect society.

A further avenue for the conspiracy theory must lie in those who benefit most from the manufacture of pharmaceutical products. With whom do they conspire? One of the problems that besets major manufacturers is the fact that of every thousand products that start life in their research laboratory, only two or three will eventually reach the pharmacist's shelf. Of those three, only one will be a major moneymaker. Depressive disorders as an area of pharmaceutical research interest are relatively recent and for a few major producers they have proven to be massively profitable. The money earned is not siphoned off into profits. Indeed, the current returns to shareholders in this sector, whilst steady, are not spectacular. The research component of their work is fearfully expensive which is why any manufacturer of a new product has at least seven years of protection against thousands of small companies who do no research but merely copy. It is how they do the research that begs the question.

Depressive disorders, for pharmaceutical companies, have to be seen as some sort of chemical imbalance, abnormality or dysfunction, which may then be remedied by another chemical. That is perhaps an oversimplification of their approach but it does describe their intervention in this field. Serotonin diminution and Prozac are a typical example. This means that their research has to treat the depression as a reaction to something else, e.g. diminished serotonin, and that something else has got to be treatable by one of their products.

In terms of classical research method this implies that the depression is a dependent variable that can be explained by the occurrence of the abnormality. For treatment the sequence is reversed. The depression is now the independent variable that can be influenced by a dependent variable – the pharmaceutical preparation. This is not a conspiracy but rather the way in which ethical pharmaceutical products are developed. If the rules of scientific research are not followed, dangerous drugs, with unknown side effects, will come onto the market and years of litigation may ensue, as Distillers Company found out.

Where there may be a conspiracy lies in the possibility that the depression and the pharmaceutical product might both be variables of the same kind. If the depression itself has occurred as a result of events outside the sufferer, fear of the future, loneliness, isolation, rejection, then a pill is not going to remedy the problem. You cannot take a pill to change the behaviour of an uncaring partner, but no pharmaceutical company is ever going to investigate such a cause of depression. If it were possible to prove conclusively that serotonin diminution occurs after something else, and if were possible to prove that a pharmaceutical company knew this, then the conspiracy theory is proven.

For the present, the possibility of the 'cock up theory' has to be borne in mind.

There appear to be a set of events, some of which were put in place over a century ago and some, particularly economic and social changes, are much more recent. Some years ago Milton Friedman, the arch guru of monetarism was addressing a group of Chinese businessmen in Singapore, advocating the dismantling of state controls on industry and commerce and espousing the theory that 'the market' could take care of any eventuality. A young doctor stood up and asked Friedman if he would extend that theory to the pharmaceutical industry. Friedman was not able to provide an answer (Long, 2000, personal communication).

State control of the pharmaceutical industry is a feature of every developed country but it is not worldwide. It is imposed because it is believed to be essential that states protect their citizens against some of the risks of life. For exactly the same reason speed limits are imposed on the roads. That being the case, it has to be accepted that the distribution of some pharmaceutical products is going to be the professional preserve of the medical profession. Much of a medical student's training involves developing the expertise to select a drug and to control its dosage. The administration of a drug carries with it the legal responsibility and liability that a doctor has to accept. The Medical Defence Union will insure him or her but they will not offer that protection to anyone else. If a depressed mother presents herself in the surgery then the doctor must attempt to deal with the depression. If the doctor knows that an antidepressant drug will ease the condition, then his own humanity may lead him to prescribe it.

There will always be some women who, for a variety of reasons, are more prone to depression than others. This may be a justification for the fact that, in their training, doctors are taught about depression. However, the teaching of 'consulting skills' is relatively recent and far from widespread. As far back as 1976 Byrne & Long demonstrated the sort of mess a GP could get into with an inept approach to this problem. They also commented that the pressure of a morning or evening surgery is not conducive to this sort of analysis.

Yet there is evidence that indicates that the management of the doctor/patient consultation, coupled with certain prescribed medications, does have a positive effect before the medication is claimed to 'kick-in'. It has also produced evidence that suggests that the human intervention, by voluntary or statutory agencies, does have a beneficial effect, as demonstrated by Gruen (1990), Eliott (1990) and Pitts (1995) in their advocacy of support groups.

Western societies differ from nearly every other form of human society in that they can be classified as 'individualist'. Initially, at the time of the Reformation, this was seen as a description of each person's relationship with his or her God. It was one of the key theological issues that prompted the split with Rome. Later that concept was to apply more and more to every aspect of our lives, finding a near complete expression in the current interpretation of the constitution of the USA. Western European societies have, arguably, not progressed so far down that road, but in the main they are individualist. In Britain this philosophy probably reached its peak towards the end of the nineteenth century, when it was claimed by a senior civil servant at the Board of Trade that an '*unemployed, able bodied labourer was not only idle but sinful.*' (Bruce, 1960). Even after 75 years of 'welfareism' a senior member of the Thatcher government was still talking about '*getting on your bike*'.

Until the 1950s the working woman was really a wartime phenomenon. During both World Wars it became necessary for women to take over the work previously done by men. After the carnage of World War I, and the influenza epidemic of 1919–1920, women remained at work because there were fewer men. That was the age of female emancipation. It was not for another generation that the full benefit of that emancipation became apparent because it took a generation for the benefits of higher and professional education to give women the opportunity to sell their labour competitively in the marketplace.

The problem identified may well derive from that 'freedom'. After the stringent years of post-war recovery, particularly during the period of the Macmillan Government, the distribution of wealth started to change and despite the fact that there remains comparative poverty, Western Europe and North America have experienced a period of individual prosperity that has never been known before. This might well have started in Britain with the notion of a 'property-owning democracy' (something that is still not so common in either France or Germany) and to buy a property all you need is money. You get money by going to work. Thus, it can be argued that it is our level of consumption that makes us poor. Women went to work in unprecedented numbers in order to better their lives. The simple problem of consumerism is that it costs a lot of money to buy a house or a car but the things then have to be maintained or replaced.

Therefore more money is needed. Society has been led to believe that we need holidays, to go out socialising, own mobile telephones and there is a seemingly endless supply of new products for people to buy to 'enjoy the good life'. To the young it may feel like a long vacation but it comes to an end when a baby appears. Perhaps the root causes of poor perinatal mental health may be found here, rather than in the supply of serotonin.

A period of relative freedom has been enjoyed, which contrasts favourably with being at school or being at home. A woman may have married simply to cement her freedom from home. Freedom is not simply economic liberation, it is also social liberation. One of the consequences can mean a pregnancy, either accidental or deliberate. If that pregnancy is not terminated, itself a traumatic decision that sometimes has equally horrible consequences, then within nine months a child is going to appear.

The number of women who suffer sufficiently from perinatal ill health to need help, is estimated at around one in ten. This raises the question about the other 90%. Today it is possible to plan a pregnancy and therefore a large number of women will have made a conscious decision to become pregnant. In making that decision they have already started the process of preparing for motherhood. Before becoming pregnant they are likely to have considered the economic and occupational consequences. They may also have considered the pattern of care they propose to provide. There is still no guarantee that they will not suffer from a perinatal mental disorder.

The mother is now looking at the future knowing that she has to care for her child. If she wishes to continue to work she must consider the problem of who is going to care for her child. If her parents and grandparents have to work and her husband has to work there may be little choice, if only because childcare is expensive. If she goes to work she will be seen as a mother who has abandoned her social responsibility to her own child and she is only likely to earn enough money to pay for the childcare. All the freedom she has enjoyed is now in jeopardy and even if she is married, she might still be on her own.

Again, it must be recognised that some women will rise above this and quite probably psychologists and personality theorists will be able to explain why this occurs. They might have other forms of support or personal reserves that give them the ability to face the problem. It is even possible that they really want to become mothers. There remain those who do not have these reserves and do not know where to look for support and if we are looking for an explanation of where feelings of loneliness or isolation begin, surely it is here. For the single mother-to-be, the experience of family anger and rejection only compound the problem.

As the pregnancy continues the mother-to-be is going to experience more and more withdrawal from what has previously been a normal life. Quite apart from the psychological and physiological changes that normally accompany a pregnancy, the mother-to-be is going to find that all sorts of other limitations are being placed upon her. Movement and the performance of simple tasks are going to become more difficult. If she has taken advantage of any antenatal care her diet is going to have to change and she will have to limit both her pleasures, especially alcohol and tobacco, and her activities. Resting routines will be advised and she will not be able to take part in many social activities. She will have to give up work, if only for a while and towards the end of her pregnancy will not be allowed to fly and will probably be advised to limit her travel. All of this is going to take place during a period of increasing isolation. A partner who is working long hours, or is not prepared to help, simply compounds the problem. What is happening to this woman is increasing social isolation which might well lead to the feeling that she has been abandoned. She may now be alone for many hours in the day and might be unable to come to terms with what is happening. All of this can happen before the baby is born.

The next event occurs when the baby arrives. For most women the experience is that they go home to a caring and supportive environment, if only provided by a caring partner. For some, however, the picture is not so good. In the first place they are now discharged from hospital much earlier than was the case fifty years ago. There do not appear to be too many clinical viewpoints that can support this practice but it does increase the rate of bed occupancy. There might well be problems in the hospital but they are nothing compared to what awaits her at home.

She is not in hospital therefore she must be 'better'. She might be alone for most of the day, but now her time is increasingly focused upon an infant who has to be fed, watered and cleaned every few hours. For many of the women there was the expectation that they would quickly resume their domestic duties. For months sleep is going to be interrupted by a demanding child and normal routines are impossible. If there is no one to look after the child her social life will be limited to a visit to the supermarket.

There is also the fact that her life has been changed by the arrival of the infant. The nine months of an increasingly uncomfortable pregnancy have resulted in a pattern of demands, especially in the case of a firstborn child, that were not there before. The routines of cleaning, feeding and comforting all demand time and attention and for those without immediate family support, the mother's previous life has come to a sudden end. It is what happens next that might give us a different insight. The constant demands of the baby have to be seen in the light of a perfectly reasonable desire to resume some of the activities of her previous life. But for most women, it is not possible to take the baby to work, or to the pub or the cinema. The social life she might have previously enjoyed is no longer available. Arguably, this is the point at which the natural onset of baby blues can develop into something else.

It is also at this point that her condition might be detected by the health visitor or indeed she might decide to seek the help of her general practitioner. If the symptoms are going to be treated there is the strong possibility that she will be given some form of medication that will mask some of the symptoms, but the baby will not go away.

Then there is the problem of how to present her problem to the general practitioner. There are strong deep-rooted fears about being labelled 'mad', which means that she may well not present what she really feels. The GP has to start with the evidence /s/he is given and even though they may well suspect what is happening they must start with whatever symptoms the mother decides to disclose. If s/he does prescribe an antidepressant then at one level a diagnosis has been made, but it is quite probable that the experienced practitioner will know that this is not a 'cure'.

It is at this point that perhaps, once more, some of the literature should be reviewed. Over thirty years ago Shaw (1976) working on the therapeutic values of 'groups' found that relationships formed in his groups led to social interactions that helped to satisfy a basic need to affiliate with others. Shaw was working in the field of depressive management but not specifically focused on postnatal depression. In 1990, Elliot took things much closer to our concern by claiming that group work appeared to reduce the prevalence of depression in new mothers and he made the recommendation that all health professionals should continue to provide education and support for mothers. In 1996, Meager & Milgrom published their findings about the value of a ten-week treatment programme, which contained educational and social support as well as cognitive behavioural components, again aimed at depressed mothers. They found a 'significant improvement in mood-state'.

In 1997, Morgan reported upon the outcome of cognitive behavioural group work for depressed mothers and their partners. They found an increase in self-esteem and a decrease in stress levels. This is seen in similar work by Appleby. His original contribution (1991) noted that there was a high risk of relapse in women if the course of antidepressants was discontinued. However, by 1997 Appleby had moved on to examine the value of behavioural counselling, coupled with the use of an antidepressant. In a very complicated set of experiments, such as fluoxetine with counselling, fluoxetine without counselling, fluoxetine on its own, counselling on its own, he found that all of his groups showed a similar level of improvement. '*Women with postnatal depression can be effectively treated with fluoxetine, which is as effective as a course of cognitive behavioural counselling in the short term*' (Hoffbrand *et al.*, 2001, p. 1). The one factor common to all of these experiments was the presence of the researcher.

The work of Elkin *et al.* (1989) offers a particularly interesting insight. He was concerned with the efficacy of tricyclics and found that they were not effective with mild levels of PND. They were effective with severe forms, indeed the greater the severity the more effective was the drug. This ties in well with Scott's (1988) finding that most forms of depression tend to resolve themselves, but about 12–15% of sufferers remained depressed after two years.

There is a great deal of evidence about the efficacy of groups and group work that is relevant here. Gordon *et al.* (1995) found that group work produced an improved self-esteem and mood state. May (1995) found, almost by accident, that within groups who were ostensibly meeting for exercise and relaxation techniques 'discussion', as an activity, was rated higher than both. Pitts (1995) had found that groups were effective and cost efficient in the management of PND. In the same year Stamp *et al.* (1995) reported that antenatal groups for prospective depressed mothers were effective in relieving their depression. Gestalt psychologists such as Braid (1996) noted that 'here and now' therapy in the presence of the therapist, offered new hope in the management of depression. All this evidence suggests that the intervention of the human being and human contact appears to have a beneficial effect on most, but not all, depressive mothers.

It is reasonable to claim that most women can suffer a mild depression at the end of a pregnancy but most get over it very quickly. Although there is argument over the actual percentages, about 10% do not. Of this 10% only a very small fraction will progress into puerperal psychosis. It is the proportion who do not suffer that terrible progression that are of interest here.

The theory, therefore, seems to be that human beings facing a change in the normal pattern of their lives also face the possibility of encountering a depressive disorder. That depressive disorder may occur if the person is enjoying or deriving satisfaction from their current lifestyle and sees no ability to control the threatened change or has no support to assimilate it. In those circumstances some people will develop a reaction to their immediate environment, which is labelled 'depression'. The majority of women who fall prey to this condition will quickly defeat the problem either on their own or with support. For others, it will continue and may require support, both societally and pharmaceutically before recovery sets in. In the small minority, the depressive disorder will continue and mothers may descend into puerperal psychosis or may try to end their lives. The problem with this theory is that it is best tested by examining its effective treatment.

It may thus be pertinent to suggest that, to some extent, poor perinatal mental health is a consequence of social deterioration, as is postulated by the theorists of functional analysis, rather than a purely physical reaction to the situation of motherhood. It appears that for many women societal factors may be an attempt on the part of society to rein in, and therefore control women; this may exacerbate their experience if they refuse or cannot conform to the standards set by that society. For example, women may be on the one hand constrained by common beliefs and facts that belong to a bygone age, that is from a functional perspective they may believe that they should stay at home to care for the child. On the other hand they may feel obliged to agree with modern day feminist thinking regarding their 'rights' to freedom and the need to accept the triple role of wife, mother and worker. Whichever way they turn it appears that women will find themselves disadvantaged.

Poor perinatal mental health was, interestingly, uncommon in past years, only coming to the fore during the past thirty years. Those same thirty years have seen significant, and in some cases, detrimental changes to Western family structure and values. It is probable that women in a previous era would have felt the same pressures and stresses had they shared the same lifestyles of today's women. However, Western women have redefined their role in society in past years and as a result there may be gains and losses which may inevitably affect childcare responsibilities and partnerships between mothers and fathers. It would appear from this study that some women cannot cope with the undue stresses and expectations of today's society.

It appears to be acceptable to suffer from postnatal 'blues', which is thought to be self-limiting and acceptable behaviour for a new mother. However, society has limits on the amount of non-coping it can accept, and will castigate the woman who is unable to cope with her position as a mother. Those who fail to cope are given the label of postnatal depression or perinatal mental health disorder. As a result, such mothers may be regarded as deviant and have to assume the sick role to enable them to seek out the support, medical and social help that is required to place them back into society. The majority of mothers do not appear to intentionally put themselves in the sick role, although they are unable to function in an accepted manner. However, most mothers would admit to identifying with the condition when questioned by a health professional and are, in the main, receptive to the 'label' when the 'diagnosis' is made. Scheff (1986) argues that such a label would emphasise the long-term negative effect of a being a 'psychiatric case'. In adverse social circumstances women are sometimes forced to negotiate their condition by adopting the label in order that society will accept that something is amiss and respond with appropriate resources.

This lack of support for women does not appear to be intentional and, whether one accepts the critical theoretical perspective or not, there may be a number of factors conspiring to disadvantage new mothers. These have been identified as a medicalisation of normal life events; current patterns of health care organisation (e.g. early hospital discharge); professional ideologies, such as regarding the importance of accepting childbirth as a natural event; societal change in which families have been fragmented and become less supportive; new forms of social organisation in which all women are expected to work to maintain standards of living and ideologies of equality in which women have sought to build a meaningful life for themselves outside the home. They had little choice about working because their financial situation dictated that their income was of prime importance to the family. Working outside the family home usually isolated mothers from the home environment. In many cases women were unfamiliar with their female counterparts in the community and were placed in the unenviable position of being forced to rely on support outside their normal social circles. Previous support systems appear to have deteriorated, as statistics show that 4.7 million of the workforce have dependent children and the majority of the workforce in the older age bracket are women. As a result, some women appear to have more commitment to the workplace than the home.

There is evidence to suggest that working mothers experience significant stress from the tensions arising from straddling the separate spheres of home and work. This may explain, in part, why most women with schoolage children prefer to work part time, if they have to work at all. Attempts to dilute and devolve this responsibility for the home sphere, as in the case of childcare facilities, have sometimes proved to be expensive and difficult. However, it is not always the case that affordable child care would encourage mothers back to work, as research by Dex & Rowthorn (1997) indicated that very few mothers express the desire to work. Perhaps it is time that women challenged the perpetual theories of the Government regarding the working woman and questioned the validity of their usefulness, not just to the State but for their children. There is frequent debate in Government about taxable allowances for childcare and politicians seem aware of the impact working women make on society. Politicians advocate that 90% of women want to work (Department of Health & Social Security, 1997), but this statistic may belie the truth. This figure, however, may relate to women who wish to work *at some point in their lives*. Mothers work, grandmothers work, aunties work, sisters work, indeed most women, in today's society, work. There is probably a sound argument for rethinking paternity leave and substituting it with 'grandmother leave'.

The process of their depression or condition has made some of the women re-evaluate their lifestyle and some have made significant changes, which included ceasing full-time employment or re-examining their family construction. This raises the question of why women should be forced to such extremes before they are able to instigate radical changes in their lives. Perhaps there is a need to re-examine the existing supportive social structures and find out why their function has been radically diminished. Certainly it would appear that further research could be encouraged to reveal why so many factors may be preventing women from seeing the poverty of their daily lives.

The existing knowledge of perinatal mental health is usually the accepted domain of the health professional. There has been extensive research into the causes, effects and treatment of the condition, and efforts appear to have been made to increase the public awareness of how the condition may manifest itself. However, the findings of this study show that despite these efforts, women are still largely ignorant about the effects an infant could have on their psychological and emotional health. Even if they were knowledgeable on the subject, it appeared from this study that despite modern living there were few naturally occurring resources easily available to the mother to enable her to cope with the demands of her infant. It is only when she succumbed to the medicalisation of her condition that health professionals initiated help. This help also extended to enlisting help from within the family. This may account for women being willing to accept the label as the only means of extricating themselves from a dilemma. If this is the case it would appear that the labelling process may disguise many adverse socio-structural factors which disadvantage women.

The period of stability is over, the future is apparently grim and there is little or no support. Possibly there is also the belief by the woman facing this scenario that she has little or no control over what is going to happen. At this point, the depressive disorder becomes apparent.

Should these women appear in the GP's surgery, the doctor will be forced into a situation in which some form of antidepressant will be prescribed. It is not unreasonable to suggest that most women, that is 90%, cope by coming to terms with their new role. It is the 10% who are unable to adapt who seem to suffer the most.

The literature suggests that mothers seem to cope better when some form of social support is provided. It might take the form of a health visitor, or a counsellor or a voluntary agency, but whatever it is it seems to work.

Some last thoughts . . .

Are we outliving our corporeal capacity? After all humans were not supposed to have been long in this world, just for the threescore years and ten. The term 'bless you' presumed your life was about to be terminated and a blessing was in order. Is all this clean living by default? Are we really moving more towards our natural state of original sin? Human beings need to quantify and codify their thoughts and feelings. There may be reasons why there is a need to be prosaic, and analyse and compartmentalise, but most do not like being in 'free fall'. It appears we need an emotional compass, to help us to keep on track and be aligned with the world. New mothers are no exception. Today the compass, which is both spiritual and emotional, is lacking because we have traded them for material comforts as we desire more and more.

References

Abdullah, M., Al-Waili, N., Baban, N., Butler, G. & Sultan, L. (2006) Postsurgical psychosis: case report and review of literature. *Advances in Therapy*, **23** (2), 325–331.

Abercrombie, N., Hill, S. & Turner, B.S. (1984) *Dictionary of Sociology*. London: Penguin Books.

Abramowitz, J.S., Schwartz, S.A., Moore, K.M. & Luenzmann, K.R. (2003) Obsessive-compulsive symptoms in pregnancy and the puerperium: a review of the literature. *J Anxiety Disord*, **17**, 461–478.

Adams, C. (2008) Lack of support for postnatal depression. *Community Practitioner*, **81** (8), 10.

Agarwal, K.N., Gupta, A., Pushkarna, R., Bhargava, S.K., Faridi, M.M.A. & Prabhu, M.K. (2000) Effects of massage and use of oil on growth, blood flow and sleep patterns in infants. *Indian Journal of Medical Research*, **112**, 212–217.

Ahokas, A., Kaukoranta, J., Wahlbeck, K. & Aito, M. (2001) Estrogen deficiency in severe postpartum psychosis: a pilot study. *J Clinical Psychiatry*, **61**, 166–169.

Aitken, P. & Jacobson, R. (1997) Knowledge of the Edinburgh Postnatal Depression Scale amongst psychiatrists and general practitioners. *Psychiatric Bulletin*, **21** (9), 550.

Akiskal, H.S. (2006) Special issue on circular insanity and beyond: historic contributions of French psychiatry to contemporary concepts and research on bipolar disorder. *Journal of Affective Disorders*, **96** (3) 141–143.

Akman, I., Ku çu, K., Özdemir, N., *et al*. (2006) Mothers' postpartum psychological adjustment and infantile colic. *Archives of Disease in Childhood*, **91**, 417–419.

Alder, C. & Polk, K. (2001) *Child Victims of Homicide*. Cambridge: Cambridge University Press.

Alwan, S., Reefhuis, J., Ramussen, S. *et al.* (2005) Maternal use of selective serotonin re-uptake inhibitors and risk for birth defects. Birth Defects Research (Part A) *Clinical and Molecular Teratology*, **731**, 291.

Alwan, S., Reefhuis, J., Rasmussen, S., Olney, R. & Friedman, J. (2007) Use of selective serotonin-reuptake inhibitors in pregnancy and the risk of birth defects. *New England Journal of Medicine*, **356**, 2684–2692.

American Psychiatric Association (1994) *Diagnostic and Statistical Manual of Mental Disorders* (DSM-IV-TR)(2000), fourthth edition, text revision. Washington, DC: American Psychiatric Association.

American Psychiatric Association (2000) *Diagnostic and Statistical Manual of Mental Disorders* (DSM-IV-TR)(2000) fourth edition, text revision. Washington, DC: American Psychiatric Association.

Anderson, E.A., Kohler, J.K. & Letiecq, B.L. (2005) Predictors of depression among low-income, non-residential fathers. *Journal of Family Issues*, **26** (5), 547–567.

Annesi, J. & Westcott, W. (2004) Relationship of feeling states after exercise and total mood disturbance over 10 weeks in formerly sedentary women. *Perceptual & Motor Skills*, **99** (1), 107–115.

Appleby, L. (1991) Suicide during pregnancy and in the first postnatal year. *British Journal of Psychiatry*, **302**, 137–140.

Appleby, L. (2000) Suicide in women. *The Lancet*, **355** (9211), 1203–1204.

Appleby, L., Warner, R., Whitton, A. & Faragher, B. (1997) A controlled study of fluoxetine and cognitive behavioural counselling in the treatment of postnatal depression. *British Medical Journal*, **29**, 314 (7085), 932–936.

Arendt, M., Rosenberg, R., Foldager, L., Peto, G. & Munk-Jorgensen, P. (2005) Cannabis-induced psychosis and subsequent schizophrenia-spectrum disorders: follow-up study of 535 incident cases. *British Journal of Psychiatry*, Dec, **187**, 510–515.

Armstrong, D. (1983) *The Political Anatomy of the Body*. Cambridge: University Press.

Armstrong, E. (1997) Rehabilitating troubled doctors. *BMJ*, **314**, 2.

Armstrong, K. & Edwards, H. (2004) The effectiveness of a pram-walking exercise programme in reducing depressive symptomatology for postnatal women. *International Journal of Nursing Practice*, **10** (4), 177–194.

Arnold, P.D., Rosenberg, D.R., Mundo, E., Tharmalingam, S., Kennedy, J.L. & Richter, M.A. (2004) Association of a glutamate (NMDA) subunit receptor gene (GRIN2B) with obsessive-compulsive disorder: a preliminary study. *Psychopharmacology*, **174**, 530–538.

Arroll, B., Goodyear-Smith, F., Kerse, N., *et al.* (2005) Effect of the addition of a 'help' question to two screening questions on specificity for diagnosis of depression in the general public: diagnostic validity study. *BMJ*, **331**, 884.

Atlantis, E. & Baker, M. (2008) Obesity effects on depression: a systematic review of epidemiological studies. *International Journal of Obesity* (London), 15 April.

Austin, M. & Lumley, J. (2003) Antenatal screening for postnatal depression: a systematic review. *Acta Psychiatrica Scandinavica*, **107** (1).

Baker, F. & Mackinlay, E. (2006) Sing, soothe and sleep: a lullaby education programme for first-time mothers. *B.J. Music*, **23** (2), 147–160.

Ball, J. & All, J. (1987) *Reactions to Motherhood, the Role of Postnatal Care*. Cambridge: Cambridge University Press.

Ballard, C.G., Davis, R., Cullen, P.C., Mohan, R.N. & Dean, C. (1994) Prevalence of postnatal psychiatric morbidity in mothers and fathers. *The British Journal of Psychiatry*, **164**, 782–788.

Barbash, I. & Taylor, L. (1997) *Cross-Cultural Filmmaking*. London: University of California Press.

Barr, R. (1998) Management of clinical problems and emotional care. Colic and crying syndromes in infants. *Pediatrics*, **102** (5), 1282–1286.

Battachaya, D. Pagalami (1986) *Europsychiatric Knowledge in Bengal*. New York: Syracuse University Press.

Beck, C.T. (1998) A checklist to identify women at risk from developing postpartum depression. *Journal of Obstetric and Gynecological Neonatal Nursing*, **21** (1), 39–46.

Beck, C.T. (2001) Predictors of postpartum depression: an update. *Nursing Research*, **50**, 275–285.

Beck, C. & Gable, R. (2001) Further validation of the postpartum depression screening scale, *Nurs Res*, **50**, 155–164.

Bennet, H., Einarson, A, Taddio, A., *et al.* (2004) Prevalance of depression during pregnancy: systematic review. *Obst.Gynec*, **103** (6), 698–709.

Biddle, S.K.H. (2000) Emotion, mood and physical activity. In *Physical Activity and Psychological Well-being* (eds S.K.H. Biddle, K.R. Fox & S.H. Boutcher), pp. 63–87. London: Routledge.

Blehar, M.C., Liberman, A.F. & Ainsworth, M.D. (1977) Early face-to-face interaction and its relation to later mother-infant attachment *Child Development*, **48** (7), 182–194.

Bloch, M., Daly, R.C. & Rubinow, D.R. (2003) Endocrine factors in the etiology of postpartum depression. *Comprehensive Psychiatry*, **44**, 234–246.

Bodnar, L., Wisner, K. & Hanusa, B. (2006) Plasma vitamin C concentrations in pregnant woman with major mood disorders. Marcé Society International Biennial Scientific meeting.

Bolton, H.L., Hughes, P.M., Turton, P. & Sedgwick, P. (1998) Incidence and demographic correlates of depressive symptoms during pregnancy in an inner London population. *Journal of Psychosomatic Obstetrics and Gynaecology*, **19**, 202–209.

Bonari, L., Bennett, H., Einarson, A., & Koren, G. (2004) Risks of untreated depression during pregnancy. *Can Fam Physician*, **50**, 37–39.

Bonnar, J. (1981) Venous thrombo-embolism and pregnancy. *Clin Obstet Gynaecol*, **8**: 455–473.

Boscalglia, N., Skouteris, H. & Werthein, E.H. (2003) Changes in body image satisfaction during pregnancy: comparison of high exercising and low exercising women. *Australia and New Zealand Journal of Obstetrics and Gynae*, **43**, 41–45.

Bowlby, J. (1973) *Attachment and Loss* (Vol 2) *Separation: Anxiety and Anger*. New York: Basic Books (reissued 1999).

Bowlby, J. (1980) *Attachment and Loss* (Vol 3) *Loss, Sadness and Depression*. New York: Basic Books.

Boyce, P. (2003) Risk factors for postnatal depression: a review and risk factors in Australian populations. *Archives of Women's Mental Health*, **6** (2), 1434–1861.

Braid, R. (1996) *Working with Postnatally Depressed Mothers, Using Gestalt Therapeutic Approach*. Paper submitted at the Marcé Society Biennial Scientific Meeting. Cambridge University. Sept.

Breggin, P. (2001) *The Antidepressant Fact Book*. Cambridge, MA: Perseus Books.

Breggin, P. (2003) Suicidality, violence and mania caused by selective serotonin reuptake inhibitors (SSRIs): a review and analysis. *Ethical Human and Social Services*, 5, 225–246.

Brians, P., Gallway, M., Hughes, D., *et al.* (1999) *Reading About the World* (Vol 2). Chestnut Hill, MA: Harcourt Brace Custom Publishing.

Briscoe, M. (1986) Identification of emotional problems in postpartum women by health visitors. *British Medical Journal*, 292, 1245–1247.

Brockington, I. (1998) Puerperal disorders. *Advances in Psychiatric Treatment*, 4, 312–319.

Brockington, I. (2006) Psychosis complicating Chorea gravidarum. *Archives of Women's Mental Health*, 9 (2), 113–114.

Brockington, I.F. & Kumar, R. (eds) (1982) *Motherhood and Mental Illness* (Vol 1). London: Academic Press.

Brown, G.W. & Harris, T. (1978) *Social Origins of Depression: a Study of Psychiatric Disorders in Women*. London: Tavistock.

Brown, H. & Bacigalupo, R. (2006) Health visitors and postnatal depression: identification and practice. *Community Practitioner*, 79 (2), 49–52.

Bruce, M. (1960) *Able Body Works. The Coming of the Welfare State*. London: Tavistock.

Buist, A. & Barnett, B. (1995) Childhood sexual abuse: a risk for postpartum depression? *Australian & New Zealand Journal of Psychiatry*, 29 (4), 604–608.

Buist, A. & Janson, H. (2001) Childhood sexual abuse, parenting and post-partum depression – a 3-year follow-up study. *Child Abuse and Neglect*, 25 (7), 909–921.

Buist, A., Morse, C. A. & Durkin, S. (2003) Men's adjustment to fatherhood: implications for obstetric health care. *Journal of Obstetric, Gynecologic, & Neonatal Nursing*, 32 (2), 172–180. March/April.

Buist, A., Condon, J., Brooks, J., *et al.* (2006) Acceptability of routine screening for perinatal depression. *Journal of Affective Disorders*, 93 (1–3), 233–237.

Buka, S., Tsuang, M., Fuller Torrey, E., Klebanoff, M., Berstein, M. & Yolken, R. (2001) Maternal infections and subsequent psychosis among offspring. *Arch Gen Psychiatry*, 58, 1032–1037.

Burdette, H., Whitaker, R., Kahn, R. & Harvey-Berino, J. (2003) Association of maternal obesity and depressive symptoms with television-viewing time in low-income preschool children. *Arch Pediatr Adolesc Med*, 157, 894–899.

Burr, J. (2002) Providing a contrasting view to evolutionary psychology's hypothesis on depression: using a 'material discursive' approach to interpret the experiences of depression from South Asian communities. *Psychology, Evolution and Gender*, 4 (1), 93–113.

Byrne, P.S. & Long, B.E. (1976) *Doctors Talking to Patients. A Study of the Verbal Behaviour of General Practitioners Consulting their Surgeries*. London: Her Majesty's Stationery Office.

Care Services Improvement Partnership (CSIP) (2008) The National Perinatal and Infant Mental Health (PIMH) network for England (http://www.csip.org.uk/~cypf/camhs/perinatal-and-infant-mental-health.html).

Cawley, S., Griffiths, L., Briers, G. & Salib, E. (1999) Who needs a mother and baby unit? *Nursing Standard*, **13** (46), 33–36.

Chaaya, M., Campbell, O.M.R., El Kak, F., Shaar, D., Harb, H. & Kaddour, A. (2002) Postpartum depression: prevalence and determinants in Lebanon. *Arch Women's Mental Health*, **5** (2) 65–72.

Charles, N. (1993) *Gender Divisions and Social Change*. London: Harvester Wheatsheaf, Barnes and Noble.

Children's Act (2004) *Every Child Matters* (www.everychildmatters.gov.uk).

Clay, E.C. & Seehusen, D.A. (2004) A review of postpartum depression for the primary care physician. *Southern Medical Journal*, **97**, 157–161.

Cohen, L., Altshuler, L., Harlow, B., *et al*. (2006) Relapse of major depression during pregnancy in women who maintain or discontinue antidepressant treatment. *Journal of American Medicine*, **295**, 449–507.

Colombo, C., Lucca, A., Benedetti, F., Barbini, B., Campori, E. & Smeraldi, E. (2000) Total sleep deprivation combined with lithium and light therapy in the treatment of bipolar depression: replication of main effects and interaction. *Psychiatry Res*, **95**, 43–53.

Condon, J.T., Boyce, P. & Corkindale, C.J. (2004) The first-time fathers study: a prospective study of the mental health and well-being of men during the transition to parenthood. *Australian and New Zealand Journal of Psychiatry*, **38** (1–2), 56–64.

Cox, J.L. (1986) *Postnatal Depression, a Guide for Health Professionals*. Edinburgh: Churchill Livingstone.

Cox, J.L. & Holden, J.M. (1986) Taking postnatal depression seriously. *Health Visitor*, **59**, 180.

Cox, J. & Holden, J. (eds) (1994) *Perinatal Psychiatry: Use and Misuse of the Edinburgh Postnatal Depression Scale*. London: Gaskell.

Cox, J., Connor, Y. & Kendell, R. (1982) Prospective study of the psychiatric disorders of childbirth. *British Journal of Psychiatry*, **140**, 111–117.

Cox, J., Holden, J. & Sagovsky, R. (1987) Detection of postnatal depression. Development of the ten-item Edinburgh, Postnatal Depression Scale. *British Journal of Psychiatry*, **150**, 182–186.

Coyle, N., Jones, I., Robertson, E., Lendon, C. & Craddock, N. (2000) Variation at the serotonin transporter gene influences susceptibility to bipolar affective puerperal psychosis. *Lancet*, **356**, 1490–1491.

Craft, A. & Hall, D. (2004) Munchausen syndrome by proxy and sudden infant death. *BMJ*, **328**, 1309–1312.

Craft, L.L. & Landers, D.M. (1998) The effects of exercise on clinical depression and depression resulting from mental illness: a meta-regression analysis. *J Sport Exerc Psychol*, **20**, 339–357.

Craig, M. (2004) Perinatal risk factors for neonaticide and infant homicide: can we identify those at risk? *R Soc Med*, **97** (2), 57–61.

Crawford, P. (1993) *The Nordic Eye*. Denmark: International Press.

Crisp, A.H., Lacey, J.H. & Crutchfield, M. (1987) Clomipramine and 'drive' in people with anorexia nervosa: an inpatient study. *Br J Psychiatry*, **150**, 355–358.

Crockenberg, S. & Leerkes, E. (2003) Developmental history, partner relationships and infant reactivity as predictors of postpartum depression and maternal sensitivity. *Journal of Family Psychology*, **17**, 1–14.

Crowe, D.M. (1996) *A History of the Gypsies of Eastern Europe and Russia*. New York: St Martins Griffin.

Cubison, J. (2007) Infanticide: just a thought or a real risk, Marcé Biennial Conference Abstracts (2006). *Archives of Women's Mental Health*, **10**, 1.

Cubison, J. & Munro, J. (2005) Acceptability of using the EPDS as a screening tool for depression in the postnatal period. In: *Screening for Perinatal Depression* (eds C. Henshaw and S. Elliot). London: Jessica Kingsley Publishers.

Currie, J. (2001) Pram-walking as postnatal exercise and support: an evaluation of the stroll your way to well-being program and supporting resources in terms of individual participation rates and community group formation. *The Australian Journal of Midwifery*, **14** (2), 21–25.

Custodero, L., Britto, P. & Brooks-Gunn, J. (2003) Musical lives: a collective portrait of American parents and their young children. *Journal of Applied Developmental Psychology*, **24** (5), 553–572.

Cypert, S.A. (1987) *Believe and Achieve*. New York: Dodd, Mead & Co.

Czarnocka, J. & Slade, P. (2000) Prevalance and predictors of post-traumatic stress symptoms following childbirth. *Br J Clin Psychol*, **39**, 35–51.

Dalton, K. (1980) *Depression After Childbirth*. New York: Oxford University Press.

Dalton, K. (1985) Progesterone prophylaxis used successfully in postnatal depression. *Practitioner*, **229**, 507–508.

Dalton, K. (1995) Progesterone prophylaxis for postnatal depression. *International Journal of Prenatal and Perinatal Psychology and Medicine*, 7, 447–450.

Danaci, A.E., Gönül Dinç, G., Deveci, A., Şen, F.S. & İçelli, I. (2002) Postnatal depression in Turkey: epidemiological and cultural aspects. Social Psychiatry and *Psychiatric Epiodemiology*, **37** (3), 125–129.

Darwin, C. (1872) *The Expression of the Emotions in Man and Animals*. London: John Murray.

Darzi, A. (2008) *High Quality Care for All. NHS Next stage review. Final Report*. London: Department of Health.

Davey, S., Dziurawiec, S. & O'Brien-Malone, A. (2006) *Men's Voices: Postnatal Depression From the Perspective of Male Partners Qualitative Health Research*, **16** (2), 206–220. Sage Publications.

Deal, L. & Holt, V. (1998) Young maternal age and depressive symptoms: results from the 1988 national maternal and infant health survey. *American Journal of Public Health*, **88**, 226–270.

Deater-Deckard, K., Pickering, K., Dunn, J. & Golding, J. (1998) Family structure and depressive symptoms in men preceding and following the birth of a child. *Am J Psychiatry*, **155**, 818–823.

Defeat Depression Campaign (1992) *Defeat Depression in the Workplace*. A national campaign organised by the Royal College of Psychiatrists and the Royal College of General Practitioners.

Dement, W. & Vaughan, C. (1999)*The Promise of Sleep*. London: Pan Books.

Denzin, N.K. (1992) Symbolic *Interactionism and Cultural Studies: The Politics of Interpretation*. Oxford: Blackwell.

Department of Education (2008) *Comprehensive Spending Review*. London: HM Treasury.

Department of Health (1999) *National Service Framework for Mental Health (1999)*. London: The Stationery Office.

Department of Health (2003) *Mental Health Act England and Wales 2003*. London: Department of Health.

Department of Health (2008) *Care Services Improvement Partnership (2008) Improving Access to Psychological Therapies – Implementation Plan: National Guidelines for Regional Delivery*. London: Department of Health Publications.

Department of Social Security (1997) *The New Deal for Lone Parents*. London: HM Treasury.

Descartes, R. (1988) *Selected Philosophical Writings*. Cambridge: Cambridge University Press.

Deuchar, N. & Brockington, I. (1998) Brief protocol for an international investigation of menstrual psychosis. *Archives of Women's Mental Health*, **1** (1), 3–50.

Dex, S. & Rowthorne, R. (1997) The case for a ministry of the family. In: *Rewriting the Sexual Contract* (ed. G. Dench), pp. 192–206. London: Institute for Community Studies/Joseph Rowntree Trust.

Dissanayake, E. (2000) Antecedents of the temporal arts in early mother-infant interaction. In: *The Origins of Music* (eds N.L. Wallin, B. Merker & S. Brown). Cambridge, MA: MIT Press. pp. 389–410.

Draper, J. (2002) 'It's the first scientific evidence': men's experience of pregnancy confirmation. *Journal of Advanced Nursing*, **39** (6), 563–570.

Driving Vehicle Licensing Authority (DVLA) (2002) Minutes of 'At a Glance' advice. Section 6.

Driving Vehicle Licensing Authority DVLA (2008) *For Medical Practitioners. At a Glance. Guide to Current Medical Standards of Fitness to Drive. Drivers Medical Group*. Swansea Driver and Vehicle Licensing Authority (DVLA) (www.dvla.gov.uk/publications).

Drummond, S., Brown, G., Gillin, C., Stricker, J., Wong, E. & Buxton, R. (2000) Altered brain response to verbal learning following sleep deprivation. *Nature*, **403**, 655–657.

Duncan, D. & Taylor, D. (1995) Which antidepressants are safe to use in breast feeding mothers? *Psychiatric Bulletin*, **19**, 551–552.

Duncan, D. & Taylor, D. (1996) Chlormethiazole or chlordiazepoxide in alcohol detoxification. *Psychiatric Bulletin*, **20**, 599–601.

Eberhard-Gran, M., Eskild, A., Tambs, K., Samuelsen, S.O. & Opjordsmoen, S. (2002) Depression in postpartum and non-postpartum women: prevalence and risk factors. *Activa Psychiarica Scandinavia*, **106** (6) 426–433.

Edhborg, M., Lundh, W., Seimyr, L. & Widstrom, A.M. (2003) The parent-child relationship in the context of maternal depressive mood. *Archives of Women's Mental Health*, **6** (3), 211–216.

Edwards, B., Galletly, C., Semmler-Booth, T. & Dekker, G. (2008) Does antenatal screening for psychosocial risk factors predict postnatal depression? A follow-up study of 154 women in Adelaide, South Australia. *Australian and New Zealand Journal of Psychiatry*, (1), 51–55.

Elkin, I., Shea, M.T., Watkins, J.L. *et al.* (1989) General effectiveness of treatments. *Archives of General Psychiatry*, **46**, 971–982.

Ellis, A. (1987) The evolution of rational – emotive therapy and cognitive behaviour therapy. In: *The Evolution of Psychotherapy* (ed. J.K. Zeig). New York: Brunner/ Mazel.

Elliot, S. (1990) Commentary on 'Childbirth as a Life Event'. *J. Repr. and Infant Psychology*, **8**, 147–159.

Ellis, A. & Dryden, W. (1987) *The Practice of Rational-emotive Therapy*. New York: Springer.

Evans, J., Heron, J., Francomb, H., Oke, S. & Golding, J. (2001) Cohort study of depressed mood during pregnancy and after childbirth. *BMJ*, **323**, 257–260.

Everingham, C. (2006) *The Trusted Confidante: a Model for Supporting Parents. Pilot Program Results*. A University of Newcastle and Home-Start National Inc. Collaborative Research Project.

Favazza, A. (1998) The coming of age of self-mutilation. *Journal of Nervous and Mental Disease Volume*, **186** (5), 259–268.

Feldman, R., Eidelman, A., Sirota, L. & Weller, A. (2002) Comparison of skin-to-skin (Kangaroo) and traditional care: parenting outcomes and preterm infant development. *Pediatrics*, **110**, (1), 26.

Ferber, S.G. & Makhoul, R.I. (2004) The effect of skin-to-skin contact (Kangaroo care) shortly after birth on neurobehavioral responses of the term newborn: a randomized control trial. *Pediatrics*, **113**, 858–865.

Ferber, S.G., Kuint, J., Weller, A., Dolberg, S. & Arbek Koheler, D. (2002) Massage therapy by mother enhances the adjustment of the circadian rhythm to the nocturnal period in full term infants. *Journal of Developmental & Behavioral Pediatrics*, **23** (6), 410–415.

Ferketich, S.I. & Mercer, R.T. (1995) Predictors of paternal role competence by risk status. *Nursing Research*, **44**, 89–95.

Field, T. (1998) Maternal depression effects on infants and early interventions. *Preventive Medicine*, **27** (2), 200–203.

Field, T., Grizzle, N., Scaffidi, F., *et al.* (1996) Massage therapy for infants of depressed mothers. *Infant Behaviour and Development*, **19** (107), 112.

Fink, G. Sumner, B.E., Rosie, R., Grace, O. & Quinne, J.P. (1996) Estrogen control of central neurotransmission: effect on mood, mental state, and memory. *Cell Molecular Neurobiology*, **16** (3), 325 –344.

Fisher, J., Hammarberg, H. & Baker, H. (2005) Assisted conception is a risk factor for postnatal mood disturbance and early parenting difficulties. *Fertility and Sterility*, **84** (2), 426–430.

Fitness, J. & Parker, V. (2003) Breaking the rules: exploring the causes and consequences of perceived rule violations by family members. *32nd Annual Meeting of the Society of Australasian Social Psychologists*, Sydney, Australia.

Fitness, J. & Williams, K. (2005) *Social Outcast: Ostracism, Social Exclusion, Rejection, and Bullying*. New York: Psychology Press.

Fordyce, M.W. (1983) A program to increase happiness: further studies. *Journal of Counselling Psychology*, **30** (4), 483–498.

Foucalt, M. (1973) *Mental Illness and Psychology*. New York: Harper.

Fox, K., Biddle, S., Edmunds, L., Bowler, I. & Killoran, A.L. (1997) Physical activity promotion through primary health care in England. *Br J Gen Pract*, **47**, 367–369.

Franco, D.L., Blais, M.A., Becker, A.E., *et al.* (2001) Pregnancy complications and neonatal outcomes in women with eating disorders. *Am J Psychiatry*, **158**, 1461–1466.

Franco, P., Seret, N., Van Hees, J.N., Scaillet, S., Groswasser, J. & Kahn, A. (2005) Influence of swaddling on sleep and arousal characteristics of healthy infants. *Pediatrics*, **115** (5), 1307–1311.

Fraser, C. (2006) A description of pregnant women's perceptions and abstract drawings of being pregnant. *Journal of Prenatal & Perinatal Psychology & Health*, **21**, (1), 25–55.

Friedman, S. & Resnick, P. (2007) Child murder by mothers: pattern and prevention. *World Psychiatry*, **6** (3), 137–141.

Friedman, S.H., Hrouda, D.R., Holden. C.E., et al. (2005) Filicide-suicide: common factors among parents who kill their children and themselves. J Am Acad Psychiatry Law, 33, 496–504.

Friedson, E. (1970) *The Profession of Medicine*. New York: Aldine Pub Co.

Fujita, F., Diener, E. & Sandvik, E. (1991) Gender differences in negative effect and well-being: the emotional case for emotional intensity. *Journal of Personality and Social Psychology*, **61**, 427–434.

Fujita, M., Endoh, Y., Saimon, N. & Yamaguchi, S. (2006) Effect of massaging babies on mothers: pilot study on the changes in mood states and salivary cortisol level. *Complementary Therapies in Clinical Practice*, **12** (3), 181–185.

Garcia-Esteve, L., Ascaso, C., Ojuel, J. & Novarro, P. (2003) Validation of the Edinburgh Postnatal Depression Scale (EPDS) in Spanish Mothers. *Journal of Affective Disorders*, **75**, 71–76.

Garcia-Esteve, L., Ascaso, C., Gelabert, E. & Martín-Santos, R. (2008) Family caregiver role and premenstrual syndrome as associated factors for postnatal depression. *Archives of Women's Mental Health*, **11** (3), 193–200.

Gaskin, K. & James, H. (2006) Using the Edinburgh Postnatal Depression Scale with learning disabled mothers. *Community Practitioner*, **79** (12), 396.

Gerard, C., Harris, A. & Thach, B. (2002) Spontaneous arousals in supine infants while swaddled and unswaddled during rapid eye movement and quiet sleep. *Pediatrics*, **110** (6), 70.

Gerhardt, U. (1989) *Ideas About Illness*. Basingstoke: Macmillan.

Gerrard, J., Holden, J.M., Elliot, S., McKenzie, J. & Cox, J. (1993) A trainer's perspective of an innovative programme teaching health visitors about the detection, treatment and prevention of postnatal depression. *Journal of Advanced Nursing*, **18**, 1825–1832.

Giddens, A. (2006) *Sociology*. Cambridge: Polity Press.

Gjerdingen, D. & Center, A. (2003) First-time parents' prenatal to postpartum changes in health, and the relation of postpartum health to work and partner characteristics. *Journal of the American Board of Family Practice*, **16**, 304–311.

Glenmullen, J. (2000) *Prozac Backlash: Overcoming the Dangers of Prozac, Zoloft, Paxil, and other Antidepressants with Safe, Effective Alternatives*. New York: Simon & Schuster.

Glover, V. (1992) Do biochemical factors play a part in postnatal depression? *Neuropsychopharmacol Biol Psychiatry*, **16** (5), 605–615.

Goldstein, J. (1987) *Console and Classify: the French Psychiatric Profession in the Nineteenth Century*. Cambridge: Cambridge University Press.

Goodwin, G.M. (2003) Evidence based guidelines for treating bipolar disorder: recommendations from the British Association for Psychopharmacology. *Journal of Psychopharmacology*, **17** (92), 149–173.

Goodwin, J.M., Cheeves, K. & Connel, V. (1990) Borderline and other severe symptoms in adult survivors of incestuous abuse. *Psychiatric Annals*, **20**, 22–32.

Gordon, J., Swan, M. & Robertson, R. (1995) 'Babies don't come with a set of instructions': running support groups for mothers. *Health Visitor*, **68** (4), April, 155–156.

Gotlib, I.H. & Hammen, C.L. (1996) *Psychological Aspects of Depression*. Chichester: John Wiley & Sons.

Gotts, E.E. (1988). The right to quality child care. *Childhood Education*, **64**, 269–273.

Greenberg, B.D., Ziemann, U., Cora-Locatelli, G., *et al.* (2000) Altered cortical excitability in obsessive-compulsive disorder. *Neurology*, **54**, 142–147.

Gregoire, A.J., Kumar, R., Everitt, B., Henderson, A.F. & Studd, J.W. (1996) Transdermal oestrogen for treatment of severe postnatal depression. *Lancet*, **347** (9006), 930–933.

Grocke, D., Bloch, S. & Castle, D. (2006) Music therapy soothes mental illness. *Music Therapy*, **11**.

Gruen, D. (1990) Post-partum depression: a debilitating yet often unassessed problem. *Health and Social Work*, **15** (4), 261–269.

Guscott, R.G.M. & Steiner, M. (1991). A multidisciplinary treatment approach to postpartum psychoses. *Can J Psychiatry*, **36** (8), 551–556.

Gutteridge, K. (2001) The Tamworth Postnatal Depression support group. *MIDIRS Midwifery Digest*, **11**, 17–19.

Haapasalo, J. & Petaja, S. (1999) Mothers who killed or attempted to kill their child: life circumstances, childhood abuse, and types of killing. *Violence Vict*, **14**, 219–239.

Haberg, M. & Matheson, I. (1997) Antidepressive agents and breast feeding. *Tidsskr Nor Laegeforen*, **10**, 117 (27), 2952–3955.

Hackney, M. & Sherlock, P. (2006) Digging their way out of a black hole: women's accounts of postnatal depression. Marcé Biennial Scientific International Conference Abstracts. *Archives of Women's Mental Health*.

Hakkarainen, R., Johansson, C., Kieseppa, T., *et al.* (2003) Seasonal changes, sleep length and circadian preference among twins with bipolar disorder. *BMC Psychiatry*, **3**, 6.

Hall, L. & Cohn, L. (1999) *Bulimia: a guide to Recovery*. Carlsbald, CA: Gruze Books.

Hall, L.A., Kotch, J.B., Browne, D. & Raynes, D. (1996) Self-esteem as a mediator of the effects of stressors and social resources on depressive symptoms in postpartum mothers. *Nursing Research*, **45** (4), 231–238.

Hallberg, P. & Sjoblom, V. (2005) The use of selective serotonin reuptake inhibitors during pregnancy and breast-feeding: a review and clinical aspects. *J. Clin Psychopharmacology*, **25**, 59–73.

Hamilton, J.A. (1962) *Post partum psychiatric problems*. St Louis: Mosby.

Hamilton, J.A. (1977) Puerperal psychosis. *Gynaecology and Obstetrics*, **2**, 1–8.

Hanley, J. (2001) *Postnatal depression in three cultures*. Unpublished PhD thesis. Swansea University.

Hanley, J. & Long, B. (2006) A study of Welsh mothers' experiences of postnatal depression. *Midwifery*, **22** (2), June, 147–157.

Hanley, J., Cox, J. & Taylor, B. (2007) A critical analysis of video tapes on postnatal depression. *Contemporary Nurse*, **24**, (1), 52– 64.

Hansard (HL) Vol 108, col 292 (22nd March 1938).

Haralambos, M. (1990) *Sociology, Themes and Perspectives*. Cambridge: University Tutorial Press.

Hardy, B. & Parke, S. (1996) Postnatal health: cooperation in the community. *Brit J, of Community Nursing*, **1** (7), 415–420.

Harris, B., Othman, S., Davies, J.A., *et al.* (1992) Association between postpartum thyroid dysfunction and thyroid antibodies and depression. *BMJ*, **18** (305) (6846), 152–156.

Harris, B., Lovett, L., Newcombe, R.G., Read, G.F., Walker, R. & Riad-Fahmy, D. (1994) Maternity blues and major endocrine changes: Cardiff puerperal mood and hormone study II. *BMJ*, **308**, 949–953.

Harvey, I., Nelson, S.J., Lyons, R.A., *et al.* (1998) A randomized controlled trial and economic evaluation of counselling in primary care. *Br J Gen Pract*, **48** (428), March, 1043–1048.

Hawkins, J. DAS Clinical Advisory Group Member (2005) (www.goodmedicine.org.uk).

Hawton, K., Arensman, E., Townsend, E., *et al.* (1998) Deliberate self-harm: systematic review of efficacy of psychosocial and pharmacological treatments in preventing repetition. *BMJ*, **317**, 441–447.

Hay, D.F. & Kumar, R. (1995) Interpreting the effects of mother's postnatal; depression on children's intelligence: a critique and re-analysis. *Child Psychiatry and Human Development*, **25** (3), 165–181.

Hay, D., Pawlby, S., Sharp, D., Asten, P., Mills, A. & Kumar, K. (2001) Intellectual problems shown by 11-year-old children whose mothers had postnatal depression. *Journal of Child Psychology and Psychiatry*, **42** (7), 871–889.

Healthcare Commission (2008) *Towards Better Births: a Review of Maternity Services in England*. July. (www.healthcarecommission.org.uk).

Hearne, G., Iliff, A., Kirby, A., et al. (1998) Postnatal depression in the community. British Journal of General Practice, 48, 1064– 1066.

Heh, S.S. (2001) The association between depressive symptoms and social support in Taiwanese women during the month. *International Journal of Nursing Studies*, **41** (5), 573–579.

Heila, H., Isometsa, A., Henriksson, K.V., *et al.* (1997) Suicide and schizophrenia: a nationwide psychological autopsy study on age and sex specific clinical characteristics of 92 suicide victims with schizophrenia. *American Journal of Psychiatry*, **154**, 1235–1242.

Hemels, M.E., Einarson, A., Koren, G., *et al.* (2005) Antidepressant use during pregnancy and the rates of spontaneous abortions: a meta-analysis. *Ann Pharmcother*, **39**, 803–809.

Henderson, J. (2007) Vagal nerve stimulation verses deep brain stimulation for treatment resistant depression: show me the data. *Clinical Neurosugery*, **54**, 88–90.

Hendrick, V. (2003) Treatment of postnatal depression. *BMJ*, **327**, 1003–1004.

Henshaw, C. (2003) Mood disturbance in the early puerperium: a review. *Archives of Women's Mental Health*, **6**, 33–42.

Her Majesty's Prison Service (2008) Women Prisoners Prison Service Order PSO 4800 and Standard 35. London: HMSO (www.hmprisonservice.gov.uk).

Heron, J., O'Connor, T.G., Evans, J., Golding, G. & Glover, V. (2004) The course of anxiety and depression throughout pregnancy and the postpartum in a community sample *J. Affec Disord*, **80**, 65–73.

Herrera, N.C., Zajonc, R.B., Wieczorkowska, G. & Cichomski, B. (2003) Beliefs about birth rank and their reflections in reality. *Journal of Personality and Social Psychology*, **85**, 142–150.

Hickey, A.R., Boyce, P.M., Elllwood, D. & Morris-Yates, A.D. (1997) Early discharge and risk for postnatal depression. *Medical Journal of Australia*, **1**, 167 (5), Sept, 244–247.

Higgins, M., St James Roberts, I. & Glover, V. (2007) Postnatal depression and mother and infant outcomes after infant massage *Journal of Affective Disord*, **15**.

Hildebrandt Karraker, K. & Young, M. (2007) Night waking in 6-month-old infants and maternal depressive symptoms. *Journal of Applied Developmental Psychology*, **28**, 5–6, 493–498.

Hiltunen, P., Raudaskoski, T., Ebeling, H. & Moilanen, I. (2004) Does pain relief during delivery decrease the risk of postnatal depression? *Acta Obstet Gynecol Scand*, **83** (3), March, 257–61.

Hiscock, H. & Wake, M. (2002) Randomised controlled trial of behavioural infant sleep intervention to improve infant sleep and maternal mood. *BMJ*, **324**, 4 May, 1062–1065.

Hofberg, K. & Brockington, I.F. (2000) Tokophobia: an unreasoning dread of childbirth: a series of 26 cases. *The British Journal of Psychiatry*, **176**, 83–85.

Hoffbrand, S., Howard, L. & Crawley, H. (2002) Antidepressant treatment for postnatal depression. *Cochrane Review, The Cochrane Library*, **4**, 12 January.

Holden, J.M. (1991) Postnatal depression: its nature, effects and identification using the Edinburgh Postnatal Depression Scale. *Birth*, **18** (4) 211–21.

Holden, J.M., Sagovsky, R. & Cox, J.L. (1989) Counselling in a general practice setting: controlled study of health visitor intervention in treatment of postnatal depression. *BMJ*, **298**, 223– 226.

Hollyman, J.A., Freeling, P. & Paykel, E.S. (1988) Double-blind placebo-controlled trial of amitriptyline among depressed patients in general practice. *J R Coll Gen. Prac*, **38**, 393–397.

Hook, E.B. (1978) Dietary cravings and aversions during pregnancy. *Am J Clin Nutr*, **31**, 1355–1362.

Horowitz, A.V. (1982) The *Social Control of Mental Illness. Studies on Law and Social Control*. London: Academic Press.

Horowitz, J.A., Bell, M., Trybulski, J., *et al.* (2001) Promoting responsiveness between mothers with depressive symptoms and their infants. *Journal of Nursing Scholarship*, **33**, 323–329.

Hostetter, A., Stowe, Z.N., Altshuler, L., Hwang, S., Lee, E. & Haynes, D. (2006) Dose of selective serotonin reuptake inhibitors across pregnancy: clinical implications. *Depression and Anxiety*, **11**, 51–57.

Howard, L. & Hannam, M. (2003) Sudden infant death syndrome and psychiatric disorders. *The British Journal of Psychiatry*, 182, 379–380.

Howard, M., Battle, C.L., Pearlstein, T. & Rosene-Montella, K. (2006) A psychiatric mother-baby day hospital for pregnant and postpartum women. *Arch. Of Women's Mental Health*, 9, 213–218.

Howard, L.M., Kirkwood, G. & Latinovic, R. (2007) Sudden infant death syndrome and maternal depression. *J Clin Psychiatry*, 68, 1279–1283.

Huang, C.C. & Warner, L.A. (2005). Relationship characteristics and depression among fathers with newborns. *Social Service Review*, 79, 95–118.

Huang, Y.C. & Mathers, N.J. (2006) A comparison of sexual satisfaction and post-natal depression in the UK and Taiwan. *International Nursing Review* , 53 (3), 197–204.

Hussain, F. & Cochrane, R. (2002) Depression in South Asian women: Asian women's beliefs on causes and cures. *Mental Health, Religion and Culture*, 5 (3).

Hypericum Depression Trial Study Group (2002) Effects of *Hypericum perforatum* (St John's Wort) in major depressive disorder: a randomized controlled trial. *Journal of the American Medical Association*, 287 (14), 1807–1814.

Jacob, R., Clare, I.C.H., Holland, A., Watson, P.C., Maimaris, C. & Gunn, M. (2005) Self-harm, capacity, and refusal of treatment: implications for emergency medical practice. A prospective observational study. *Emergency Medicine Journal*, 22, 799–802.

Jadresic, E. & Araya, R. (1995) Prevalence of postpartum depression and associated factors in Santiago de Chile. *Rev Med Chil*, 123, 694–699.

Jebali, C. (1993) A feminist perspective on postnatal depression. *Health Visitor*, 66, 2, 59–60.

Jefferson, G. (2005) Video websites pop up, invite postings. *USA Today*. 21 November. Gannett Co. Inc.

Johanson, R., Chapman, G. Murray, D. Johnson, I. & Cox, J. (2000) The North Staffordshire Maternity Hospital prospective study of pregnancy associated depression. *Journal of Psychosomatic Obstetrics and Gynecology*, 21, 93–97.

Johnstone, S., Boyce, P., Hickey, A. Morris-Yates, A. & Harris, M. (2001) Obstetric risk factors for postnatal depression in urban and rural community samples. *Australian and New Zealand Journal of Psychiatry*, 35 (1), 69–74.

Jones, C. (2002) *Traditional Postpartum Rituals of India, North Africa and the Middle East*. Ohio: Kent State University.

Jones, I. & Craddock, N. (2001) Molecular genetics of bipolar disorder. *The British Journal of Psychiatry*, 178, 128–133.

Judd, L.L., Akiskal, H.S., Schlettler, P.J., *et al.* (2002) The long-term natural history of the weekly symptomatic status of bipolar 1 disorder. *Archives of General Psychiatry*, 59, 530–537.

Kallen, B. (2004) Neonate characteristics after maternal use of antidepressants in late pregnancy. *Archives of Pediatric Adolescent Medicine*, 158, 312–316.

Kallen, B. & Otterblad Olausson, P. (2006) Antidepressant drugs during pregnancy and infant congenital heart defect. *Reproductive Toxicology*, 21, 221.

Kalliomaki, M., Laippala, P., Korvenranta, H., Kero, P. & Lsolauri, E. (2001) Extent of fussing and colic type crying preceding atopic disease. *Arch Dis Child*, 84, 349–350.

Kalra, H., Tandon, R., Trivedi, J. & Janca, A. (2005) Pregnancy-induced obsessive compulsive disorder: a case report. *Annals of General Psychiatry*, **4**, 12.

Kammerer, M. Taylor, A. & Glover, V. (2006) The HPA axis and perinatal depression: a hypothesis. *Archives of Womens' Mental Health*, **9**, 187–196.

Kaplan, P.S., Dungan, J.K. & Zinser, M.C. (2004) Infants of chronically depressed mothers learn in response to male, but not female, infant-directed speech. *Developmental Psychology*, **40**, 140–148.

Kauppi, A., Kumpulainen, K., Vanamo, T., Merikanto, J. & Karkola, K. (2008) Maternal depression and filicide – case study of ten mothers. *Archives of Women's Mental Health*, **11** (3), 1434–1816.

Kawamura, K., Ichikawa, Y., Nakano, M., *et al.* (1999) Stressed parents with infants: reassessing physical abuse risk factors – child, parent, and family dysfunction. *Child Abuse and Neglect*, **23** (9) September, 845–853.

Kaye, W.H., Bulik, C.M.,Thornton, L., *et al.* (2004) Comorbidity of anxiety disorders with anorexia and bulimia nervosa. *Am J Psychiatry*, **161**, December, 2215–2221.

Kelly, A. (1994) Management of postnatal psychological disturbances. *J. of Psychiatry in Practice*, **13** (2), 13–15.

King, M., Sibbald, B., Ward, E., *et al.* (2000) Randomised controlled trial of non-directive counselling, cognitive behaviour therapy and usual general practitioner care in the management of depression as well as mixed anxiety and depression in primary care. *Health Technology Assessment*, **4** (19).

Kirsch, I., Moore, T., Scoboria, A. & Nicholls, S. (2002). The emperor's new drugs: an analysis of antidepressant medication data submitted to the US Food and Drug Administration. *Prevention & Treatment*, **5** (23).

Kleinke, C., Staneski, R. & Mason, J. (1982) Sex differences in coping with depression. *Sex Roles*, 8 (8), 877–889.

Klerman, G.L., Weissman, M.M., Rounsaville, B.J. & Chevron, E.S. (1984) *Interpersonal Psychotherapy for Depression*. New York: Basic Books.

Klonsky, E.D. & Moyer, A. (2008) Childhood sexual abuse and non-suicidal self-injury: meta-analysis. *The British Journal of Psychiatry*, **192**, 166–170.

Kukil, K.V. (ed.) (2000) *The Journals of Sylvia Plath 1950–1962*. London: Faber and Faber Ltd.

Kumar, R. (1994) Postnatal depression. *Maternal and Child Health*, **19** (11), 354–358.

Kumar, R. & Robson, K. (1984) A prospective study of emotional disorders in childbearing women. *Br J. Psychiatry*, **144**, 35–47.

Kurstjens, S. & Wolke, D. (2001) Effects of maternal depression on cognitive development of children over the first 7 years of life. *Journal of Child Psychology and Psychiatry*, **42** (5), 623–636.

Lacey, J.H. & Smith, G. (1987) Bulimia nervosa: the impact of pregnancy on mother and baby. *Br J Psychiatry*, **150**, 777–781.

La Coursiere, D.Y., Baksh, L., Bloebaum, l. & Varner, M.W. (2006) Maternal body mass index and self-reported postpartum depressive symptoms. *Maternal Child Health*, 8 Aug.

Laine, K., Heikkinene, T., Ekblad, U. & Kero, P. (2003) Effects of exposure to selective serotonin reuptake inhibitors during pregnancy on seroteonergic symptoms in newborn and cord blood monoamine and prolactin concentrations. *Archives of General Psychiatry*, **60**, 720–726.

Laing, R.D. (1969) *The Divided Self*. New York: Pantheon Books.

Lam, D., Watkins, E., Hayward, P., *et al.* (2003) A randomised controlled study of cognitive therapy of relapse prevention for bipolar affective disorder – outcome of the first year. *Archives of General Psychiatry*, 60, 145–152.

Lau, A. (2005) The case for inclusion: mental health and the NSF for long-term conditions. *Advances in Psychiatric Treatment*, 11, 385–387.

LaValle, J.B., Krinsky, D.L., Hawkins, E.B., *et al.* (2000) *Natural Therapeutics Pocket Guide*. Hudson, OH: LexiComp. pp. 387–388.

Law Commissions Act (1965) Chapter 22 (www.lawcom.gov.uk/publications.htm).

Lawlor, D. & Hooker, S. (2001) The effectiveness of exercise as an intervention in the management of depression: systematic review and meta-regression analysis of randomised controlled trials. *BMJ*, 3 (322), 763.

Lawrence, M. (1969) *The Tunnel*. London: Granada Publishing.

Leary, M. (2003) *Interpersonal Rejection*. New York: Oxford University Press.

Leask, S.J., Jones, P.B., Done, D.J., Crow, T.J. & Richards, M. (2000) No association between breast-feeding and adult psychosis in two national birth cohorts. *The British Journal of Psychiatry*, 177, 218–221.

Leviston, A. & Downs, M. (1999) When instinct is not enough. *Community Practitioner*, 2 (6), 184–185.

Levison-Castiel, R. (2006) Infants and antidepressant withdrawal. *Archives of Pediatric and Adolescent Medicine*, 160, 173–176.

Levison-Castiel, R., Merlob, P., Linder, N., Sirota, L. & Klinger, G. (2006) Neonatal abstinence syndrome after in utero exposure to selective serotonin reuptake inhibitors in term infants. *Archives of Pediatrics & Adolescent Medicine*, 160, 173–176.

Lewis, C. & Lamb, M.E. (2003) Father's influences on children's development. The evidence from two-parent families. *European Journal of Psychology of Education*, 18, 211–228.

Limosin, F., Rouillon, F., Payan, C., Cohen, J.-M. & Strub, N. (2003) Prenatal exposure to influenza as a risk factor for adult schizophrenia. *Acta Psyvhiatrica Scandinavica*, 107 (5), 331–335.

Linde, K. & Mulrow, C.D. (2004) St John's Wort for depression (Cochrane review). In: The Cochrane Library, Issue 3, 2004. Chichester, UK: Wiley.

Litchfield, P. (1993) Depression in the workplace. *Defeat Depression Campaign Literature*. London: Royal College of Psychiatry.

Littlewood, J. & McHugh, N. (1997) *Maternal Distress and Postnatal Depression: the Myth of Madonna*. London: MacMillan Press.

Livingstone, J.E., Macleod, P.M. & Applegarth, D.A. (1978) Vitamin B6 status in women with post- partum depression. *American Journal of Clinical Nutrition*, 31, 886–891.

Llorente, A.M., Jensen, C.L., Voigt, R.C., *et al.* (2003) Effect of maternal docosahexaenoic acid supplementation on post-partum depression and information processing. *American Journal of Obstetrics and Gynecology*, 188, 1345–1353.

Lloyd, G.E.R. (ed.) (1978*) Hippocrates. Hippocratic Writings*. Harmondsworth: Penguin Books.

Louik, C., Lin, A., Werler, M., Hernandez-Diaz, S. & Mitchell, A. (2007) First-trimester use of selective serotonin-reuptake inhibitors and the risk of birth defects. *New England Journal of Medicine*, 356, 2675–2683.

Lovestone, S. & Kumar, R. (1993) Postnatal psychiatric illness: the impact on partners. *British Journal of Psychiatry*, **163**, 210–216.

Lucas, A. & St James Roberts, I. (1998) Crying, fussing and colic behaviour in breast- and bottle-fed infants. *Early Human Development*, **53** (1), 9–18.

Ma, L., Tan, Q., Wang, Z., *et al.* (2007) Lower levels of whole blood serotonin in obsessive-compulsive disorder and in schizophrenia with obsessive-compulsive symptoms. *Psychiatry Research*, **150** (1), 61–69.

Macdonald-Milner, T. (2002) *The Marks and Spencer Programme. Stress Management in Retail*. Harrogate: Marks and Spencer.

Mackenzie, B. & Levitan, R. (2005) Psychic and somatic anxiety differentially predict response to light therapy in women with seasonal affective disorder. *Journal of Affective Disorders*, **88** (2), 163–166.

Main, M., Tomasini, L. & Tolan, W. (1979) Differences among mothers of infants judged to differ in security. *Development Psychology*, **15** (7), 472– 473.

Manber, R., Allen, J.J. & Morris, M.M. (2002) Alternative treatments for depression: empirical support and relevance to women. *J Clin Psychiatry*, **63**, 628–40.

Marcus, S.M., Flynn, H.A., Blow, F. & Barry, K. (2005) A screening study of antidepressant treatment rates and mood symptoms in pregnancy. *Archives of Women's Mental Health*, **8**, 25–27.

Marcuse, H. (1964) One *Dimensional Man*. Boston: Beacon Press.

Markowitz, S. & Friedman Rutgers, M.S. (2008) Understanding the relationship between obesity and depression: casual mechanisms and implications for treatment. *Clinical Psychology: Science and Practice*, **15** (1).

Marks, C.R. (1996) *Relation of marital violence, parenting self-efficacy, and child adjustment*. Unpublished doctoral dissertation, University of Southern California, Los Angeles.

Marks, M.N. & Kumar, R. (1993) Infanticide in England and Wales. *Med Sci Law*, **33**, 329–339.

Marks, M.N. & Kumar, R. (1996) Infanticide in Scotland. *Med Sci Law*, **36**, 201–204.

Martin, J., Hiscock, H., Hardy, P., Davey, B. & Wake, M. (2007) Adverse associations of infant and child sleep problems and parent health: an Australian population study. *Pediatrics*, **119** (5), 947–955.

Marzuk, P.M., Tardiff, K., Leon, A.C., *et al.* (1997) Lower risk of suicide during pregnancy. *Am J Psychiatry*, **154** (1), 122–123.

Masden, S.A. & Juhl, T. (2007) Paternal depression in the postnatal period assessed with traditional and male depression scales. *The Journal of Men's Health & Gender*, **4** (1), 26–31.

Masefield, John (1910) *CLM*.

Matthews, K. & Eljamel, M.K. (2003) Status of neurosurgery for mental disorder in Scotland. *Br J Psychiatry*, **182**, 404–411.

Matthey, S., Barnett, B., Kavanagh, D.J. & Howie, P. (2001) Validation of the Edinburgh Postnatal Depression Scale for men, and comparison of item endorsement with their partners. *Journal of Affective Disorders*, **64** (2–3), 175–184.

Matthey, S., Kavanagh, D.J., Howie, P., Barnett, B. & Charles, M. (2004) Prevention of postnatal distress or depression: an evaluation of an intervention at preparation for parenthood classes. *Journal of Affective Disorders*, **79** (1–3), 113–126.

May, A. (1995) Using exercise to tackle postnatal depression. *Health Visitor*, 4, 146–147.

McClure, R., Davis, P. & Meadow, S. (1996) Epidemiology of Munchausen syndrome by proxy. *Arch Dis Child*, 75, 57–61.

McMunn, A., Bartley, M., Hardy, R. & Kuh, D. (2006) Life course social roles and women's health in mid-life: causation or selection? *Journal of Epidemiology and Community Health*, 60, 484–489.

Mead, G.H. (1934) *Mind, Self and Society*. Chicago: Chicago University Press.

Meadow, S.R. (1977) Munchausen syndrome by proxy: the hinterland of child abuse. *Lancet*, 2, 343–345.

Meager, I. & Milgrom, J. (1996) Group treatment for postpartum depression: a pilot study. *Australian & New Zealand Journal of Psychiatry*, 30 (6), Dec, 852–860.

Meichenbaum, D. & Genest, M. (1987) Cognitive behavioural modification: an integration of cognitive and behavioural methods. In: *Helping People Change: a Text Book of Methods* (eds F.H. Kanfer & A.P. Golstein) second edn. New York: Pergamon Press.

Meyer, C.L. Oberman, M. (2001) *Mothers who Kill their Children: Understanding the Acts of Moms from Susan Smith to the 'Prom Mom'*. New York: New York University Press.

Milgrom, J., Negri, L., Gemmill, A., McNeil, M. & Martin, P.R. (2005) A randomized control trial of psychological interventions for postnatal depression. *British Journal of Clinical Psychology*, 44 (4), 529–542.

Mind (2006) New mums failed by services. Report posted on Monday 15 May (Survey was commissioned by M. Oates & I. Rotheroe. *Out of the Blue? Motherhood and Depression*). Brighton and Hove: Mind Publications.

Misri, S., Kostaras, X., Fox, D. & Kostaras, D. (2000) The impact of partner support in the treatment of postpartum depression. *Canadian Journal of Psychiatry*, 45 (6), 554–558.

Mitchell, E.A., Taylor, B.J., Ford, R.K., *et al.* (1992) Four modifiable and other major risk factors for cot death: the New Zealand Study. *Journal of Paediatric Child Health*, 28 (suppl 1), S3–S8.

Mittendorfer-Rutz, E., Rasmussen, F. & Wasserman, D. (2005) Restricted fetal growth and adverse maternal psychosocial and socioeconomic conditions as risk factors for suicidal behavior of offspring: a cohort study. *Obstetrical & Gynecological Survey*, 60 (3), 152–153.

Moncrieff, J. & Kirsch, I. (2005) Efficacy of antidepressants in adults. *British Medical Journal*, 331, 155–157.

Morgan, P. (1996) Who *Needs Parents?* London: Institute of Economic Affairs.

Morgan, M. (1997) A group programme for postnatally depressed women and their partners. *Journal of Advanced Nursing*, 26 (5), 913–920.

Morgan, W.P. & Goldston, S.E. (1987) *Exercise and Mental Health*. Washington: Hemisphere Publishing.

Morgan, M., Calnan, M. & Manning, N. (1991) *Sociological Approaches to Health and Medicine*. London: Routledge.

Morgan, J.F., Lacey, J.H. & Sedgwick, P.M. (1999) Impact of pregnancy on bulimia nervosa. *Br J Psychiatry*, 174, 135–140.

Morgan, J., Hubert Lacey, J. & Chung, E. (2006) Risk of postnatal depression, miscarriage, and preterm birth in bulimia nervosa: retrospective controlled study. *Psychosomatic Medicine*, **68**, 487–492.

Murray, L. (2001) *How Postnatal Depression can Affect Children and their Families*. CPHVA conference proceedings, 20–23 October.

Murray, L. & Carothers, A.D. (1990) The validation of the Edinburgh Postnatal Depression Scale on a community sample. *British Journal of Psychiatry*, **157**, 288–290.

Murray, L., Stanley, C., Hooper, R., *et al.* (1996a) The role of infant factors in postnatal depression and mother infant interactions. *Developmental Medicine and Child Neurology*, **38**, 109–119.

Murray, L., Fiori-Cowley, A., Hooper, R. & Cooper, P.J. (1996b) The impact of postnatal depression and associated adversity on early mother infant interactions and late infant outcome. *Child Development*, **67** (5), 2512–2526.

National Center for Complementary and Alternative Medicine (2005) St John's Wort fact sheet. July. Available at http://nccam.nih.gov/health/stjohnswort

National Institute for Clinical Excellence (2003) *Guidelines for Antenatal Care*. London: NICE.

National Institute for Clinical Excellence (2004) *Depression: Management of Depression in Primary and Secondary Care*. Clinical practice guideline No. 23. London: NICE.

National Institute for Clinical Excellence (2005a) *Guidelines for Depression in Children and Young People*. London: NICE.

National Institute Clinical Excellence (2005b) *National Institute Clinical Excellence Guidelines on Self-harm*. No. CG16. London: NICE.

National Institute for Clinical Excellence (2007) *Antenatal and Postnatal Mental Health*. Clinical practice guideline No. 45. London: NICE.

National Screening Committee for Postnatal Depression (2002) *Use of the Edinburgh Postnatal Depression Screening Scale*. London: Department of Health.

Netmums (2007) A Mum's Life. http://www.netmums.com

Neziek, J.B. (1995) Social construction, gender/sex similarity and social interaction in close personal relationships. *Journal of Social and Personal Relationships*, **12** (4), 503–520. Sage Publications.

Nicholas, S. (2007) Are you a tokophobic? *Daily Mail*. 27 October.

Niebuhr, D., Millikan, A., Cowan, D., Yolken, R., Yuanzhang, L. & Webber, N. (2008) Selected infectious agents and risks of schizophrenia among US military personnel. *American Journal of Psychiatry*, **165**, 99–106.

Nikolopoulou, M. & St James-Roberts, I. (2003) Preventing sleeping problems in infants who are at risk of developing them. *Archives of Disease in Childhood*, **88**, 108–111.

Nishihara, K., Horiuchi, S., Eto, H. & Uchida, S. (2002) The development of infants' circadian rest-activity rhythm and mothers' rhythm. *Physiology & Behavior*, **77**, 91–98.

Nonacs, R. & Cohen, L.S. (2002) Depression during pregnancy: diagnosis and treatment options. *J Clin Psychiatry*, **63** (S7), 24–30.

Nonacs, R. & Cohen, L. (2003) Assessment and treatment of depression during pregnancy: an update. *Psychiatric Clinics of North America*, **26** (3), 547–562.

Nusche, J. (2002) Lying in. *JAMC*, **167** (6), Sept.

Oakeshott, I. (2008) John Prescott: my secret battle with bulimia. Timesonline from *The Sunday Times*. 20 April.

Oakley, A. (1975) *Women Confined: Towards a Sociology of Childbirth*. London: Martin Robertson.

Oberlander, T.F., Warburton, W., Misri, S., Aghajanian, J. & Hertzman, C. (2006) Neonatal outcomes after prenatal exposure to selective serotonin reuptake inhibitor antidepressants and maternal depression using population-based linked health data. *Arch Gen Psychiatry*, **63**, 898–906.

O'Connor, T.G., Heron, J., Glover, V. & the ALSPAC Team (2002a) Antenatal anxiety predicts child behavioral/emotional problems independently of postnatal depression, *J. Am. Acad. Child Adolesc. Psych*, **41**, 1470–1477.

O'Conner, T.G., Heron, J., Golding, J., Beveridge, M. & Glover, V. (2002b) Maternal antenatal anxiety and children's behavioural/emotional problems at 4 years: report from the ALSPAC. *British Journal of Psychiatry*, **180**, 502–508.

O'Hara, M.W. & Swain, A.M. (1996) Rates and risk of postpartum depression: a meta-analysis. *International Review of Psychiatry*, **8**, 37–54.

Olausson, P.O., Cnattingius, S. & Haglund, B. (1999) Teenage pregnancies and risk of late fetal death and infant mortality. *Br J Obstet Gynaecol*, 106, 116–121.

Olausson, P.O., Cnattingius, S. & Haglund, B. (2001) Does the increased risk of preterm delivery in teenagers persist in pregnancies after the teenage period? *Br J Obstet Gynaecol*, **108**, 721–725.

Oldershaw, A., Richards, C. & Schmidt, U. (2008) Parents' perspectives on adolescent self-harm: qualitative study. *The British Journal of Psychiatry*, **193**, 140–144.

Olds, D., Eckenrode, J. & Henderson, C.R. (1997) Long-term effects of home visitation on maternal life course and child abuse and neglect: fifteen year follow-up of a randomized trial. *JAMA*, **278**, 637–643.

Oren, D., Wisner, K., Spinelli, M., *et al.* (2002) An open trial of morning light therapy for treatment of antepartum depression. *Am J Psychiatry*, **159**, 666–669,

Orr, J. & Luker, K. (1992) *Health Visiting Towards Community Health Nursing*. London: Blackwell Scientific Publications.

Owen, T. (1987) *Welsh Folk Customs*. Llandysul: Gomer.

Palmero, G. (2002) Murderous parents *International Journal of Offender Therapy and Comparative Criminology*, **46** (2), 123–143.

Palermo, M.T. (2003) Preventing filicide in families with autistic children. *Int J Offender Ther Comp Criminol*, **47** (1), 47–57.

Papoušek, M. (1996) Intuitive parenting. A hidden source of musical stimulation in infancy. In: I. Deliège & J. Sloboda (eds) *Musical Beginnings and Development of Musical Competence*. pp. 88–112. Oxford: Oxford University Press.

Pariante, C., Thomas, S., Lovestone, S., Makoff, A. & Kerwin, R. (2004) Do antidepressants regulate how cortisol affects the brain? *Psychoneuroendocrinology*, **29** (4), 423–447.

Parsons, T. (1951) *The Social System*. Glencoe, Ill: The Free Press.

Paulson, J., Dauber, S. & Leiferman, J.A. (2006) Individual and combined effects of postpartum depression in mothers and fathers on parenting behavior. *Pediatrics*, **1818** (2), 659–668.

Pawlby, S.J., Hay, D.F. & Sharp, D.J. (2001) The effects of postnatal depression on the development of boys. *Archives of Women's Mental Health*, **3** (suppl 2), 5.

Pearlstein, T., Zlotnick, C., Battle, C., *et al.* (2006) Patient choice of treatment for postpartum depression: a pilot study. *Archives of Women's Mental Health*, **9**, 303–309.

Pearson, P. (1997) *She Was Bad: Violent Women and the Myth of Innocence*. Toronto: Random House of Canada.

Peindle, K.S. (1995) Effects of postpartum psychiatric illness on family planning. *International Journal of Psychiatric Medicine*, **25** (3), 291–300.

Perlis, M., Jungquist, C., Smith, M. & Posner, D. (2005) *Cognitive Behavioral Treatment of Insomnia: a Session-by-session Guide*. New York: Springer.

Phillips, M. (1997) The *Sex Change State*. London: Social Market Foundation Memorandum. No. 30.

Pink, S. (2001) *Doing Visual Ethnography*. London: Sage Publications.

Pitt, B. (1968) 'Atypical' depression following childbirth. *The British Journal of Psychiatry*, **114**, 1325–1335.

Pitt, B. (1993) Down *with GLOOM or How to Defeat Depression*. London: Gaskell.

Pitts, F. (1995) Comrades in adversity: the group approach. *Health Visitor*, **68** (4), 144–145.

Pitts, F. (1999) The Monday group: postnatal depression revisited. *Community Practitioner*, **72** (10), 327–329.

Plath, S. (1963) *The Bell Jar*. London: Faber and Faber Ltd.

Plath, S. (2000) *The Journals of Sylvia Plath (1950–1962)*. (ed. K. Kukil) London: Faber and Faber Ltd.

Poole, H., Mason, L. & Osborne, T. (2006) Women's views of being screened for postnatal depression. *Community Practitioner*, **79** (11), 363–367.

Powell, J. & Clarke, A. (2002) The www of the world wide web: who, what, and why? *J Med Internet Res*, **4** (1), e4.

Pretty, J., Peacock, J., Hine, R., Sellens, M., South, N. & Griffin, M. (2007) Green exercise in the UK countryside: effects on health and psychological well-being, and implications for policy and planning. *Journal of Environmental Planning and Management*, **50** (2), 211–231.

Priya, J.V. (1992) *Birth Traditions and Modern Pregnancy Care*. Shaftesbury: Element.

Profet, M. (1995) *Protecting your Baby-to-be: Preventing Birth Defects in the First Trimester*. Reading, MA: Addison-Wesley.

de Quincy, Thomas (1821) Confessions of an opium eater. *London Magazine*.

Rachman, S. (1993) Obsessions, responsibility and guilt. *Behav Res Therapy*, **31**, 149–154.

Rade-Yarrow, M., Cummings, E.M. & Kuczinsky, L. (1985) Patterns of attachment in two and three-year-olds in normal families with parental depression. *Child Development*, **56**, 884–893.

Ramchandani, P., Stein, A., Evans, J., O'Connor, T. and the ALSPAC study team (2005) Paternal depression in the postnatal period and child development: a prospective population study. *Lancet*, **365** (9478), 2201–2205.

Raphael, D. (1996) *Pre-term Birth and Good Obstetric Practice*. Marcé Society. Biennial International Scientific Plenary lecture. Cambridge.

Raymont, V. (2001) Suicide in schizophrenia – how can research influence training and clinical practice? *Psychiatric Bulletin*, **25**, 46–50.

Read, J. (1999) Sexual problems associated with infertility, pregnancy and ageing. *BMJ*, **318**, 587–589.

Reid, I.A., Morris, B.J. & Gangong, W.F. (1977) The Renin-angiotensin system. *Annual Review of Physiology*, **40**, 377–398.

Resnick, P.J. (1970) Murder of the newborn: a psychiatric review of neonaticide. *American Journal of Psychiatry*, **126**, 58–64.

Reynolds, J.L. (1997) Post-traumatic stress disorder after childbirth: the phenomenon of traumatic birth. *CMAJ*, **15** (6), 831–835.

Rhodes, P. & Nocon, A. (2003) A problem of communication? Diabetes care among diabetic Bangladeshis in Bradford. *Health and Social Care in the Community*, **11** (2), 45–54.

Rice, R. (1997) Neurophysiological development in premature infants following stimulation. *Developmental Psychology*, **13** (69), 76.

Riemann, D., Hohagen, F., König, A., et al. (1996) Advanced versus normal sleep timing: effects on depressed mood after response to sleep deprivation in patients with a major depressive disorder. *J Aff Disord*, **37**.

Riemann, D., Berger, M. & Voderholzer, U. (2001) Sleep and depression – results from psychobiological studies: an overview. *Biological Psychology*, **57** (1–3), 67–103.

Risco, L., Jadresic, E., Galleguillos, T., et al. (2002) Depresión post parto: alta frecuencia en puérperas chilenas, detección precoz, seguimiento y factores de riesgo. *Psiquiatría y Salud Integral*, **2**, 61–66.

Robertson, E., Grace, S., Wallington, T. & Steward, D.E. (2004) Antenatal risk factors for post-partum depression: a synthesis of recent literature. *Gen Hosp Psych*, **26**, 289–295.

Robertson, S., Grace, T., Wallington, D. & Stewart, E. (2006) Antenatal risk factors for postpartum depression: a synthesis of recent literature. *General Hospital Psychiatry*, **26** (4), 289–295.

Robinson, J. (2003) Postnatal depression: why women lie. *British Journal of Midwifery*, **11** (11), 679.

Rogers, C. (1957) The necessary and sufficient conditions of therapeutic personality change. *Journal of Consulting Psychology*, **21** (2), 95–103.

Rondo, P.H., Ferreira, R.F., Nogueira, F., Ribeiro, M.C., Lobert, H. & Artes, R. (2003) Maternal psychological stress and distress as predictors of low birthweight, prematurity and intrauterine growth retardation. *Eur J Clin Nutr*, **57**, 266–272.

Rony, F.T. (1996) *The Third Eye. Race, Cinema and Ethnographic Spectacle*. Durham and London: Duke University Press.

Ross, L.E., Murray, B.J. & Steiner, M. (2005) Sleep and perinatal mood disorders: a critical review. *J Psychiatry Neurosci*, **30**, 247–256.

Rouge-Maillart, C., Jousset, N., Gaudin, A., et al. (2005) Women who kill their children. *Am J Forensic Med Pathol*, **26**, 320–326.

Rowley, C. & Dixon, L. (2002) The utility of the EPDS for health visiting practice. *Community Practitioner*, **75** (10), 385–389.

Royal College of Obstetricians and Gynaecologists (2002) *Confidential Enquiry into Maternal Deaths in the United Kingdom (1997–1999) Why Mothers Die*. London: Royal College of Obstetricians and Gynaecologists.

Royal College of Obstetricians and Gynaecologists (2003) *Confidential Enquiry into Maternal deaths in the United Kingdom (2003–2005) Saving Mothers' Lives: Reviewing Maternal Deaths to Make Motherhood Safer.* London: Royal College of Obstetricians and Gynaecologists.

Royal College of Psychiatrists (2000) *Perinatal Maternal Mental Health Services.* Council Report CR88. London: Royal College of Psychiatrists.

Rubertsson, C., Waldenstrom, U. & Wickberg G, (2003) Depressive mood in early pregnancy: prevalence and women at risk in a national Swedish sample. *Journal of Reproductive and Infant Psychology,* **21** (2), 113–123.

Ryan, M. (1995) *Postnatal Depression, Relationships and Men* Presentation at the First International Congress on Men. Ottowa Cited George M. paper in the HVA/NCH National Conference 1996.

Sanderson, C.A., Cowden, B., Hall, D.M.B., Taylor, E.M., Carpenter, R.G. & Cox, J.L. (2002) Is postnatal depression a risk factor for sudden infant death? *British Journal of General Practice,* **52,** 636–640.

Scaffidi, F., Field, T., Schanberg, S., *et al.* (1990) Massage stimulates growth in preterm infants: a replication. *Infant Behav Dev,* 13, 69–76.

Scheff, T. (1986) *Being Mentally Ill: a Sociological Theory.* Chicago: Adline.

Scholl, T.O., Miller, L.K., Salmon, R.W., Cofsky, M.C. & Shearer, J. (1987) Prenatal care adequacy and the outcome of adolescent pregnancy: effects on weight gain, preterm delivery and birth weight. *Obstet Gynecol,* **69,** 312–316.

Scholl, T.O., Hediger, M.L. & Belsky, D.H. (1994) Prenatal care and maternal health during adolescent pregnancy: a review and meta-analysis. *Journal of Adolescent Health,* **15,** 444–456.

Scottish Intercollegiate Guideline Network (SIGN) (2002) *Guidelines for Postnatal Depression and Puerperal Psychosis: a National Clinical Guideline.* SIGN Publication No. 60. Edinburgh.

Scott, J. (1988) Chronic Depression. *Br J Psych,* **153,** 287–297.

Scott, C. (2005) Diagnosing childhood conditions: have you considered[e]...? *Medical Protection Society Casebook,* **13,** 22–25.

Scott, J. & Colom, F. (2005) Psychosocial treatments for bipolar disorders. *Psychiatric Clinics of North America,* **28,** 371–384.

Scott, J., Paykel, E., Morriss, R., Bentall, R., Kinderman, P. & Johnson, T. (2006) Cognitive–behavioural therapy for bipolar disorder *The British Journal of Psychiatry,* **188,** 488–489.

Seeley, S. (2001) Strengths and limitations of the Edinburgh Postnatal Depression Scale *CPHVA Conference Proceedings,* October, 16–19.

Semple, D.M., McIntosh, A.M. & Lawrie, S.M. (2005) Cannabis as a risk factor for psychosis: a systematic review. *Journal of Psychopharmacol,* **19** (2), March, 187–194.

Shakespeare, J., Blake, F. & Garcia, J. (2003) A qualitative study of the acceptability of routine screening of postnatal women using the Edinburgh Postnatal Depression Scale. *British Journal of General Practice,* **53,** 614–619.

Sharp, D., Hay, D.F., Pawlby, S., *et al.* (1995) The impact of postnatal depression on boys' intellectual development. *Journal of Child Psychology and Psychiatry and Allied Disciplines,* **36,** 1315 –1336.

Shaw, M.E. (1976) *Group Dynamics. The Psychology of Small Group Behavior*. Second edition. New York: McGraw Hill.

Sheard, C., Cox, S., Oates, M., Ndukwe, G. & Glazebrook, C. (2007) Impact of a multiple, IVF birth on post-partum mental health: a composite analysis. *Human Reproduction*, **1**.

Shelton, R.C., Keller, M.B., Gelenberg, A., *et al.* (2001) Effectiveness of St John's Wort in major depression: a randomized controlled trial. *Journal of the American Medical Association*, **285**, 1978–1986.

Sheppard, M. (1997) Depression in female health visitor consulters: social and demograghic facets. *Journal of Advanced Nursing*, **26** (5), 921–929.

Shi, L., Fatemi, S.H., Sidwell, R. & Patterson, P. (2003) Maternal influenza infection causes marked behavioral and pharmacological changes in the offspring. *The Journal of Neuroscience*, **23** (1), 297–302.

Shrivastava, A., Davis, P. & Davies, D.P. (1997) SIDS: parental awareness and infant care practices in contrasting socioeconomic areas in Cardiff. *Arch Dis Child*, **77**, 52–52.

Sichel, D. & Driscoll, J.W. (2000) *Women's Moods: What Every Woman Must Know About Hormones, the Brain and Emotional Health*. New York: Harper Paperbacks.

Siegel, C., Graves, P., Maloney, K., Norris, J.M., Calonge, B.N. & Lezotte, D. (1996) Mortality from intentional and unintentional injury among infants of young mothers in Colorado, 1986 to 1992. *Archives of Pediatrics & Adolescent Medicine*, **150**, 1077–1083.

Silberweig, D.A., Stern, E., Firth, C., *et al.* (1995) A functional neuroanatomy of hallucinations in schizophrenia. *Nature*, **378**, 176–179.

Sinclair, J. & Green, J. (2005) Understanding resolution of deliberate self-harm: qualitative interview study of patients' experiences. *BMJ*, **330**, 1112.

Skouteris, H., Germano, C., Wertheim, E., Paxton, S. & Milgrom, J. (2008) Sleep quality and depression during pregnancy: a prospective study. *Journal of Sleep Research*, **17** (2), 217–220.

Slater, E. & Shields, J. (1953) Psychotic and neurotic illnesses in twins: Medical Research Council Special Report, 278. London: HMSO.

Smith, S. (1999) The images of women in film: some suggestions for future. In: *Feminist Film Theory* (ed. S. Thornham). Edinburgh: Edinburgh University Press.

Smith, G.C.S. & Pell, J.P. (2001) Teenage pregnancy and risk of adverse perinatal outcomes associated with first and second births: population based retrospective cohort study. *BMJ*, **323**, 476–479.

Sobowale, A. (2003) Perinatal mental health – new resources for supporting non-English speaking women. Postnatal depression and maternal mental health in multicultural society. *CPHVA*. October, 24–28.

Spalding, F. (1988) *Stevie Smith. A Critical Biography*. London: Faber and Faber.

Spinelli, M.G. (1997) Interpersonal psychotherapy for depressed antepartum women: a pilot study. *American Journal of Psychiatry*, **154** (7), 1028–1030.

Spinelli, M.G. (2002) *Psychological and Legal Perspectives on Mothers Who Kill*. Paffenbarger and McCabe: American Psychiatric Pub.

Spinelli, M.G. (2005) Neuroendocrine effects on mood. *Reviews in Endocrine and Metabolic Disorders*, **6** (2), 109–115.

Sroufe, L.A. & Piccard Wunsch, J. (1972) The Development of Laughter in the First Year of Life. *Child Development*, **43** (4) 1326–1334.

Stamp, G.E., Williams, A.S. & Crowther, C.A. (1995) Evaluation of antenatal and postnatal depression: a randomised, controlled trial. *Birth*, **22** (3), Sept., 138–143.

Stanley, C., Murray, N. & Stein, A. (2004) The effect of postnatal depression on mother–infant interaction, infant response to the still-face perturbation, and performance on an instrumental learning task. *Developmental Psychopathology*, **16**, 1–18.

Stanley, N., Borthwick, R. & Macleod, A. (2006) Antenatal depression: mothers' awareness and professional responses. *Primary Health Care Research and Development*, 7, 257–268.

Steiger, H. & Zankor, M. (1990) Sexual traumata among eating-disordered, psychiatric, and normal female groups: comparison of prevalences and defense styles. *Journal of Interpersonal Violence*, 5, 74–86.

Stein, G., Morton, J., Marsh, A., Hatshorn, J., Ebling, J. & Desaga, U. (1984) Vasopressin and mood during the puerperium. *Biological Psychiatry*, 19, 1711–1718.

Stein, J.A., Gath, D.H., Butcher, J., Bond, A., Day, A. and Cooper, P.J. (1991) The relationship between postnatal depression and mother-child interaction. *British Journal of Psychiatry*, **158**, 46–52.

Stein, A., Woolley, H. & McPherson, K. (1999) Conflict between mothers with eating disorders and their infants during mealtimes. *Br J Psychiatry*, **175**, 455–461.

Stevenson, A. (1990) *Bitter Fame. A life of Sylvia Plath*. London: Penguin.

Stone, M., Steinmeyer, E., Dreher, J. & Krischer, M. (2005) Infanticide in female forensic patients:the view from the evolutionary standpoint. *Journal of Psychiatric Practice*, **11** (1), 35– 45.

Store, A. (1968) *Human Aggression*. Harmondsworth: Penguin books Ltd.

Stewart, C. & Henshaw, C. (2002) Role of the midwife. *British Journal of Midwifery*, **10** (2), 117–121.

St James-Roberts, I., Sleep, J., Morris, S., *et al.* (2001) Use of a behavioural programme in the first 3 months to prevent infant crying and sleeping problems. *J Paediatr Child Health*, **37**, 289–297.

Stuber, M., Hilber, S., Mintzer, L., Castaneda, M., Glover, D. & Zeltzer, L. (2007) *Laughter, Humor and Pain Perception in Children: A Pilot Study*. *eCAM Advanced Access*.

Suckling, J. (1646) *Against Fruition*. Fragmenta Aurea.

Sugawara, M., Toda, M.A., Shima, S., Mukai, T., Sakakura, K. & Kitamura, T. (1997) Premenstrual mood changes and maternal mental health in pregnancy and the postpartum period. *Journal of Clinical Psychology*, **53** (3), 225–325.

Sulloway, F. (1996) *Born to Rebel: Birth Order, Family Dynamics, and Creative Lives*. New York: Pantheon.

Swain, A.M., O'Hara, M.W., Starr, K.R. & Gorman, L.L. (1997) A prospective study of sleep, mood, and cognitive function in postpartum and nonpost-partum women. *Obstetrics & Gynecology*, **90**, 381–386.

Talge, N., Neal, C., Glover, G., *et al.* (2007) Antenatal maternal stress and long-term effects on child neurodevelopment: how and why? *J of Child Psychol and Psychiatry*, **48** (4), 245–261.

Tang, H. & Hwee Kwoon Ng, J. (2006) Googling for a diagnosis –use of Google as a diagnostic aid: Internet based study. *BMJ*, **333**, 1143–1145.

Tantum, D. & Whittaker, J. (1992) Personality disorder and self-wounding. *British J or Psych*, **161**, 451–464.

Tcixeira, J.M.A., Fisk, N.M. & Glover, V. (1999) Association between maternal anxiety in pregnancy and increased uterine artery resistance index: cohort based study. *British Medical Journal*, **318**, 153–157.

Thomas, M., Sing, H., Belenky, G., *et al*. (2000) Neural basis of alertness and cognitive performance impairments during sleepiness. I. Effects of 24 hours of sleep deprivation on waking human regional brain activity, *J Sleep Res*, **9**, 335–352.

Thompson, C. & Thompson, C.M. (1989) The prescribing of antidepressants in general practice. 11: a placebo controlled trial of low-dose dothiepin. *Hum.Psychopharmacol*, **4**, 191–204.

Thornton, C. & Russell, J. (1997) Obsessive compulsive comorbidity in the dieting disorders. *International Journal of Eating Disorders*, **21**, 83–87.

Toglia, M.R. & Weg, J.G. (1996) Venous thromboembolism during pregnancy. *N Engl J Med*, **335**, 108–114.

Tronick, E.Z. (1995) Touch in mother-infant interaction. In: *Touch in Early Development* (ed. T.M. Field), pp. 53–65. Hillsdale, NJ: Lawrence Erlbaum Associates.

Tronick, E.Z., Morelli, G. & Ivey, P. (1992) The Efe forager infant and toddlers' pattern of social relationships: multiple and simultaneous. *Developmental Psychology*, **28**, 568–577.

Tully, l., Garcia, J., Dacidson, L. & Marchant, S. (2002) Role of midwives in depression screening. *British Journal of Midwifery*, **10** (96), 374– 378.

Tweedy, J. (1980) *In the Name of Love*. London: Granada.

Uddenberg, N. & Englesson, I. (1978) Prognosis of postpartum mental disturbance: a prospective study of primiparous women and their children. *Acta Psychiatrica Scandinavica Supplementum*, **58**, 201–212.

Ugarriza, D. (2004) Group therapy and its barriers for women suffering from postpartum depression. *Archives of Psychiatric Nursing*, **18**, 39–48.

Underdown, A., Barlow, J., Chung, V. & Stewart-Brown, S. (2006) Massage intervention for promoting mental and physical health in infants aged under six months. The Cochrane Database of Systematic Reviews, 4.

UNICEF (2008) The State of the World's Children. Executive summary Dec 2007. London: UNICEF.

Van Grootheest, D.S., Cath, D.C., Beekman, A.T. & Boomsma, D.I. (2005) Twin studies on obsessive-compulsive disorder: a review. *Twin Res Hum Genet*, 8 October, 450–458.

Veale, D., Le Fevre, K., Pantelis, C., de Souza, V., Mann, A. & Sargeant, A. (1992) Aerobic exercise in the adjunctive treatment of depression: a randomized controlled trial. *Journal of the Royal Society of Medicine*, **85** (9), 541–544.

Wadhwa, P., Culhane, J., Rauh, V. & Barve, S. (2004) Stress and pre-term birth: neuroendocrine, immune/inflammatory and vascular mechanisms. *Maternal and Child Health Journal*, **5** (2), 119–125.

Wahl, O.F. (1997) *Media Madness of Public Images of Mental Illness*. Fredericksburg, PA: Rutgers University Press.

Walker, L.O. & Wilging, S. (2000) Rediscovering the 'M' in 'MCH': maternal health promotion after childbirth. *J Obstet Gynecol Neonatal Nurs*, **29**, 229–236.

Wallace, W.R. (1819–1881) *The Hand That Rules the World*.

Wan, M.W., Salmon, M.P., Riordan, D.M., Appleby, L., Webb, R. & Abel, K.M. (2007) What predicts poor mother-infant interaction in schizophrenia? *Psycho Med*, **37** (4), 537–546.

Wang, S.Y., Jiang, X.Y., Jan, W.C. & Chen, C.H. (2003) A comparative study of postnatal depression and its predictors in Taiwan and mainland China. *American Journal of Obstetrics and Gynecology*, **189** (5), 1407–1412.

Waters, M. (1994) *Modern Sociology Theory*. Sage: London.

Weissman, M.M. (1975) Wrist cutting: relationship between clinical observations and epidemiological findings. *Arch Gen Psychiatry*, **32**, 1166–1171.

Weissman, M.M. & Paykel, E.S. (1974) *The Depressed Woman: a Study of Social Relationships*. Chicago: University of Chicago Press.

Welch, S.L. & Fairburn, C.G. (1994). Sexual abuse and bulimia nervosa: three integrated case control comparisons. *American Journal of Psychiatry*, **151**, 402–407.

Welford, H. (1998) *Feelings After Birth: The NCT Book of Postnatal Depression*. London: National Childbirth Trust.

Wheatland, R. (2002) Alternative treatment considerations in anorexia nervosa. *Med Hypotheses*, **59** (6), 710–715.

Wheeldon, T.J., Robertson, C., Eagles, J.M. & Reid, I.C. (1999) The views and outcomes of consenting and non-consenting patients receiving ECT. *Psychological Medicine*, **29**, 221–223.

Whooley, M.A., Avins, A.L., Miranda, J. & Browner, W.S. (1997) Case-finding instruments for depression. two questions are as good as many. *J Gen Intern Med*, **12** (7), 439–445.

Wieck, A., Kumar, R., Hirst, A.D., Marks M.N., Campbell, I.C. & Checkley, S.A. (1991) Increased sensitivity of dopamine and recurrence of affective psychosis after childbirth. *Br Med J*, **303**, 613–616.

Williams, H. & Carmichael, A. (1985) Depression in mothers in a multi-ethnic urban industrial municipal city in Melbourne. Aetiology factors and effects on infants and preschool children. *Journal of child Psychology and Psychiatry*, **26** (2), 277–288.

Williams, K. & Koran, L. (1997) Obsessive-compulsive disorder in pregnancy, the puerperium, and the premenstrual. *J Clin Psychiatry*, **58**, 330–334.

Wisner, K., James, P. & Findling, R.L. (1997) Antidepressant treatment during breast-feeding. *Obstetrical & Gynacological Survey*, **52** (4), 223–224.

Wisner, K., Gelenberg, A., Leonard, H., Zarin, D. & Frank, E. (1999) Pharmacologic treatment of depression during pregnancy. *JAMA*, **282**, 1264–1269.

Wolkind, S., Taylor, E.M., Waite A.J., *et al.* (1993) Recurrence of unexpected infant death. *Aca Paediatr*, **82**, 873–876.

Wolman, W.L., Chalmers, B., Hofmeyr, G.J. & Nikodem, V.C. (1993) Postpartum depression and companionship in the clinical birth. *American Journal of Obstetrics & Gynecology*, 1388–1393.

World Health Organisation (1992) *The ICD-10 Classification of mental and Behavioural Disorders*. Geneva: WHO.

Yoshida, K., Smith, B. & Kumar, R. (1999) Psychotropic drugs in mother's milk: a comprehensive review of assay methods, pharmacokinetics and of safety of breast-feeding. *Journal of Psychopharmacology*, **13** (1), 64–80.

Zajicek, E. & De Sallis, B. (1979) A longitudinal study of maternal depression and child behaviour problems. *Journal of Child Psychology and Psychiatry and Allied Disciplines*, **25**, 91–109.

Zhou, S., Chan, E., Pan, S.Q., *et al.* (2004) Pharmacokinetic interactions of drugs with St John's Wort. *Journal of Psychopharmacology*, **18**, 262–276.

Zigmond, A.S. & Snaith, R.P. (1983) The Hospital Anxiety and Depression Scale. *Acta Psychiatrica Scandinavica*, **67** (6), 361–370.

Zuckerman, B., Amaro, H., Bauchner, H., *et al.* (1989) Depressive symptoms during pregnancy: relationship to poor health behaviours. *Am J Obstetr. Gynecol*, **160**, 1107–1111.

Appendix 1

CG45 Antenatal and postnatal mental health: understanding NICE guidance
http://www.nice.org.uk/guidance/index.jsp?action=download&r=true&o=30436

Contact list for organisations

Action on Puerperal Psychosis
Established at the University of Birmingham, Action on Puerperal Psychosis (APP) is a
   network of women who have suffered puerperal psychosis and who are willing to
   receive correspondence about research projects. NB project has moved to Cardiff.
Email: APP Telephone: 02920 743 242
www.neuroscience.bham.ac.uk/research/app

Ante and postnatal depression, post-partum depression
London Harley Street and Bristol Hypnotherapy Depression Clinic, provides effective
   brief therapy, CBT, analytical, for depression, clinical depression, ante and
   postnatal depression, anxiety, OCD, insomnia, panic attacks, major depressive
   disorder.
The Courtyard 11a Canford Lane, Westbury-on-Trym, Bristol BS9 3DE
Tel: 0117 968 6886 Mobile: 07811 37 37 03
http://www.depression-bristol.co.uk/page5.html

AskAMum
Askamum is the website for *Mother & Baby* and *Pregnancy & Birth* magazines.
http://www.askamum.co.uk/GLOBAL/Search-Results/?Ntt=pnd&Ntx=mode%
   20matchallpartial&id=160&Ntk=site&N=0

Association for Postnatal Depression
Provides support to mothers suffering from postnatal illness. It exists to increase
    public awareness of the illness and to encourage research into its cause and nature.
Helpline: 020 7386 0868 (10 am–2 pm Mon, Weds & Fri, 10 am–5 pm, Tues &
    Thurs)

Association for Postnatal Illness
Established in 1979 to provide support to mothers suffering from postnatal illness.
145 Dawes Road, Fulham, London SW6 7EB
Tel 020 7386 0868
www.apni.org

Babycentre
BabyCentre is all about creating a personal experience. Start by answering a few
    simple questions and you'll see the site change to reflect your stage.
http://www.babycentre.co.uk/baby/youafterthebirth/pnd/

British Association for Behavioural and Cognitive Psychotherapies (BABCP)
The Globe Centre, PO Box 9, Accrington BB5 0XB
Tel: 01254 875277
www.babcp.org.uk

British Association for Counselling and Psychotherapy
BACP House, 35–37 Albert Street, Rugby, Warwickshire CV21 2SG
Tel: 0870 443 5219
www.bacp.co.uk

CRY-SIS
Provides self-help and support for families with excessively crying and sleepless
    babies.
Helpline: 020 7404 5011 (line open 9.00 am to 10.00 pm, 365 days a year)

Depression Alliance
Website with information about depression symptoms, treatments for depression and
    self-help groups).
England Office
Depression Alliance, 212 Spitfire Studios, 63–71 Collier Street, London N1 9BE
Email: information@depressionalliance.org
http://www.depressionalliance.org

Depression-in-Pregnancy.org.uk
Personal description of mother suffering from PND.
PO Box 1144, Bedford MK42 7ZH
info@depression-in-pregnancy.org.uk.
http://www.depression-in-pregnancy.org.uk/HomePage.php?p=Aboutus.htm

Elaine Hanzak, wrote the book, *Eyes without Sparkle – a Journey Through Postnatal
    Illness*
www.elainehanzak.co.uk

Foundation for Sudden Infant Death
Artillery House, 11–19 Artillery Row, London SW1P 1RT

Helpline: 020 7233 2090
General: 020 7222 8001
Fundraising: 020 7222 8003
Media: 020 7227 5212
Fax: 020 7222 8002
office@fsid.org.uk

Home-Start
Home-Start's informal and friendly support for families with young children provides
    a lifeline to thousands of parents and children in over 337 communities across the
    UK.
Home-Start UK North West Region
Address: 6 Liverpool Road, Penwortham, Preston PR1 0AD
Telephone: 01772 752 418
Email: northwestregion@home-start.org.uk
www.home-start.org.uk

Informaworld
Child abuse prevention: studies of antenatal and postnatal services.
Antenatal and postnatal services provide an obvious focus for preventive strategies for
    child abuse.
http://www.informaworld.com/smpp/content~db=all~content=a788341985~tab
    =content

Meet-A-Mum-Association (MAMA)
Self-help groups for mothers with small children and specific help and support to
    women suffering from postnatal depression.
Helpline: 0845 120 3746 (7.00 pm to 10.00 pm weekdays)

Mental Health Foundation
24 January 2008: 'Maternity services must prioritise mental health,' says Mental
    Health Foundation (press release).
Mental Health Foundation, London Office, 9th Floor, Sea Containers House, 20
    Upper Ground, London SE1 9QB
http://www.mentalhealth.org.uk/media/news-releases/news-releases-2008/24-january-
    2008

Mindinfoline
Monday to Friday 9 am to 5 pm. Free information for lone parents on issues
    including: maintenance, tax credits, benefits, work, education, legal rights,
    childcare and holidays. Also information about other organisations and local
    groups who may be able to help.
Telephone 0845 766 0163
Lone Parent Helpline: Tel 0800 018 5026
www.oneparentfamilies.org.uk

Motherbliss
Life after birth – Postnatal depression
7 West View, Loughton, Essex IG10 1TA
http://www.mothersbliss.com/life/pnd.asp

MUMSNET
Mumsnet was set up in January 2000 by Justine Roberts, a sports journalist and
  Carrie Longton, a TV producer. We met in antenatal classes and soon discovered
  that the best source of information on everything from sleep problems to choosing
  first shoes was the other mums from our antenatal group.
http://www.mumsnet.com/Talk/2290/292209
info@mumsnet.com

National Childbirth Trust
Advice, support and counselling on all aspects of childbirth and early parenthood.
Enquiry line: 0870 444 8707
Pregnancy and Birth Line: 0870 444 8709
Breast-feeding line: 0870 444 8708

PNI ORG UK
Formerly: Veritee's Post Natal Illness Website
Post Natal Illness Support Forum – Leeds mother and baby unit
http://www.pni.org.uk/index.ht

PND Training:
Training in the detection and treatment of postnatal depression.
We provide training in the detection and management of postnatal depression to
  health visitors and other health professionals.
http://www.pndtraining.co.uk/articles/doc_refs.htm

PNI-UK: Perinatal Illness – UK
Perinatal Illness – UK is a registered charity for women and their families who have or
  think they have any type of perinatal illness (PNI).
PO BOX 4976, London WC1H 9WH
http://www.pni-uk.com

Patient UK
About one in ten mothers develop postnatal depression. Support and understanding
  from family, friends, and sometimes from a professional such as a health visitor can
  help recovery. Other treatment options include antidepressant drugs and 'talking
  treatments' such as cognitive behaviour therapy.
http://www.patient.co.uk/showdoc/23069110
(Licensing Patient UK data for your site:
http://www.patient.co.uk/licencepils.htm)

Postnatal Mental Health (The Royal College of Psychiatrists)
www.rcpsych.ac.uk/info

Talking Life Seminar – Postnatal Depression
This is an on-site seminar, which can be brought to your workplace for up to 40
  people. Costs are estimated on the distance our trainer has to travel, so for a quote
  under no obligation, please call Wendy Bennett 0151-632-0662 or email:
  wendy@talklife.u-net.com
Talking Life, 36 Birkenhead Road, Hoylake, Wirral CH47 3BW
Tel: 0151-632-0662
Fax: 0151 632 1206

Shaw Trust

A comprehensive source of advice and practical support to help employers deal with
mental ill health issues in the workplace.

Fox Talbot House, Bellinger Close, Greenways Business Park, Chippenham, Wiltshire
SN15 1BN

mentalhealth@shaw-trust.org.uk

http://www.tacklementalhealth.org.uk

The Angela Harrison Charitable Trust

This is a registered charity which aims to help women and their families by raising
awareness and to provide information on postnatal depression/illness.

Trenissick Lane, Cubert, Newquay, Cornwall TR85PN

Registered Charity 1114051

http://www.help4mums.org/asp/default.asp?pID=1

The Mental Health Helpline

This provides an information and listening service for people in Lancashire.

It is available between 7.00 pm and 11.00 pm Mondays to Fridays and from 12.00
noon until 12.00 midnight on Saturdays and Sundays.

Tel: Freephone 0500 639000

The National Childbirth Trust

Registered Charity Number 801395

Telephone: 07020 965146

Fax: 020 8330 6622

http://www.isleofely-nct.org.uk/index.php

The Samaritans

Provides confidential emotional support to any person who is suicidal or despairing.

Tel: 08457 909090 (UK) or 1850 609090 (Eire)

Email: jo@samaritans.org

Uniview

The leading supplier of psychology teaching resources. Also features educational
resources for teachers of biology, social studies, PSHE and citizenship, health and
social care, and child studies. They supply educational DVDs, videos and software
to schools and teachers internationally.

Uniview Worldwide Ltd, PO Box 20, Hoylake, Wirral CH48 7HY

Telephone: +44 (0)151 625 3453

Fax: +44 (0)151 625 3707

http://www.uniview.co.uk/acatalog/ante-postnatal-health.html

Appendix 2

Edinburgh Postnatal Depression Scale[1] (EPDS)

Name: _____   Address: _____

Your Date of Birth: _____   _____

Baby's Date of Birth: _____   Phone: _____

As you are pregnant or have recently had a baby, we would like to know how you are feeling. Please check the answer that comes closest to how you have felt **IN THE PAST 7 DAYS,** not just how you feel today.

Here is an example, already completed.

I have felt happy:
☐   Yes, all the time
☒   Yes, most of the time   This would mean: 'I have felt happy most of the time' during the
                                                past week.
☐   No, not very often   Please complete the other questions in the same way.
☐   No, not at all

In the past 7 days:

1. I have been able to laugh and see the funny   ☐ Not quite so much now
   side of things   ☐ Definitely not so much now
      ☐ As much as I always could   ☐ Not at all

[1]Source: Cox, J.L, Holden, J.M. & Sagovsky, R. (1987) Detection of postnatal depression: Development of the 10-item Edinburgh Postnatal Depression Scale. *British Journal of Psychjatry*, **150**, 782–786.

2. I have looked forward with enjoyment to things
   ☐ As much as I ever did
   ☐ Rather less than I used to
   ☐ Definitely less than I used to
   ☐ Hardly at all

*3. I have blamed myself unnecessarily when things went wrong
   ☐ Yes, most of the time
   ☐ Yes, some of the time
   ☐ Not very often
   ☐ No, never

4. I have been anxious or worried for no good reason
   ☐ No, not at all
   ☐ Hardly ever
   ☐ Yes, sometimes
   ☐ Yes, very often

*5. I have felt scared or panicky for no very good reason
   ☐ Yes, quite a lot
   ☐ Yes, sometimes
   ☐ No, not much
   ☐ No, not at all

*6. Things have been getting on top of me
   ☐ Yes, most of the time I haven't been able to cope at all
   ☐ Yes, sometimes I haven't been coping as well as usual
   ☐ No, most of the time I have coped quite well
   ☐ No, I have been coping as well as ever

*7. I have been so unhappy that I have had difficulty sleeping
   ☐ Yes, most of the time
   ☐ Yes, sometimes
   ☐ Not very often
   ☐ No, not at all

*8. I have felt sad or miserable
   ☐ Yes, most of the time
   ☐ Yes, quite often
   ☐ Not very often
   ☐ No, not at all

*9. I have been so unhappy that I have been crying
   ☐ Yes, most of the time
   ☐ Yes, quite often
   ☐ Only occasionally
   ☐ No, never

*10. The thought of harming myself has occurred to me
   ☐ Yes, quite often
   ☐ Sometimes
   ☐ Hardly ever
   ☐ Never

Administered/Reviewed by_____   Date_____

Post-partum depression is the most common complication of childbearing.[2] The ten-question Edinburgh Postnatal Depression Scale (EPDS) is a valuable and efficient way of identifying patients at risk for 'perinatal' depression. The EPDS is easy to administer and has proven to be an effective screening tool.

Mothers who score above 13 are likely to be suffering from a depressive illness of varying severity. The EPDS score should not override clinical judgement. A careful clinical assessment should be carried out to confirm the diagnosis. The scale indicates how the mother has felt *during the previous week.* In doubtful cases it may be useful to repeat the tool after two weeks. The scale will not detect mothers with anxiety neuroses, phobias or personality disorders.

Women with postpartum depression need not feel alone. They may find useful information on the web sites of the National Women's Health Information Center <www.4women.gov> and from groups such as Postpartum Support International <www.chss.iup.edu/postpartum> and Depression after Delivery <www.depressionafterdelivery.com>.

$$\boxed{\text{SCORING}}$$

QUESTIONS 1, 2 & 4 (without an *)
Are scored 0, 1, 2 or 3 with top box scored as 0 and the bottom box scored as 3.

QUESTIONS 3, 5–10 (marked with an *)
Are reverse scored, with the top box scored as a 3 and the bottom box scored as 0.

    Maximum score: 30
    Possible Depression: 10 or greater
    Always look at item 10 (suicidal thoughts)

Instructions for using the Edinburgh Postnatal Depression Scale

1. The mother is asked to check the response that comes closest to how she has been feeling in the previous seven days.
2. All the items must be completed.
3. Care should be taken to avoid the possibility of the mother discussing her answers with others. (Answers come from the mother or pregnant woman.)
4. The mother should complete the scale herself, unless she has limited English or has difficulty with reading.

---

[2]Source: Wisner, K.L., Parry, B.L., & Piontek, C.M. (2002) Postpartum Depression. *N Engl J Med*, **347** (3), July 18.

© 1987 The Royal College of Psychiatrists. The Edinburgh Postnatal Depression Scale may be photocopied by individual researchers or clinicians for their own use without seeking permission from the publishers. The scale must be copied in full and all copies must acknowledge the following source: Cox, J.L., Holden, J.M. and Sagovsky, R. (1987). Detection of postnatal depression: Development of the 10-item Edinburgh Postnatal Depression Scale. *British Journal of Psychiatry*, **150**, 782–786. Written permission must be obtained from the Royal College of Psychiatrists for copying and distribution to others or for republication (in print, online or by any other medium).

Translations of the scale, and guidance as to its use, may be found in Cox, J.L. and Holden, J. (2003) *Perinatal Mental Health: A Guide to the Edinburgh Postnatal Depression Scale*. London, Gaskell.

Index